A Colour Atlas of

Paediatric Surgical Diagnosis

Lewis Spitz
MB, Ch B, Ph D, FRCS (Edin), FRCS (Eng)

Nuffield Professor of Paediatric Surgery,
University of London

G.M. Steiner
MBBS, DCH, D Obs RCOG, FRCR, FRCP

Consultant Radiologist, Sheffield Children's Hospital

R.B. Zachary
MB, Ch B, FRCSI, FRCS (Eng)

Formerly Director, Subdepartment of Paediatric Surgery,
University of Sheffield

Wolfe Medical Publications Ltd

Copyright © L. Spitz, G.M. Steiner and R.B. Zachary, 1981
Published by Wolfe Medical Publications Ltd, 1981
Printed by Royal Smeets Offset b.v., Weert, Netherlands
ISBN 0 7234 0763 0 Cased edition
ISBN 0 7234 1611 7 Paperback edition
Paperback edition © 1989

All rights reserved. No reproduction, copy or transmission of this publication may be made without written permission.

No paragraph of this publication may be reproduced, copied or transmitted save with written permission or in accordance with the provisions of the Copyright Act 1956 (as amended), or under the terms of any licence permitting limited copying issued by the Copyright Licensing Agency, 33-34 Alfred Place, London WC1E 7DP.

Any person who does any unauthorised act in relation to this publication may be liable to criminal prosecution and civil claims for damages.

A CIP catalogue record for this book is available from the British Library.

For a full list of Wolfe Medical Atlases, plus forthcoming titles and details of our surgical, dental and veterinary Atlases, please write to Wolfe Medical Publications Ltd, 2-16 Torrington Place, London WC1E 7LT, England.

Contents

		Page
Acknowledgements		6
Preface		7
1	Transport	9
2	Perinatal injuries	10
3	Non-accidental injury (child abuse)	15
4	Accidents in childhood	19
5	Burns	23
6	The eye	25
7	The nose	29
8	The mouth	31
9	The jaws	34
10	The tongue	37
11	The ears	39
12	Face and skull	40
13	Salivary glands	43
14	Pharynx and larynx	45
15	Thyroid gland	46
16	The neck	49
17	The breast	54
18	The chest wall	56
19	The oesophagus	59
20	The mediastinum	66
21	The lungs	70
22	The diaphragm	73
23	The abdominal wall	76
24	Exomphalos (omphalocoele)	83
25	The peritoneal cavity	86
26	The stomach	89
27	The duodenum	93
28	The small intestine	96
29	The appendix	116
30	The colon	118
31	Rectum and anus	128
32	Liver and biliary tract	137
33	The pancreas	147
34	The spleen and portal hypertension	149
35	Adrenal gland	153
36	Retroperitoneal tumours	156
37	The kidney	166
38	The ureter	172
39	The bladder	176
40	The urethra	180
41	Penile disorders	182
42	Testis and scrotum	185
43	Female genital organs	189
44	Intersex	192
45	Central nervous system	194
46	Skin and subcutaneous tissue	204
47	Musculoskeletal system	210
48	Miscellaneous conditions	229

Acknowledgements

We wish to record our gratitude and indebtedness to Louise Spitz, M.A., for many hours of editorial assistance and for compiling the index; to the departments of medical illustration at The Children's Hospital and Hallamshire Hospital, Sheffield, and at the Institute of Child Health and Hospital for Sick Children, Great Ormond Street, London; to Mr P.M. Elliot for the illustrations; to Blackwell Scientific Publications Ltd., Oxford, for permission to reproduce a number of illustrations from 'Paediatric Orthopaedics and Fractures', Second Edition (1979) by W.J.W. Sharrard; and to Camera Talks Ltd. for permission to publish two slides from their series on home safety (Figs. 43 and 46).

In addition we wish to thank the following colleagues for providing slides for use in the Atlas:

- A. Atalar
- L. Chait
- M.R.Q. Davies
- R.C.W. Dinsdale
- J.L. Emery
- C. Hall
- V. Hemalatha
- R. Hoare
- M. Katzen
- E. Kiely
- B. Lake
- J. Lari
- R.K. Levick
- G.C. Lloyd-Roberts
- J. Lorber
- A.E. MacKinnon
- C. Metrovelli
- R.W.S. Miller
- R.D.G. Milner
- H.H. Nixon
- J. Pincott
- A.M.K. Rickwood
- W.J.W. Sharrard
- J.D. Shaw
- J. Stark
- C. Williams
- P. Upadhyaya

Finally, thanks to Mrs J. Billington and Miss S. Shonuga for patiently and competently typing and retyping the manuscript.

Preface

This book presents the surgery of infancy and childhood in pictorial form. We have deliberately excluded cardiothoracic conditions which we feel constitute a separate speciality. Other specialities such as otorhinolaryngology, ophthalmology and neurosurgery are only sparsely covered. The main body of the Atlas is concerned with neonatal surgery and the general surgery of the child, including urology and orthopaedics.

The Atlas is not designed as a textbook of Paediatric Surgery but as a pictorial introduction, and should be used in conjunction with one of the many textbooks on the subject.

1 Transport

Newborn infants can be transported safely over long distances provided adequate temperature homeostasis can be maintained, and the staff accompanying the infant are fully equipped and experienced in the management of cardiorespiratory emergencies.

Guidelines for the safe transfer of the surgical neonate include:

1 Availability of a transport incubator, ideally with modifications to provide monitoring facilities for heartrate, body temperature and inspired oxygen concentration.
2 Equipment for resuscitation including apparatus necessary for endotracheal intubation, suction devices, chest drainage and drugs for cardiorespiratory support.
3 Nasogastric decompression to prevent aspiration of gastric content during transfer.
4 Specimen of maternal serum for compatibility studies, should the infant require blood transfusion.
5 A valid consent form for surgery.
6 Copies of all details of the pregnancy and delivery and of the infant's progress and treatment, including special investigations, e.g. xrays and biochemical tests.

Special precautions are required to transport infants with oesophageal atresia, diaphragmatic hernia and exomphalos.

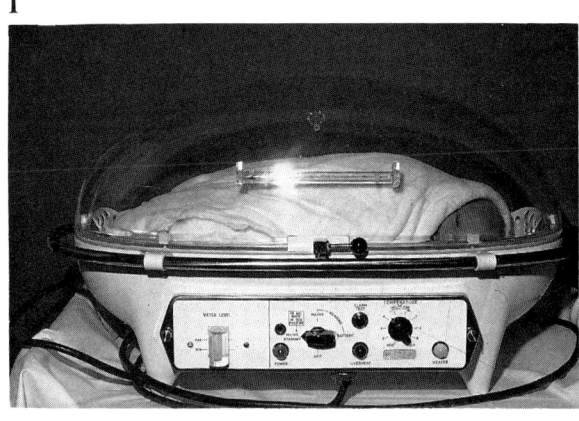

1 Simple portable incubator.

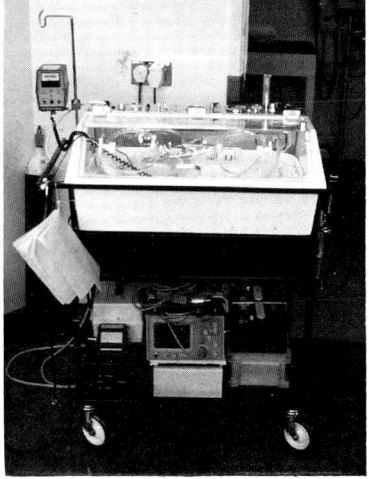

2 Portable incubator with facilities for continuous monitoring of heartrate, ECG, body temperature and inspired oxygen concentration. A self-contained infant ventilator is also visible.

2 Perinatal injuries

Injuries associated with intrauterine invasive procedures

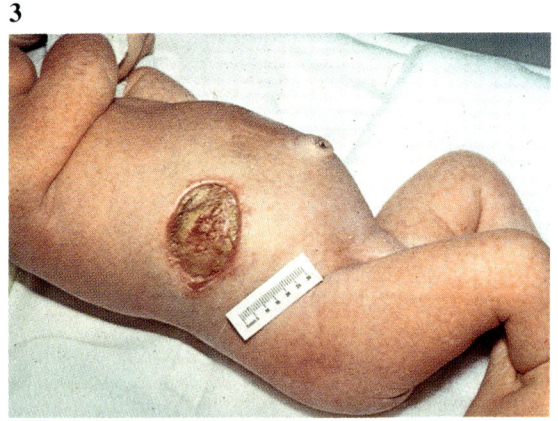

3 Soft tissue necrosis. Full-thickness necrosis of the skin in the right upper quadrant of the abdomen after subcutaneous injection of radio-opaque contrast material (iophendylate) during foetoamniography. This complication can be avoided by confirming safe positioning of the needle, as implied by free backflow of liquor amnii on aspiration, before an injection of any contrast material.

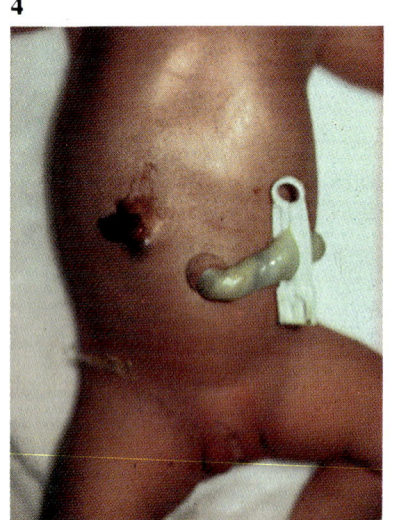

4 Intestinal fistula. The infant presented at birth with a fistula discharging meconium-stained fluid in the right hypochondrium. Laparotomy revealed an ileal atresia with the proximal intestine terminating in the fistula. It was presumed that amniocentesis performed at 18 weeks gestation caused the anomaly.

Birth trauma

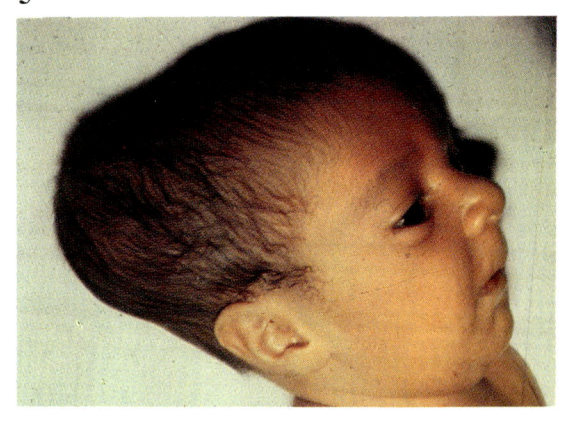

5 Caput succedaneum (extreme moulding). Interference with the venous return during delivery results in the accumulation of fluid in the subcutaneous tissue of the presenting part of the foetus. The size of the caput is proportional to the degree and duration of compression. The extent of the caput is not confined by the attachments of the periosteum. The swelling is maximal at birth and resolves within a few days.

6 Cephalhaematoma involving the right parietal region. A subperiosteal haemorrhage caused by separation of the periosteum from the underlying bone. Extent is limited by the periosteal attachments. There may be an associated skull fracture. The swelling reaches maximum girth a few days after birth and may persist for several weeks. Jaundice may develop as a result of resorption of blood from the haematoma. No treatment required.

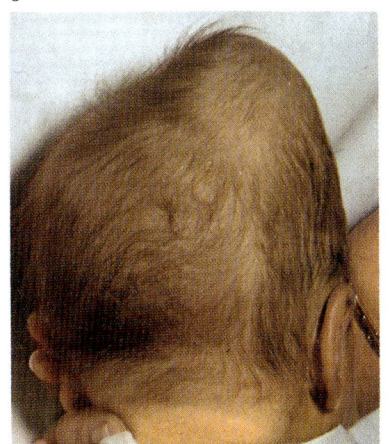

7 Cephalhaematoma: necropsy appearance. Cephalhaematoma showing the subperiosteal collection of blood. The extent is confined by the attachments of the periosteum at the sites of the suture lines.

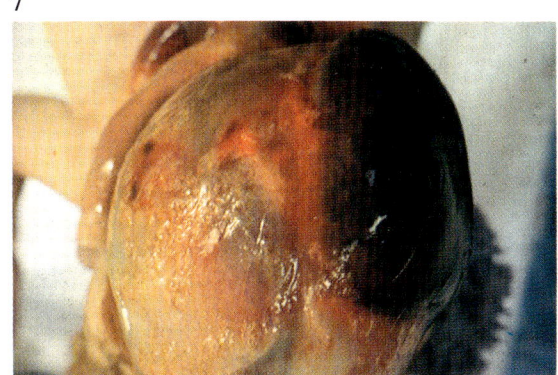

8 Bruising of the face. Extensive bruising, oedema and petechial haemorrhages incurred during a prolonged second stage of a face presentation.

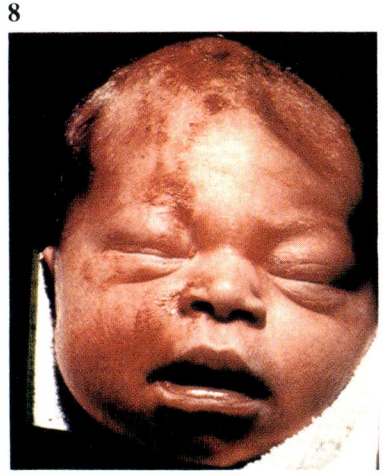

9 Bruising of the buttocks. Oedema and bruising of the left buttock (gluteal area) in a baby after a prolonged second stage of a breech delivery.

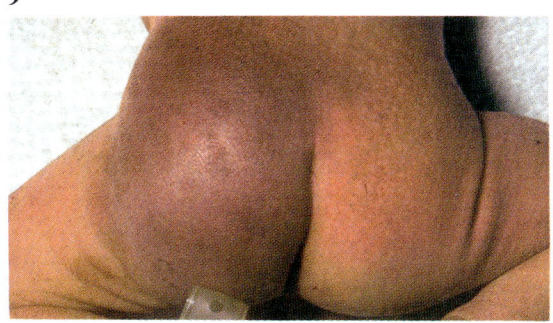

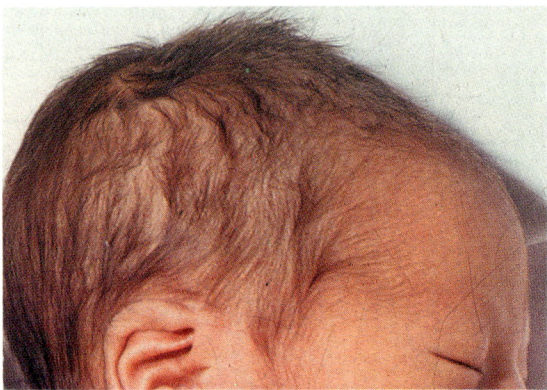

10 Depressed fracture of the skull. Depression in the posterior part of the right parietal region. This type of injury may occur during assisted deliveries, particularly those involving forceps.

11 Fractured skull. Xray of depressed fracture in the right parietal region. Surgical elevation is recommended when the depression is greater than 5 mm.

12 Vacuum extraction. Ecchymosis and bruising of the scalp after vacuum (ventouse) extraction to assist a delayed second stage of a vertex delivery. Skin necrosis indicates the site of application of the vacuum suction.

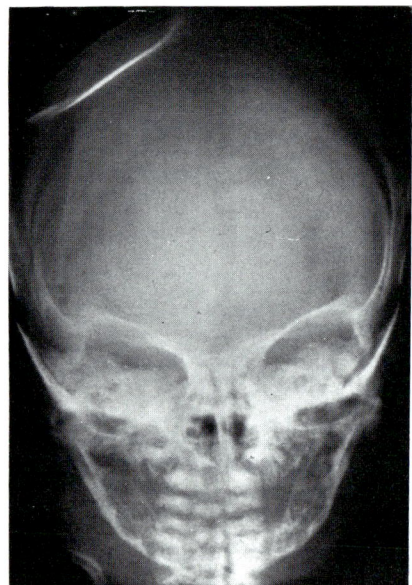

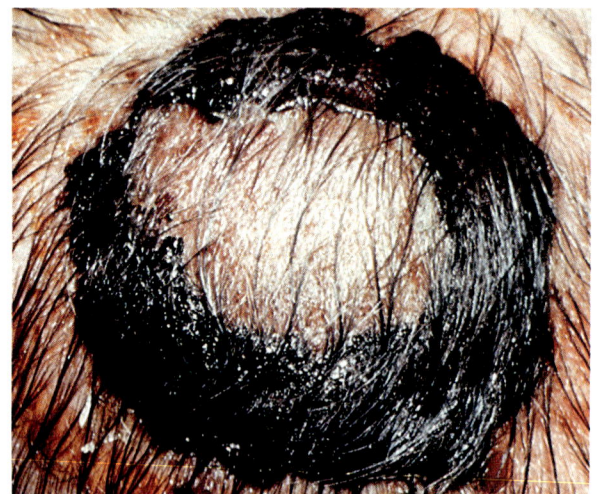

13 Facial palsy. Forceps injury to the right cheek. The infant developed a transient facial palsy. In 15 to 35 per cent of cases the facial nerve paralysis is permanent. Direct trauma to the eye, nose or ear may result from incorrect application of the forceps.

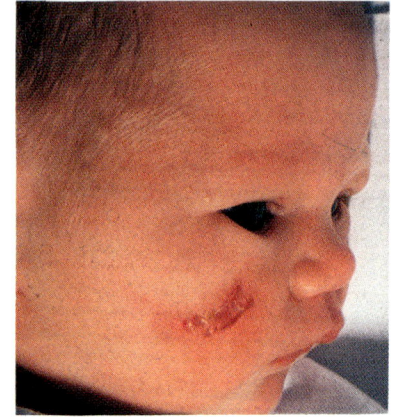

14 Intraventricular haemorrhage with extensive involvement of the left cerebral hemisphere. The condition is almost invariably associated with prematurity particularly after precipitate labour. Progressive hydrocephalus is the most common sequela in the few infants who survive.

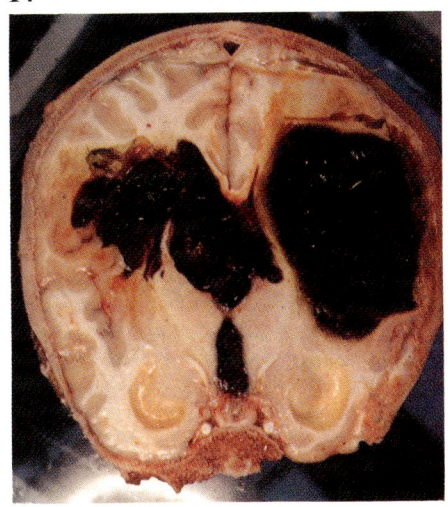

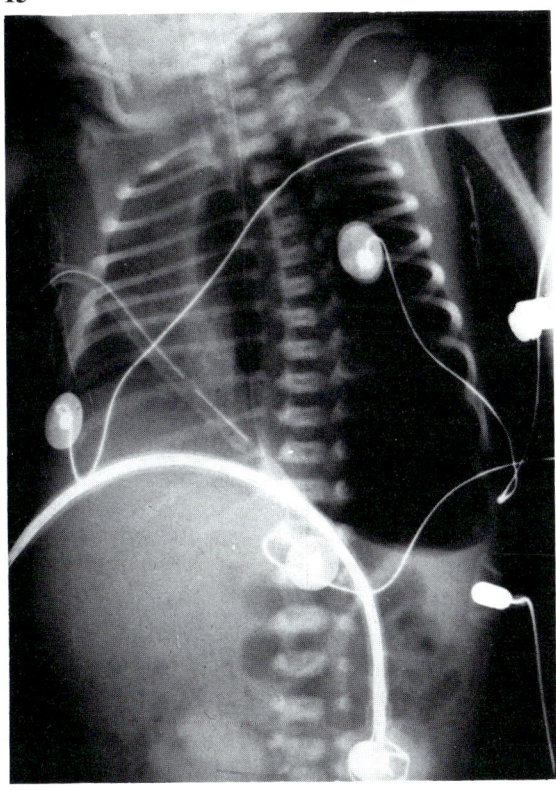

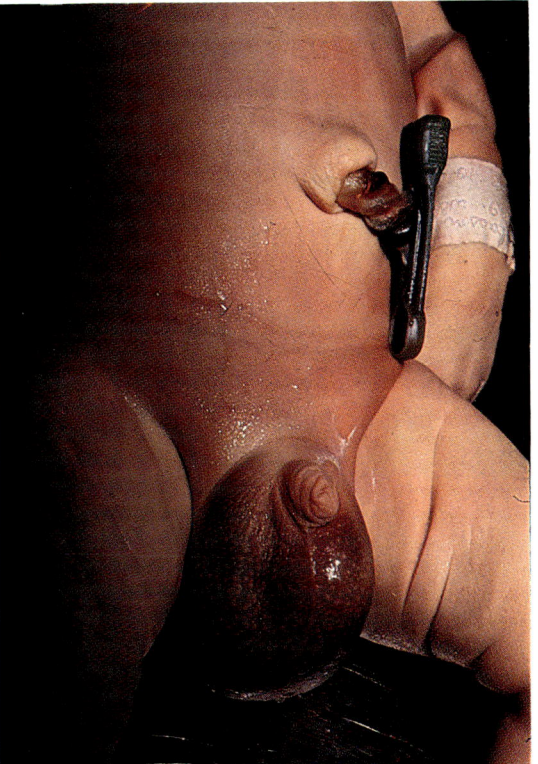

15 Tension pneumothorax may develop during respiratory resuscitation of the newborn. Incidence is particularly high in premature infants with respiratory distress syndrome already receiving ventilatory support. The chest xray shows an extensive tension pneumothorax on the left with the mediastinal structures displaced to the right. Emergency needle aspiration of the chest may be necessary before radiological confirmation of the diagnosis.

16 Abdominal visceral trauma. Injury to the abdominal viscera may occur during a difficult breech extraction. The liver is the organ most commonly involved, but the spleen or adrenal gland may also be injured. The infant presents with signs of acute blood loss. Haemoperitoneum may cause a bluish discoloration of the anterior abdominal wall or umbilicus (Cullen's sign) or in the presence of patent processus vaginalis, a scrotal haematoma (as shown in this infant).

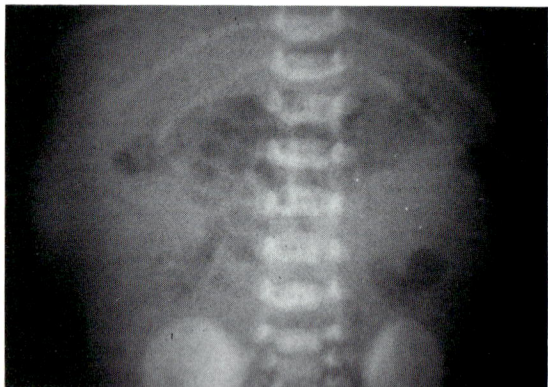

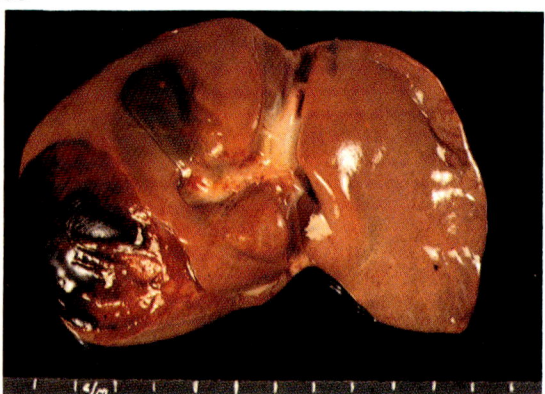

17 Ruptured viscus. Supine abdominal xray in an infant with abdominal distension and cardiovascular shock 24 hours after a 'traumatic' delivery. The bowel gas shadows are all centrally located and appear to be 'floating' on the top of free intraperitoneal fluid ('flowerpot sign').

18 Ruptured liver. A subcapsular haematoma of the right lobe of the liver sustained during a traumatic delivery, usually breech extraction or shoulder dystocia. This type of injury is more common than primary rupture of the liver. In most cases the bleeding stops spontaneously.

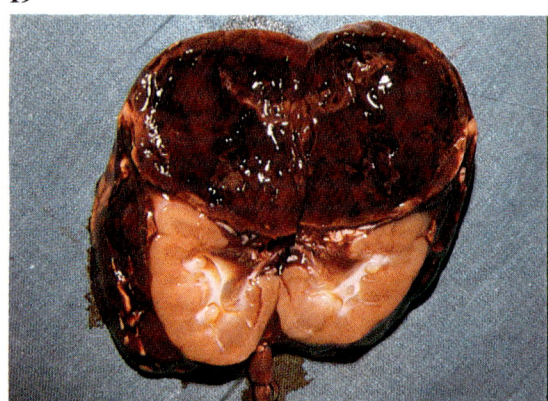

19 Adrenal haemorrhage may be caused by a traumatic delivery or develop during an episode of septicaemia. The ipsilateral kidney is displaced downwards on excretory urogram. A 'rim sign' of adrenal calcification on xray may develop within two weeks. Operative intervention is rarely required.

20 Fractures of the long bones, particularly the humerus and femur, may result from a difficult breech delivery. A fracture through the mid-shaft of the left femur as well as through the neck of the right femur. Fractures of the clavicles occasionally occur in large infants with shoulder dystocia.

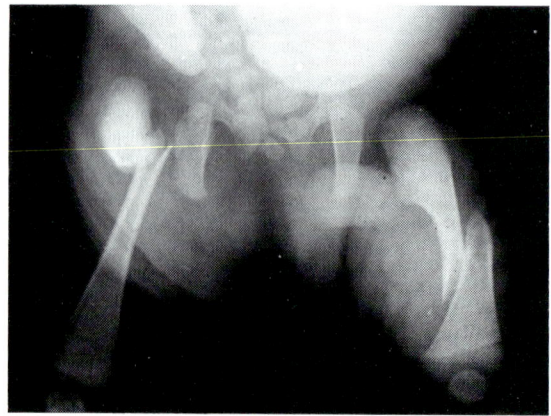

3 Non-accidental injury (child abuse)

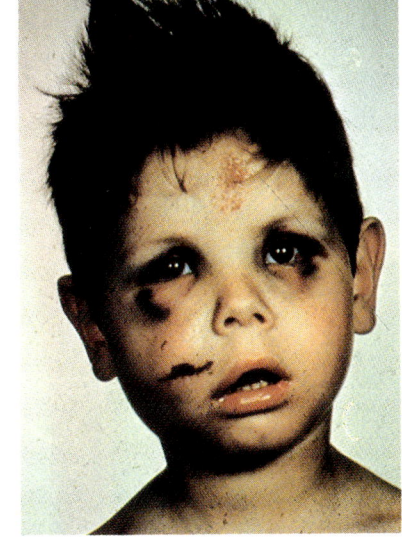

Appreciation of the magnitude of this sociomedical problem is relatively recent. Approximately ten per cent of children attending accident and emergency departments with injuries are in this category. Diagnosis should be considered carefully when there is an apparent discrepancy between the nature of the injury and the history obtained from the parent(s); a prolonged delay between the time of injury and attendance at hospital; or where there are other signs of abuse, e.g. other unexplained injuries, malnutrition, extreme anxiety in the child.

21 Bruises. Child with multiple bruises periorbitally, over the right mandible and on the upper chest wall.

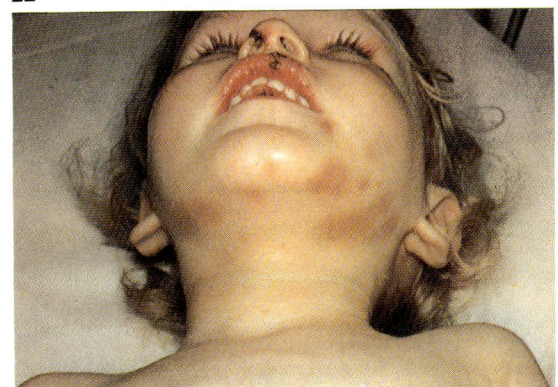

22 Attempts at strangulation. Bruises of the neck caused by pressure exerted by fingers and thumbs in an attempt to stop the child crying. Note also the laceration of the upper lip and right nostril.

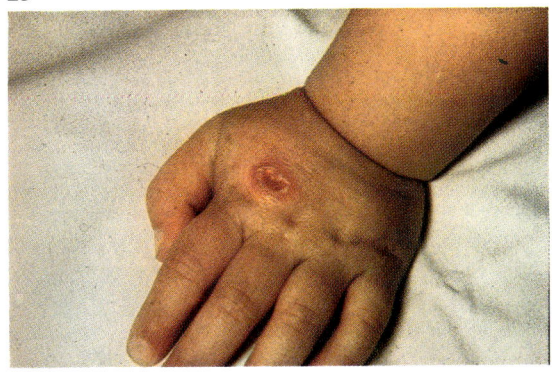

23 Cigarette burn. Typical cigarette burn on the dorsum of the hand of a young child.

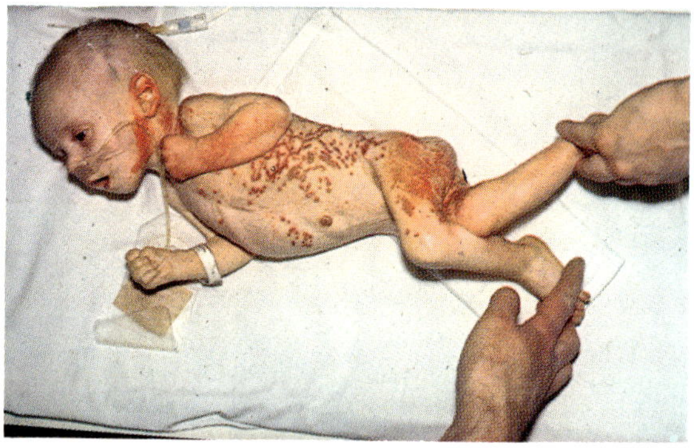

24 Malnutrition. Nutritional abuse and evidence of overall poor care with diffuse nappy rash. The infant weighed 3 kg at four months. No other evidence of physical injury was present.

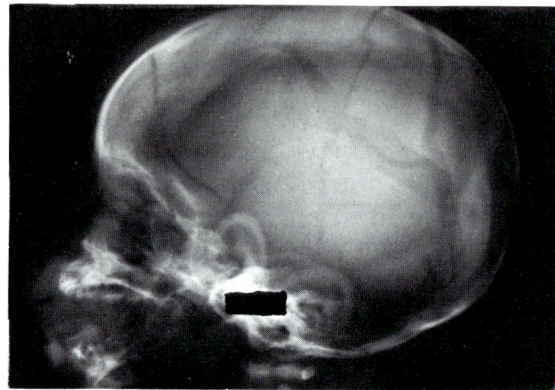

25 Fractures of the skull. Xray showing multiple linear fractures on both sides of the skull.

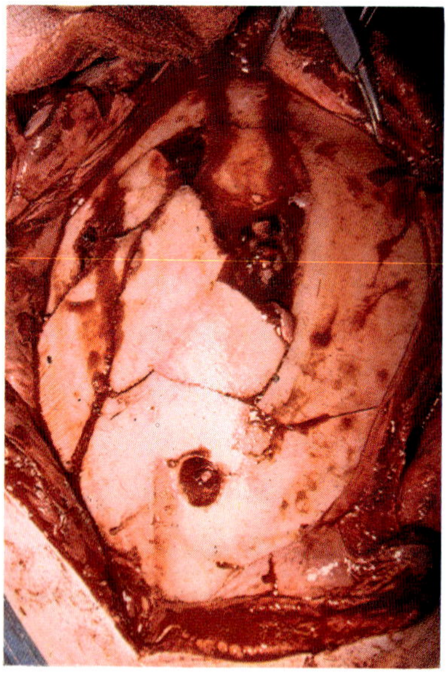

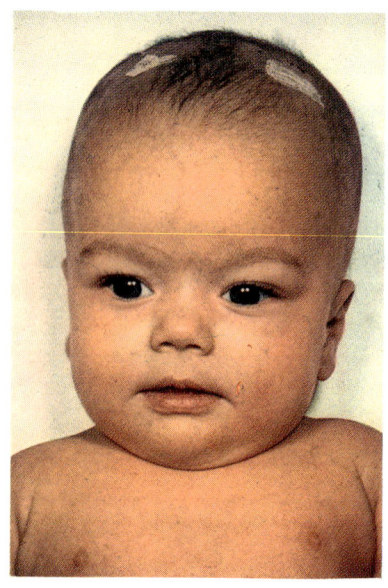

26 Skull trauma. Operative view of a child who had been attacked with an axe and had sustained numerous compound depressed fractures of the skull.

27 Subdural haematoma. Infant with bilateral subdural haematomas caused by non-accidental trauma. The infant presented with vomiting and a bulging anterior fontanelle. Note the sites through which the subdural effusions have been aspirated.

28 'Pulled elbow' in a young child. The injury occurs when the head of the radius is partially pulled out of the annular ligament. The condition is characterised by acute onset of pain in the affected elbow and the child loses the use of the arm. It usually responds well to manipulating the head of the radius back into position.

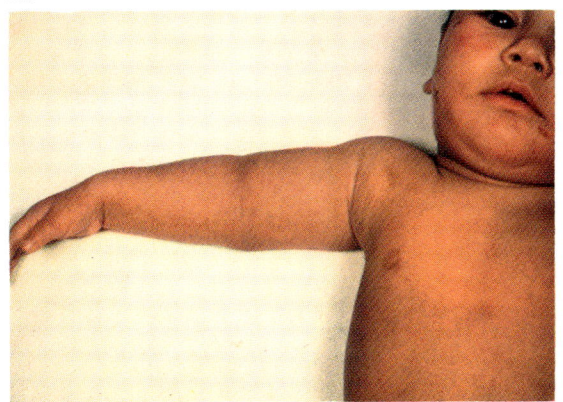

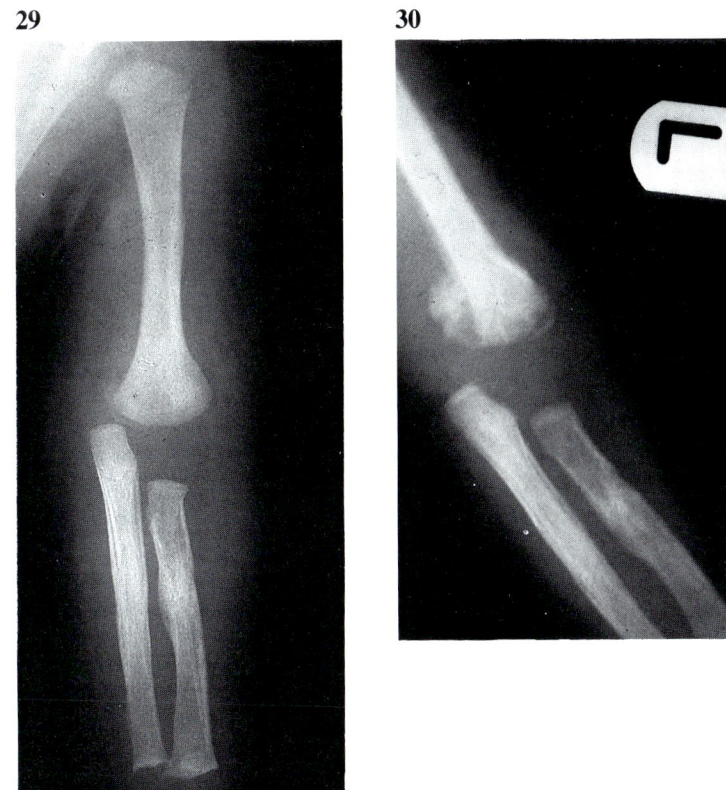

29 Fractures around the elbow. The arm of a child who presented with acute pain and swelling of the left elbow. The xray shows evidence of a healed fracture of the upper third of the radius.

30 Fractures around the elbow of the same child as in **29** taken one week later showing well-marked features of a 'bucket handle' tear of the metaphysis of the humerus.

31 Fractured ribs. Chest radiographs taken three weeks apart. The initial xray appears normal. Three weeks later multiple fractures of the ribs on both sides of the thorax are clearly visible. The site of fracture has become radiologically obvious as a result of expansion of the rib ends with callus formation during the healing process.

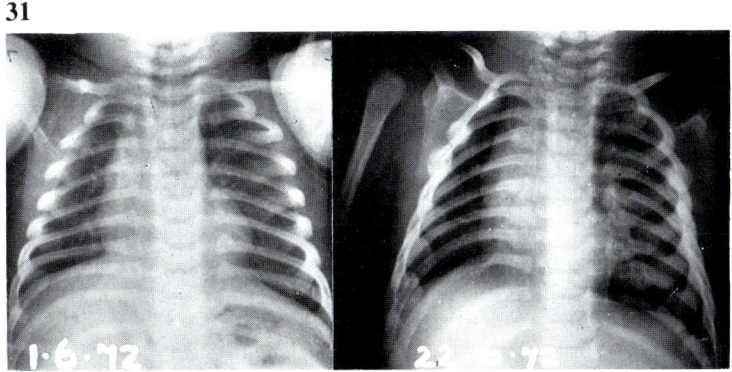

32 Tension pneumothorax. Right tension pneumothorax with subcutaneous emphysema extending into the neck. No rib fractures are seen.

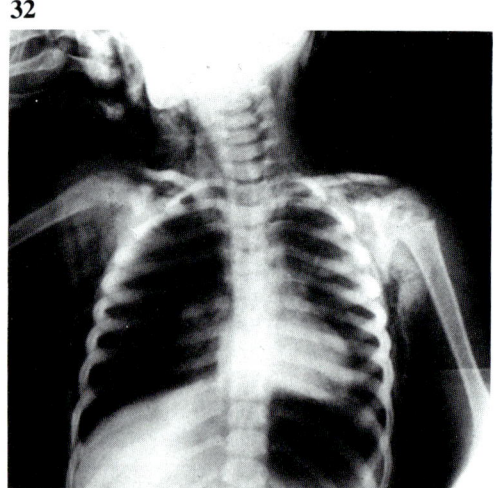

33 Mongolian spot present in 90 per cent of dark-skinned races and in one to five per cent of Caucasian infants. It consists of a bluish-grey discoloration over the lumbosacral area or buttocks. The area of discoloration usually fades during late infancy. Often confused with child abuse bruising.

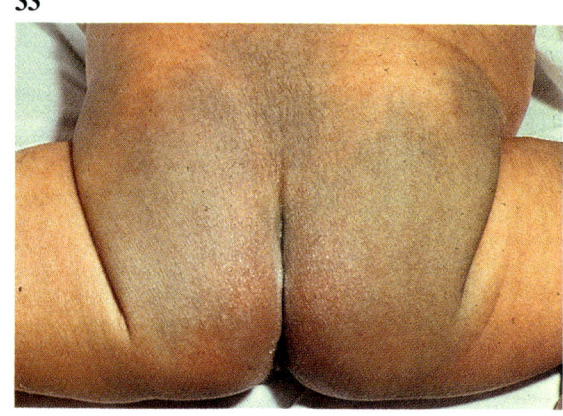

4 Accidents in childhood

Accidents are the largest single cause of death in children over the age of one year and account for one in five of all hospital admissions, and between 40 and 60 per cent of attendances at accident and emergency departments for this age group. Road accidents, predominantly involving pedestrians, account for 40 per cent of the deaths, accidents in and around the home for 35 per cent, while deaths from burns amount to ten per cent of the total. In the age range 0 to 5 years, 70 per cent of accidents occur at home and four per cent on the roads, compared with 40 per cent and 12 per cent respectively in the 6 to 16-year age group.

34 Trauma to the eye. Periorbital bruising as a result of direct trauma to the face. No underlying fracture of the facial bones was present. It is important to exclude non-accidental trauma in cases such as this, particularly if there is an implausible explanation for the injury or there are other signs of abuse.

35 Facial trauma. Extensive bruising of the face and forehead in a child who had fallen from a flat garage roof. There was a fracture of the base of the skull. Injuries of this nature may occur from falls out of trees but are particularly common in modern apartments because of faulty architectural design, e.g. inadequate protection of stairways by using horizontal bannisters, poor safety features of windows above ground-floor level allowing easy access and unsatisfactory design allowing toddlers to fall through. Playground accidents are also a common cause of this type of injury.

36 Fractured skull. Anterior fossa of the skull with periorbital bruising and subconjunctival haemorrhage. Characteristically, the posterior limit of the haemorrhage is not visible. The injury was sustained in a motor-vehicle accident in which the girl was a passenger. Children are safer in the rear seats than in the front. The use of effective child restraints reduces the severity of injuries in the event of an accident.

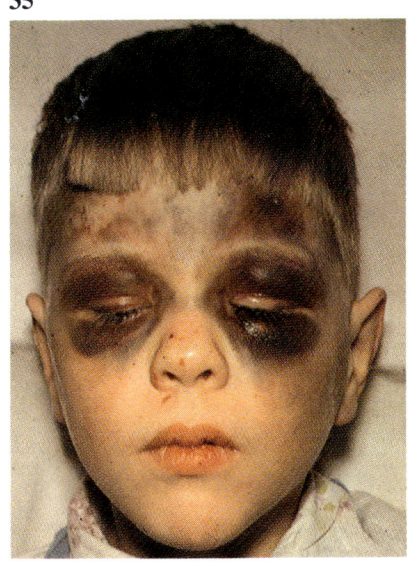

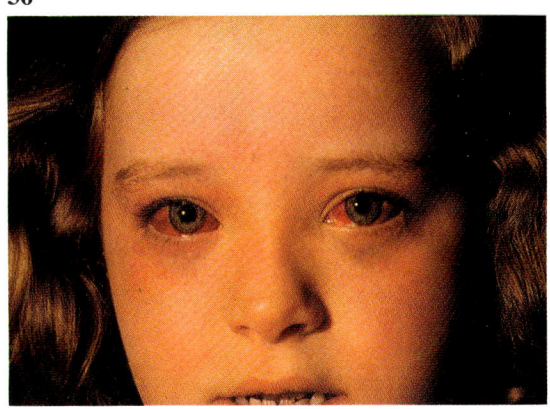

37 Head injury. Minor head injuries are extremely common. Indications for admission to hospital for observation include loss of consciousness, drowsiness and recurrent vomiting. Evidence of a skull fracture of the linear type is of no consequence but does signify the force of the injury. Extension of the fracture into paranasal air sinuses converts this type of injury into a compound fracture.

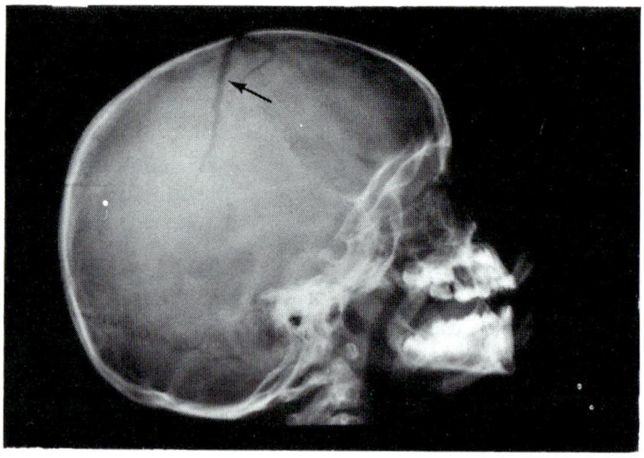

38 Compound depressed fracture of the skull may be associated with laceration of the underlying cerebral cortex. Surgical elevation of the depressed segment is required in all cases of compound depressed fractures or in the closed type where the depression is greater than 0.5 cm.

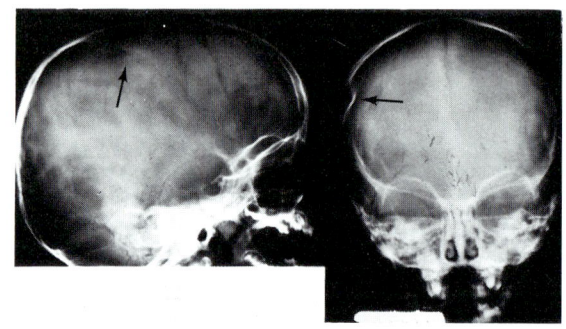

39 Subdural haematoma. Subdural haemorrhage results from rupture of the bridging veins from the brain surface to the dural sinuses as a result of a sheering force. There is frequently associated damage to the cerebral cortex. The distribution of the blood clot conforms to the convolutions of the cerebral cortex. Computerised tomography assists in accurately delineating the extent of the haematoma and in directing the surgical approach.

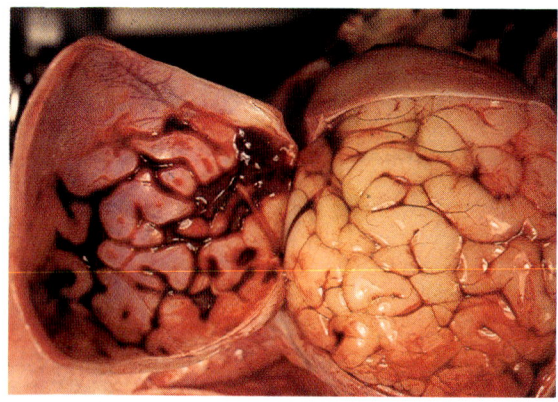

40 Extradural haematoma is uncommon in childhood. Characteristically there is a 'lucid interval' between initial and later relapse of unconsciousness. Lateralising signs e.g. ipsilateral fixed dilated pupil and contralateral muscular weakness are caused by compression of the underlying brain. Computerised tomography of the skull reveals the site and extent of the haematoma. Evacuation of the haematoma is the emergency treatment required.

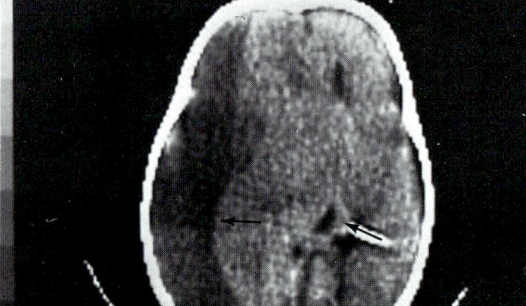

41 Suffocation injury caused by compression of the thoracic cavity impeding venous return. The child had been trapped under the wheel of a motor car. There is intense subconjunctival haemorrhage, periorbital oedema and petechiae confined to the head and neck region.

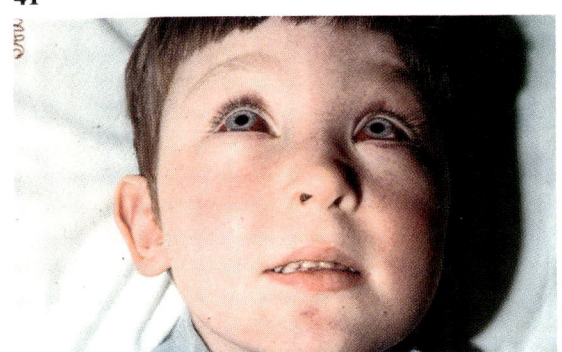

42 Accidental hanging showing the impression left by the compressing force on the neck. An emergency tracheostomy was performed for resuscitation of the child. The injury was sustained while the child was constructing a swing from a rope suspended from a branch of a tree.

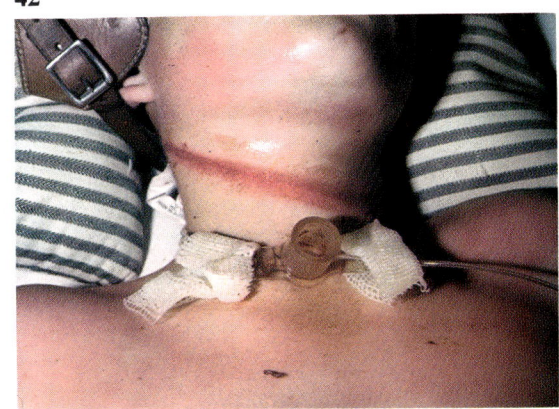

43 Lacerations of the buttocks after a fall on to an unprotected escalator grid.

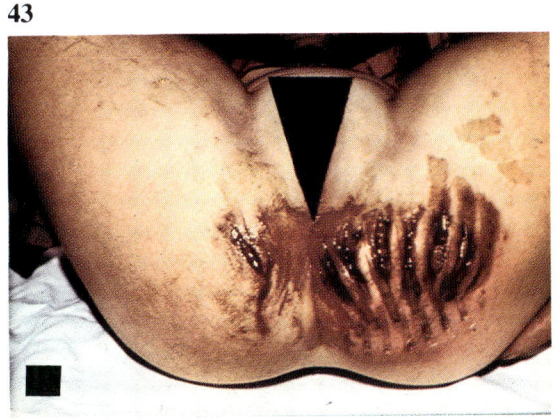

44 Dog bite of the face resulting in an extensive deep laceration of the left cheek and multiple abrasions of the face. The offending dog was a German shepherd (Alsatian). Protection against tetanus is required and the offending dog should be observed for signs of rabies.

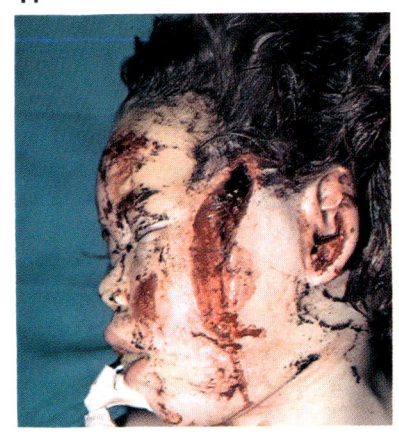

45 Wringer injury of the forearm resulting in a friction burn. The injury results from the fact that the rollers of the clothes wringer fail to open in the presence of excess pressure.

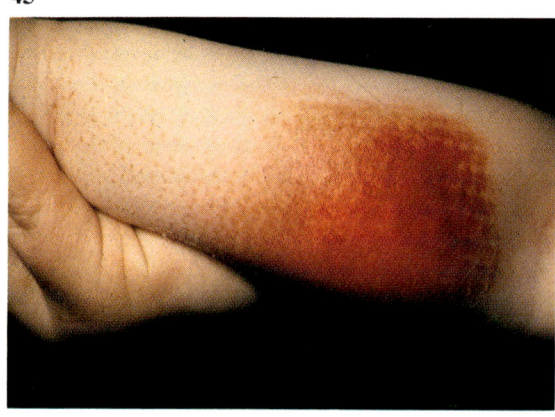

46 Wringer injury of the hand causing multiple lacerations and skin abrasions of the compressed fingers. Associated fractures are rare.

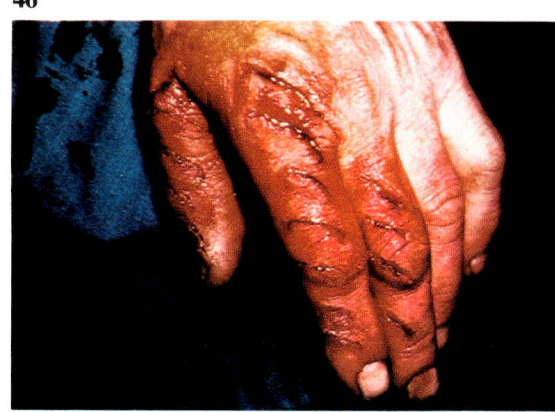

47 Pellet injury of the right cheek. The degree of penetration depends on the velocity and force of the pellet. The pellet is capable of penetrating the eyeball and of entering the thoracic or abdominal cavities causing injury to the viscera.

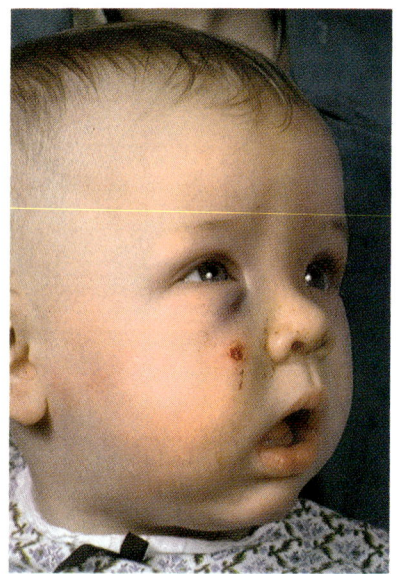

5 Burns

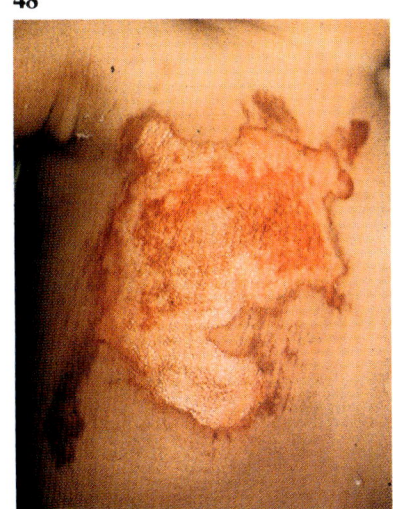

48 Scald of the chest wall. This type of burn is common in toddlers who unbalance a hot kettle or pot perched on the edge of a flat surface. The red (erythematous) area in the centre of the scald indicates full thickness skin loss.

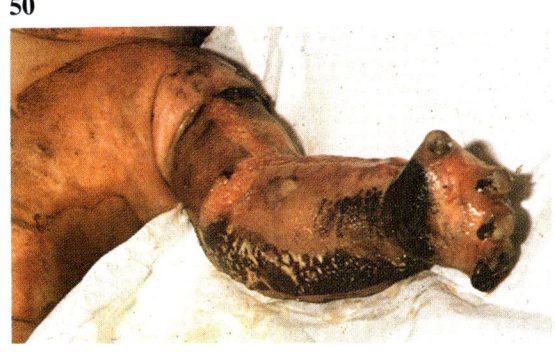

49 Scald. Extensive scald of the back, shoulders and upper arms in a two-year old who toppled a boiling kettle by grabbing the electric cord (flex). All burns involving more than ten per cent surface area of the body should be admitted to hospital.

50 Burns. Full-thickness burn of the left arm and hand in an 18-month-old baby who fell into an unguarded fire. Note the extensive soft-tissue damage to the palm of the hand and fingers.

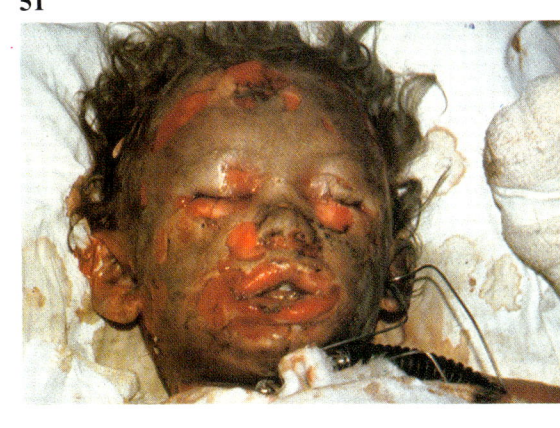

51 Fire burn. Flame burn of the face in an infant trapped in a burning room. Burns of the face may be associated with oedema of the larynx in the immediate post-burn period and endotracheal intubation may be required to provide an adequate air passage.

52 Inhalation of fumes by a victim trapped in a burning room damages the bronchial and alveolar membranes resulting in pneumonia and pulmonary oedema. Artificial ventilation may be life saving.

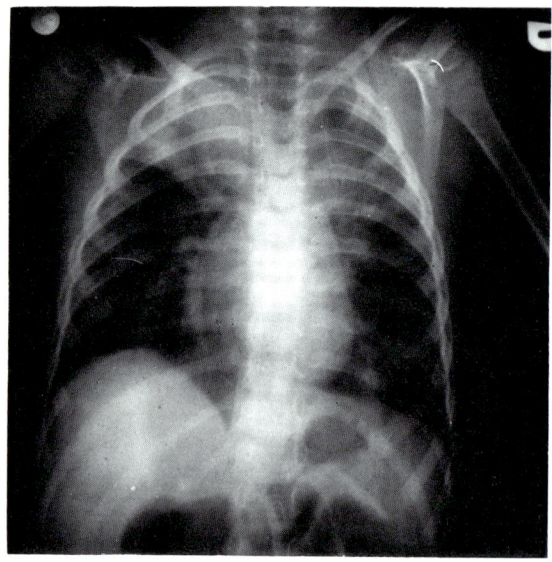

53 Electric burn of the palm of the hand. The infant grasped the bar of an electric heater. In most cases full-thickness tissue injury, which commonly involves the muscle tendons producing fixed contractures of the fingers, is sustained.

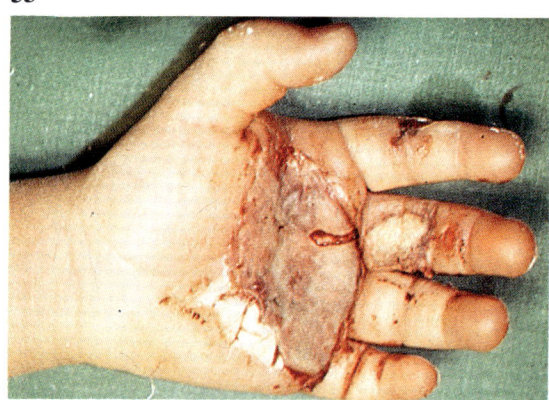

54 Electric shock caused by handling a live wire. Note the maximum damage at the site of contact with skip-lesions at the flexures of the elbow and shoulder.

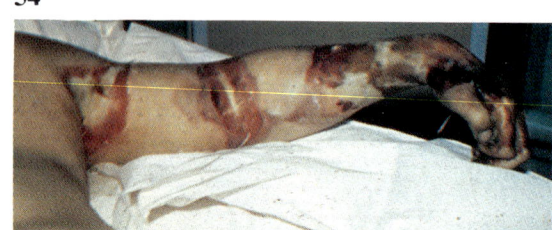

55 Electric burn of the lower lip with subsequent scarring. The infant sucked the bared flex of an electric iron plugged into the mains.

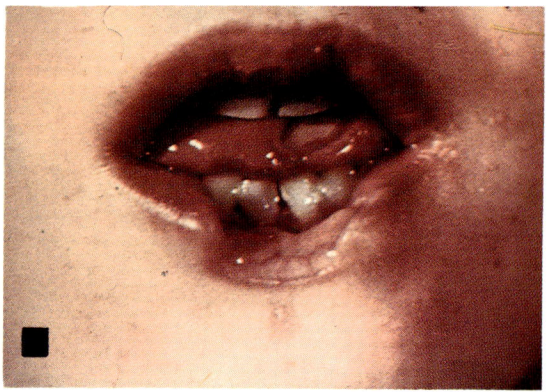

6 The eye

56 Hyphaema – blood in the anterior chamber of the eye after blunt trauma. Note also a fairly extensive subconjunctival haemorrhage. Hyphaema may also develop after a penetrating injury of the eyeball. The bleeding arises from a tear in the ciliary body.

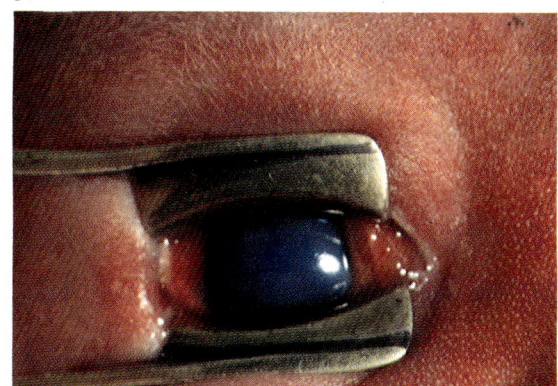

57 Orbital fractures, usually caused by blunt trauma, may involve separation of the frontozygomatic junction in the lateral wall of the orbit and result in downward displacement of the floor. Orbital blowout fractures are caused by impact from a tennis ball, a snowball or a fist. Tomography of the left orbit reveals a defect in the inferior margin. The left maxillary antrum is radiodense as a result of the prolapse of orbital contents and oedema of the antral mucosa.

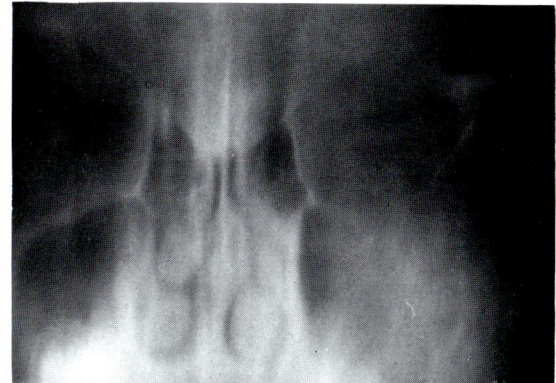

58 Adhesions of the eyelids is an uncommon congenital failure of complete separation of the upper from the lower eyelid. Simple lysis of the adhesions is all that is required.

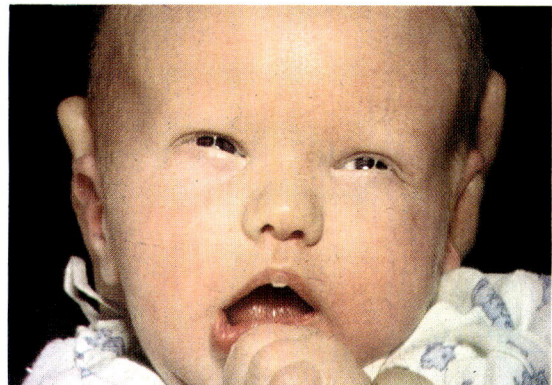

59 Coloboma, i.e. a defect in the lid margin, predominantly affects the upper lid. In this situation associated defects of the eye are uncommon. Coloboma of the lower lid may be accompanied by a defect in the iris.

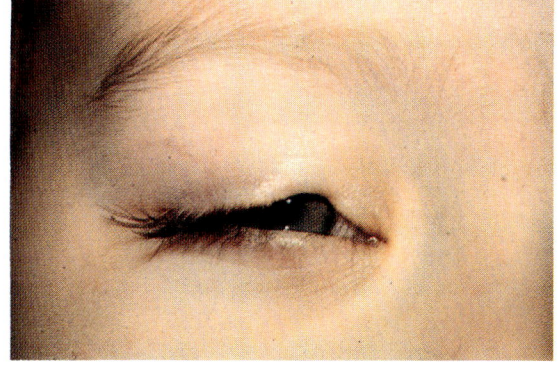

60 Congenital ptosis of the left eyelid. The condition is caused by a varying degree of localised muscular dystrophy of the levator palpebrae superioris. Treatment is by plication of the levator muscle or by excision of the redundant portion. Must be differentiated from paralytic or sympathetic ptosis and ptosis caused by neuromuscular diseases.

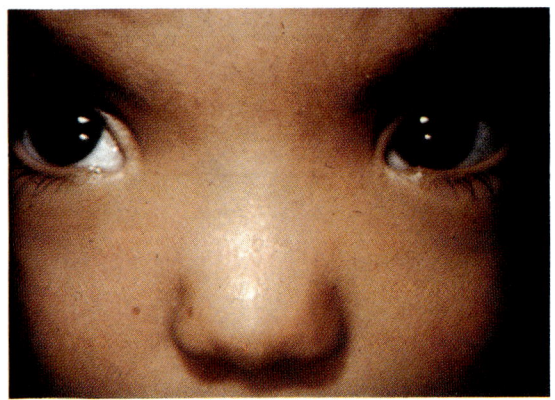

61 Hypertelorism i.e. lateral displacement of the orbits, varies in severity from a minor deformity in which the intercanthal distance measures between 30 mm and 34 mm to gross deformities in which the interorbital distance is considerably increased and where the orbits are rotated outwards. The condition may be associated with facial clefts or craniosynostosis and mental deficiency is common in the severe form.

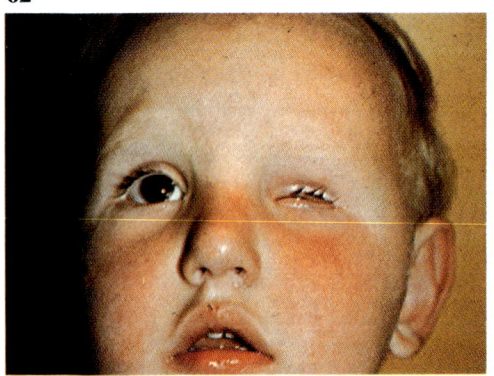

62 Congenital absence of the eye. Rarely this may represent a true anophthalmos but more commonly there is a microphthalmos in which a vestigial eyeball is present. The eye socket is usually small and requires to be deepened to retain a prosthesis.

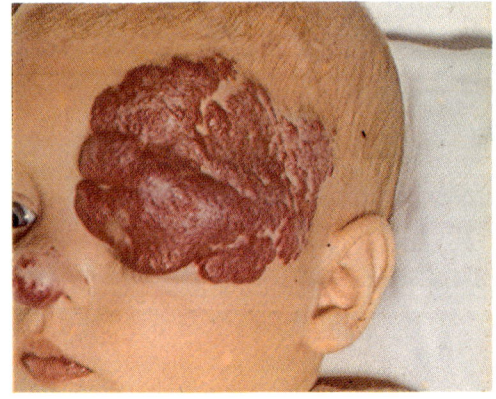

63 Haemangioma involving the left eye. The condition presents as a superficial, flat lesion at birth, but rapidly develops a deep cavernous element causing the lesion to project from the surface encasing the underlying eye. Spontaneous involution by five to seven years of age is the expected outcome, but there may be residual skin deformity.

64 Anterior encephalocoele involving the left supraorbital region. Protrusion of the meningeal sac occurred through the superior orbital fissure. Encephalocoeles are more commonly sited in the midline of the skull with posterior lesions (occipital) predominating.

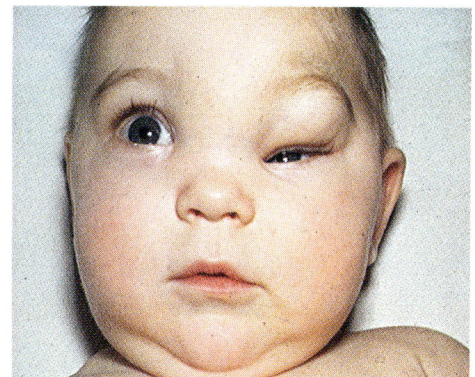

65 External angular dermoid cyst. The cyst composed of sebaceous material is generally closely adherent to the underlying periosteum and often produces a saucer-shaped depression in the frontal bone. The cyst is excised via an incision placed in the line of the eyebrow.

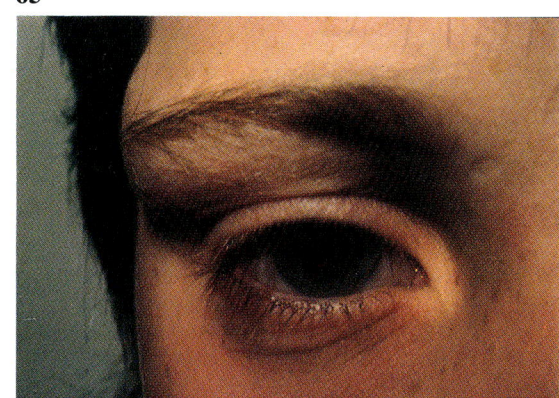

66 Acute dacrocystitis is common secondary to obstruction of the nasolacrimal duct. Usually responds to antibiotic therapy (local and systemic). Probing of the duct once the infection has been controlled may be indicated to prevent recurrent infections.

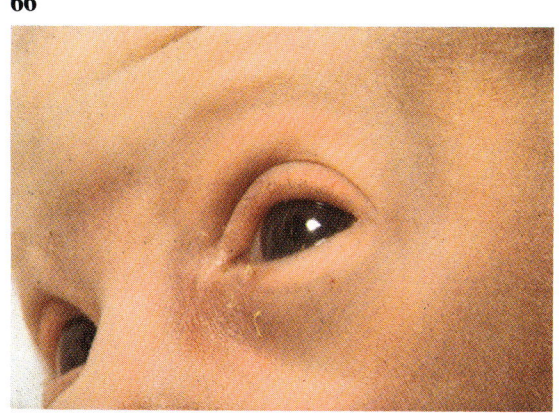

67 Strabismus (squint) is a deviation of the visual axis of one or other eye. The angle of deviation between the two visual axes remains more or less constant, irrespective of the direction in which the eyes are moved. Convergent strabismus is more common than the divergent type. Early treatment (conservative or surgical) is important if binocular vision is to be established.

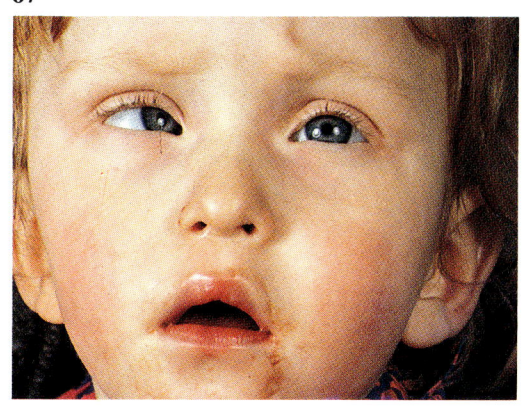

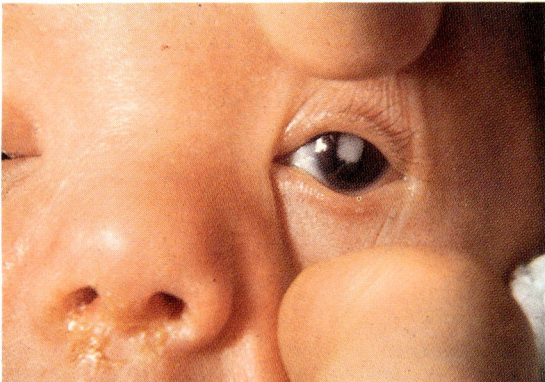

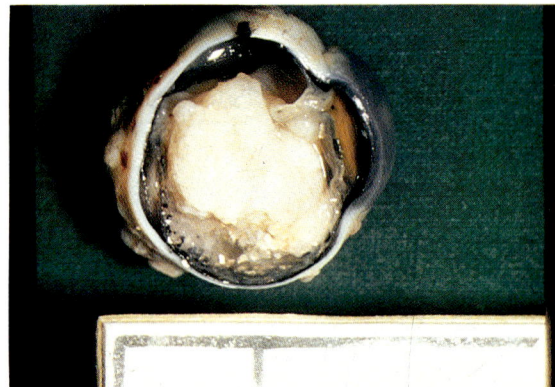

68 Cataract in an infant with congenital rubella syndrome. Usually, but not invariably bilateral. A dense white opacity is centrally located and gradually fades towards the periphery of the lens. Differentiation from the many other causes of congenital cataract is important, e.g. hereditary, chromosomal, metabolic, ocular, CNS disorders.

69 Retinoblastoma is the most common intraocular malignant tumour of childhood. Incidence: approximately 1:20,000. The diagnosis is most frequently made between 18 and 24 months of age. The presenting sign in most cases is the familiar 'cat's eye' reflex (leukokoria) first noted by the mother. Strabismus occurs in 20 per cent of cases. One-third of cases are bilateral. The disease may be familial-autosomal dominant.

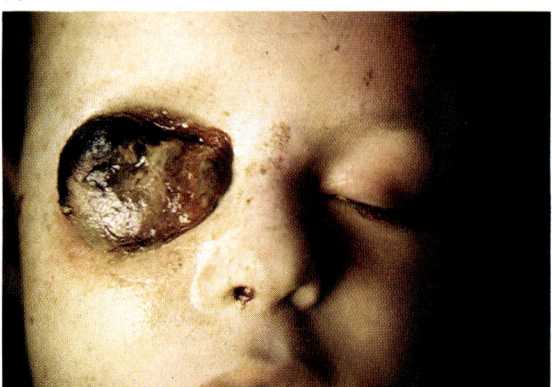

70 Rhabdomyosarcoma of the orbit in a seven-year-old boy. The presenting symptom was unilateral proptosis which progressed at an alarming rate. The prognosis depends on cell type (embryonal, alveolar or undifferentiated), stage of disease and mode of treatment. Radiotherapy and combined multiple chemotherapy have improved the outcome significantly.

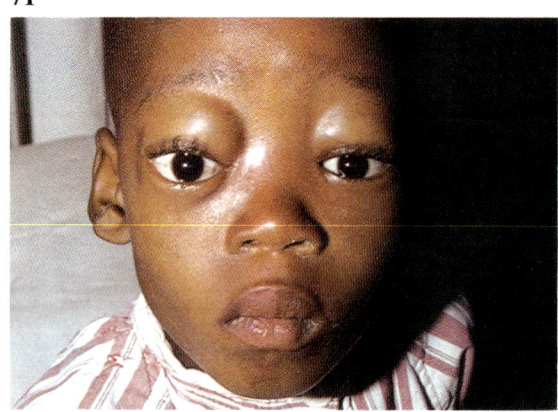

71 Proptosis. Unilateral proptosis of recent onset in a four-year-old boy. The differential diagnosis includes any space-occupying lesion of the orbit, e.g. primary and secondary neoplasm of which rhabdomyosarcoma and neuroblastoma respectively are the most common, haemangiomas, trauma and inflammatory conditions (orbital cellulitis). This child was diagnosed as having retro-orbital tuberculosis.

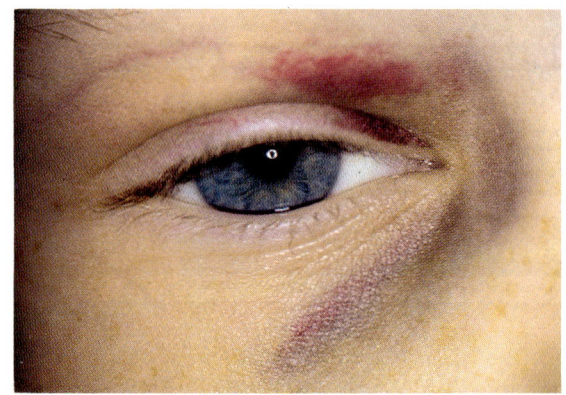

72 Neuroblastoma. Metastatic neuroblastoma to the orbit usually occurs late in the course of the disease. The primary is almost invariably abdominal in location. There is spontaneous periorbital lid ecchymosis without involvement of the eye itself. Xray may reveal metastatic involvement of the orbital bones.

7 The nose

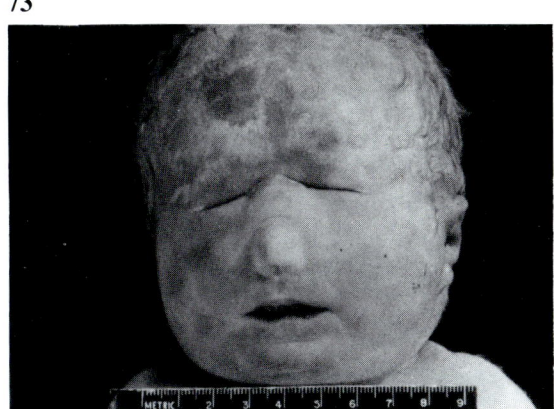

73 Anosia. Absence of the nasal cavity on both sides in a stillborn infant. This rare congenital abnormality more commonly affects one side of the nose.

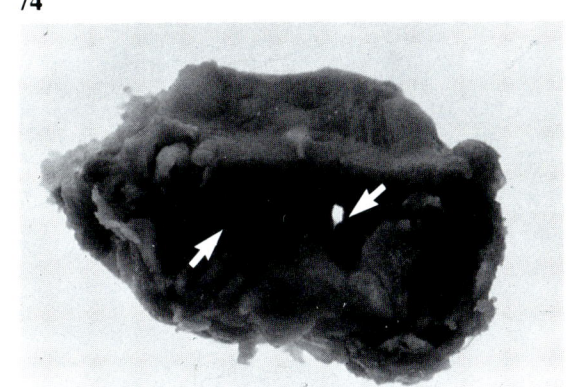

74 Choanal atresia – resected specimen of the nasopharyngeal region showing a complete block of the right and a narrow stenosis of the left nasal passage. As the newborn infant is an obligatory nose breather, bilateral choanal atresia is a life-threatening condition. Failure of a fine catheter to enter the nasopharynx through the nose is diagnostic. The diagnosis may be confirmed by instilling radio-opaque contrast material through the nose. Provision of a patent airway is urgent.

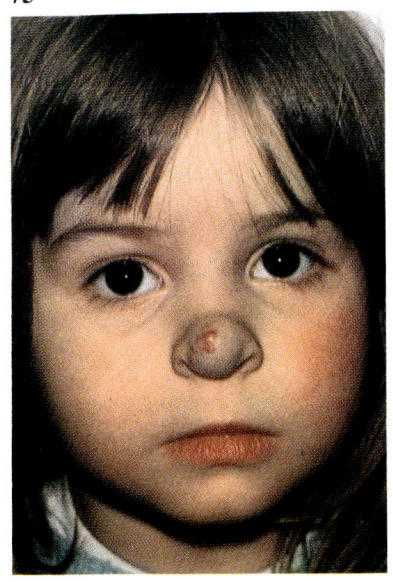

75 Haemangioma of the nose. Usually presents within a short period after birth and increases in size until 9 to 12 months of age. Thereafter, there is a lag of about five years after which rapid spontaneous regression takes place. Cosmetic surgery may be required for residual disfigurement. Surgery may be required if there is ulceration and haemorrhage or the entire lesion can be excised without excessive haemorrhage and without causing further disfigurement.

76 Nasal encephalocoele is caused by protrusion of the meninges through a defect in the frontonasal suture. These lesions have a better prognosis than the occipital encephalocoeles as herniation of brain tissue occurs less frequently. Treatment is by excision of the dural sac and repair of the defect by bone graft.

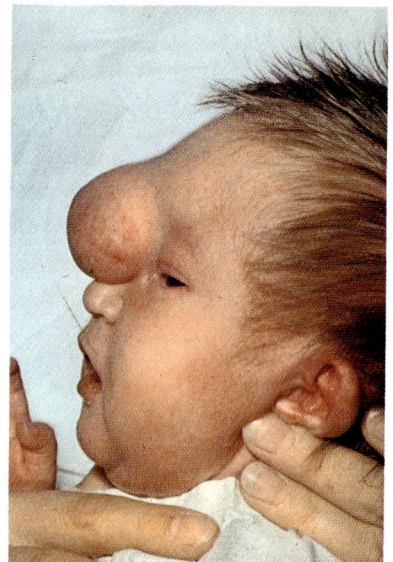

77 Cleft lip. Deformity of the right nasal cavity in association with complete unilateral cleft lip and palate. This deformity is discussed more fully in the section on the mouth.

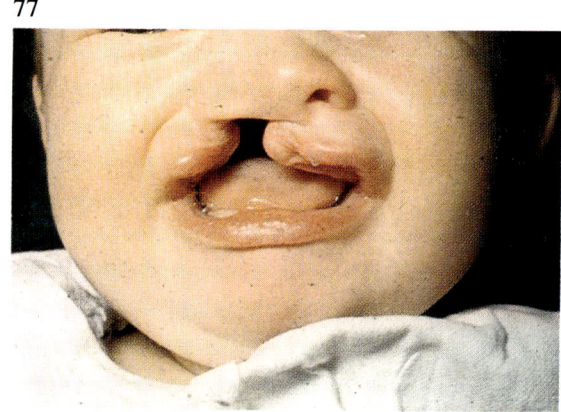

8 The mouth

78 Microstoma may be a congenital abnormality or acquired secondary to a burn, either electric or corrosive (caustic soda), or after extensive excisional lip surgery.

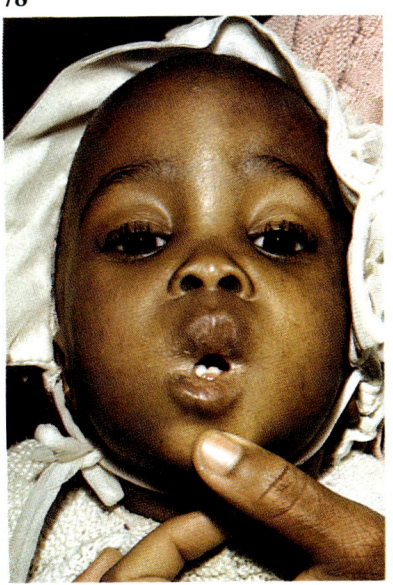

79 Macrostoma or transverse facial cleft is a crease or fissure which appears on the cheek between the developing mesoderm of the mandible and the maxillary processes. The cleft extends from the angle of the mouth for a varying distance to the region of the ear. It may be unilateral or bilateral.

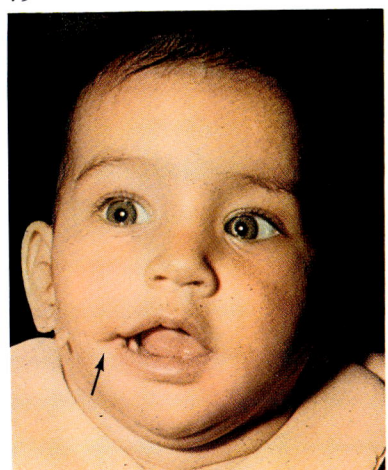

80 Haemangioma of the lower lip in a four-month-old girl. Note also the swelling of the left parotid region, also caused by a haemangioma. The lesion invariably contains a mixture of capillary and cavernous elements and usually regresses by the age of seven to eight years. Surgical excision may be indicated for the bleeding and ulcerating lesion, or where complete excision without causing disfigurement can be easily accomplished.

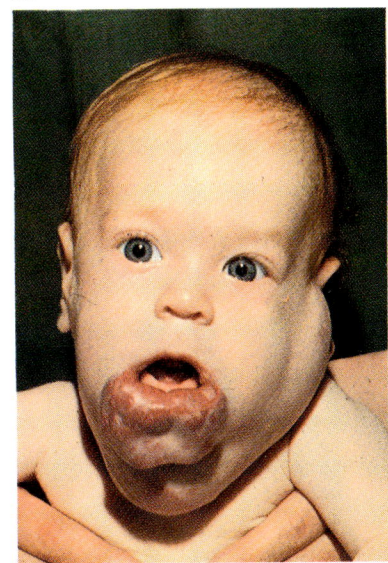

81 Frenulum of the upper lip extending on to the hard palate and causing separation of the upper central incisor teeth. Treatment is by Z-plasty lengthening of the band together with excision of the excessive submucosal tissue between the incisor teeth.

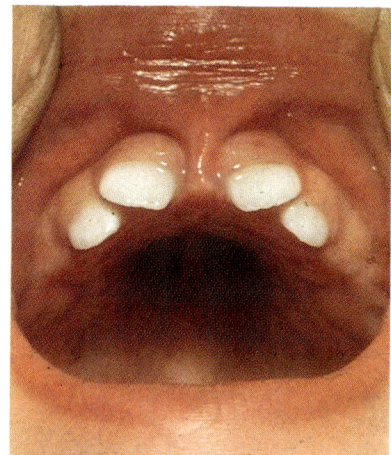

82 Mucus cyst of the lower lip. Characteristically presents as a soft bluish inframucosal painless swelling. Caused either by extravasation of mucus from or retention of mucus in a minor salivary gland. It may occur on the lips, cheeks or floor of the mouth.

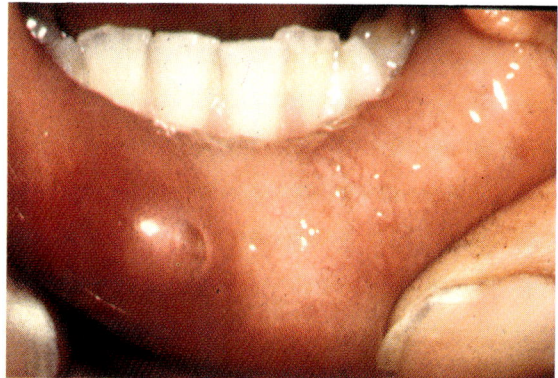

83 Ranula – a slowly enlarging, painless swelling in the floor of the mouth beneath the anterior part of the tongue. It is smooth, rounded, of fluid consistency and bluish in colour. Probably caused by retention and/or extravasation of mucus from the sublingual and/or submandibular salivary glands. Occasionally extends into the neck – 'plunging ranula'. Treatment is by marsupialisation. Excision of the sublingual gland may be required for recurrence of the lesion.

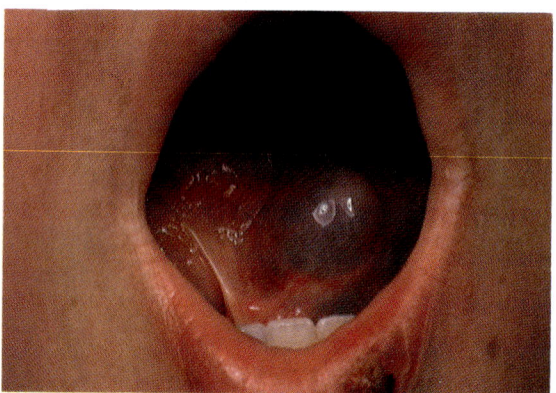

84 Ludwig's angina – rapidly spreading infection of the sublingual and submandibular spaces. Tendency to spread down into the neck and cause laryngeal oedema with stridor and dysphagia. Caused by infection, usually streptococcal, originating in an infected tooth, wound or ulcer in the floor of the mouth. Treatment is by massive broad-spectrum antibiotics with drainage of pus, where present, to relieve tissue tension.

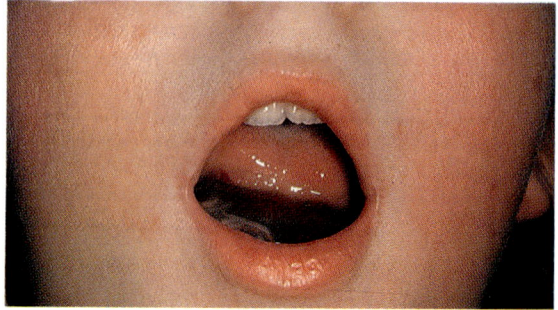

Clefts of the lip and palate

The basic embryological defect is a failure of separate mesodermal masses to meet and fuse; as a result the overlying epithelium is stretched until it separates leaving a cleft of varying degrees. The primary palate is formed by the fusion of a central mass, from which the premaxilla develops, and two lateral masses. The secondary palate i.e. the remainder of the hard palate and the soft palate, results from fusion of the lateral shelves which normally completes the separation of the oral and nasal cavities.

Three groups of clefts are recognised.
- Group 1: clefts of the anterior or primary palate
- Group 2: clefts of the anterior and posterior palate
- Group 3: clefts of the posterior or secondary palate

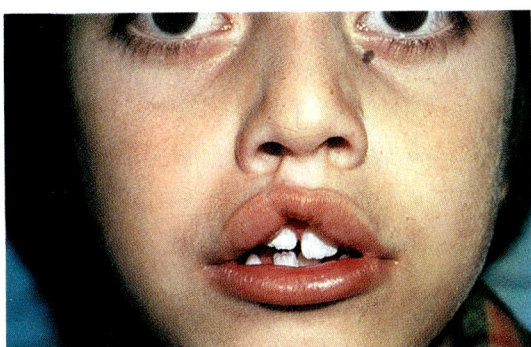

85 Minor cleft of the right upper lip. An example of a Group 1 defect.

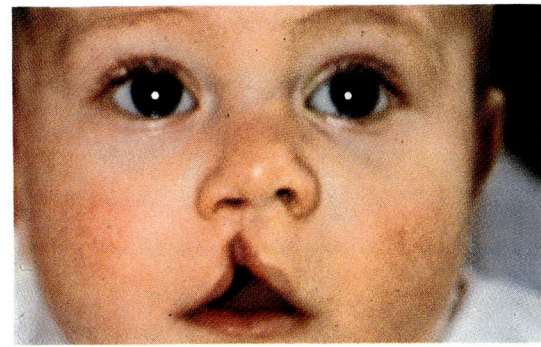

86 Partial or incomplete cleft of the left upper lip (Group 1 defect).

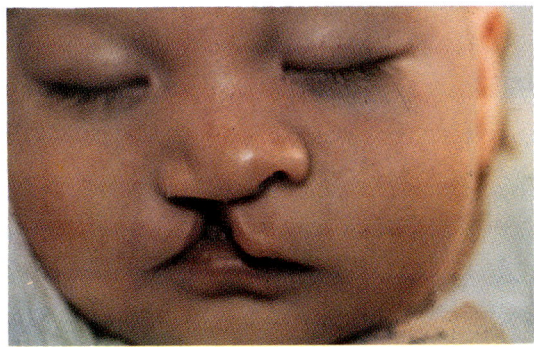

87 Complete cleft of the right upper lip without associated cleft palate (Group 1 defect).

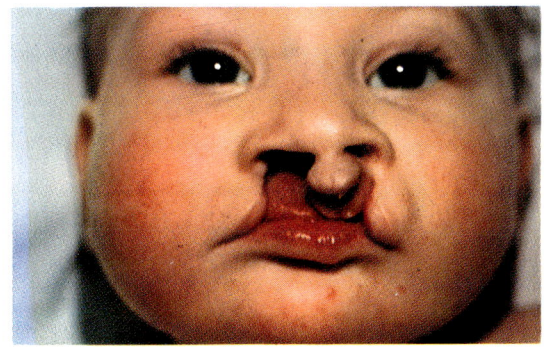

88 Bilateral cleft lip, complete left and incomplete right, in association with cleft palate (Group 2 defect).

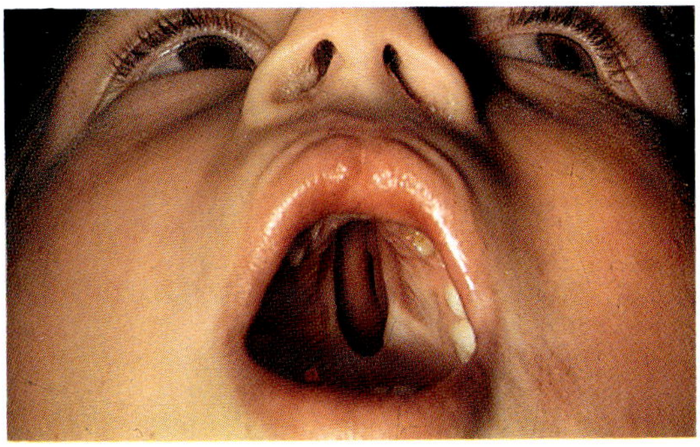

89 Isolated cleft of the hard palate extending to the posterior margin of the premaxilla. An example of a Group 3 anomaly.

33

9 The jaws

90 Pierre-Robin syndrome consists of a hypoplastic mandible in association with a cleft palate. It may result in recurrent attacks of respiratory distress in the neonatal period as a result of the tongue falling backwards and obstructing the airway. With skilful nursing and careful positioning respiratory obstruction can be prevented. Surgical intervention is rarely required. Spontaneous disappearance of the micrognathism occurs within two to three years.

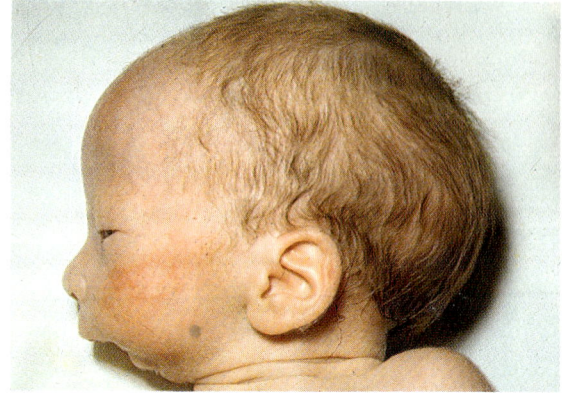

91 Eruption cyst of the upper gum margin at the site of the developing first premolar tooth. The cyst has a bluish appearance and it usually ruptures spontaneously discharging its fluid content.

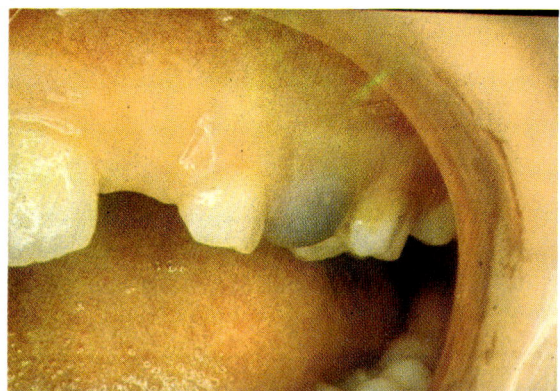

92 Congenital epulis (granular cell myoblastoma) in a newborn infant. The pedunculated lesion is covered by mucosa and arises from the anterior portion of the upper jaw. Treatment is by simple excision. Recurrence is rare.

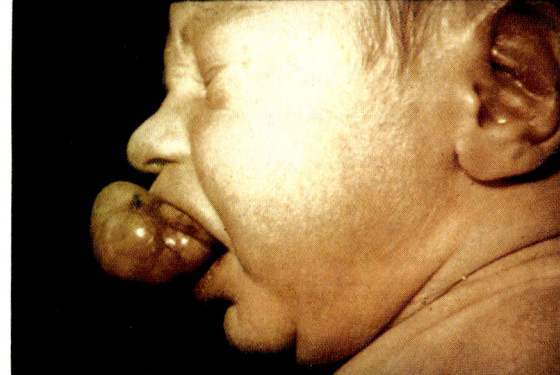

93   Giant epulis in a female newborn infant.

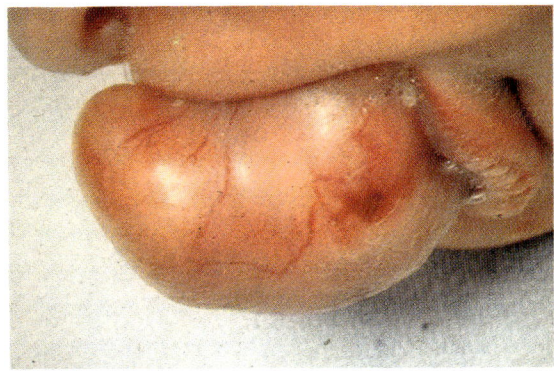

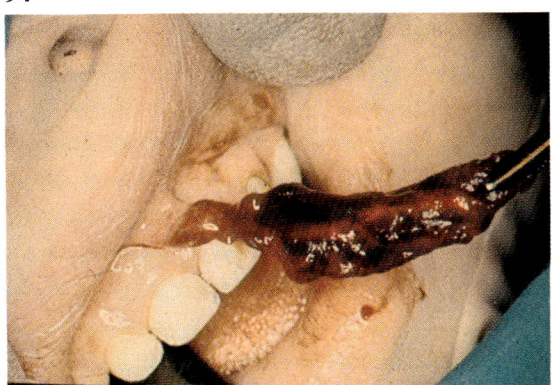

94   Haemophilia. Haemorrhage into the frenulum of the upper lip following trauma in a child with haemophilia. The frenulum is distended with blood and forms a pedunculated mass.

95   Haemangiolymphangioma. Hamartomatous malformation of the left maxillary region consisting of mixed haemangiomatous and lymphangiomatous elements. Spontaneous regression is rare although the lesion ceases to grow after puberty. Excision for cosmetic purposes is usually indicated.

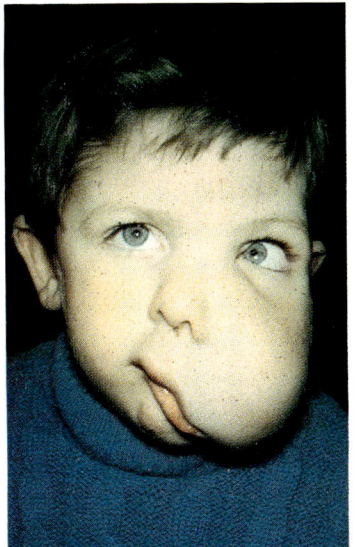

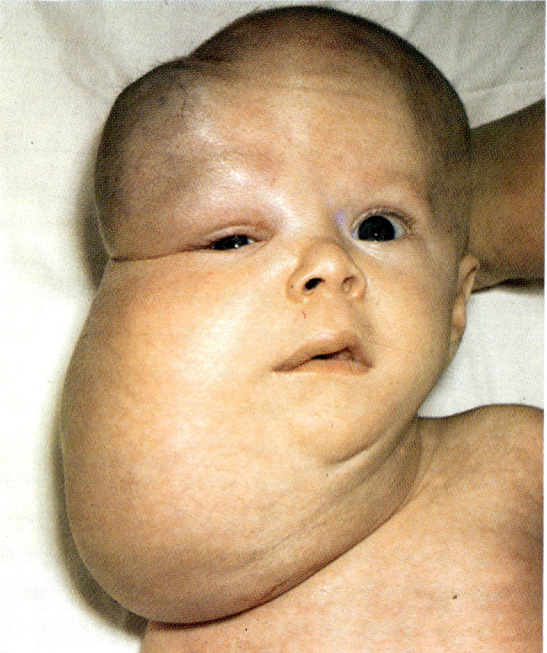

96 Haemangiolymphangioma. Extensive haemangiolymphangioma of the right submandibular region extending into the neck and upwards into the temporal region of the scalp.

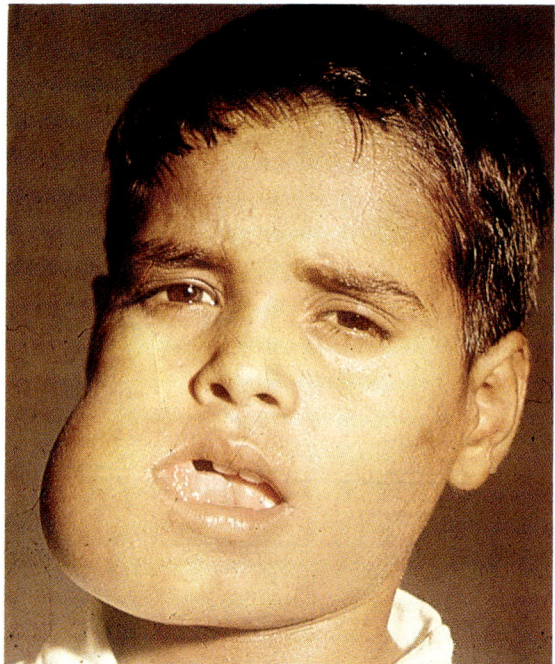

97 Ameloblastoma (adamantinoma) – multilocular tumour, usually involving the mandible, arising from the epithelium of the enamel organ. Rare in childhood. Treatment is by radical excision. Incomplete removal is responsible for the high incidence of recurrence.

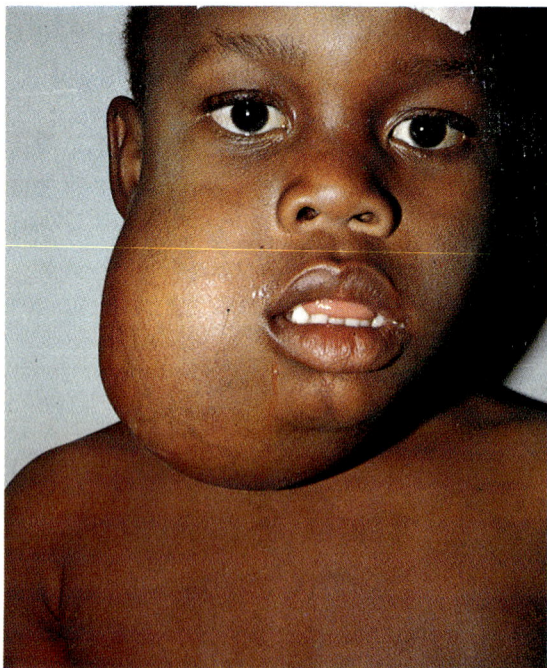

98 Burkitt's lymphoma – commonest tumour in African children. It has a striking predilection for the jaw. Earliest manifestation of jaw involvement is loosening of the teeth. The maxilla is more frequently involved than the mandible. One-third of patients present with abdominal involvement. Epstein-Barr virus has been implicated in the aetiology. Prognosis is poor.

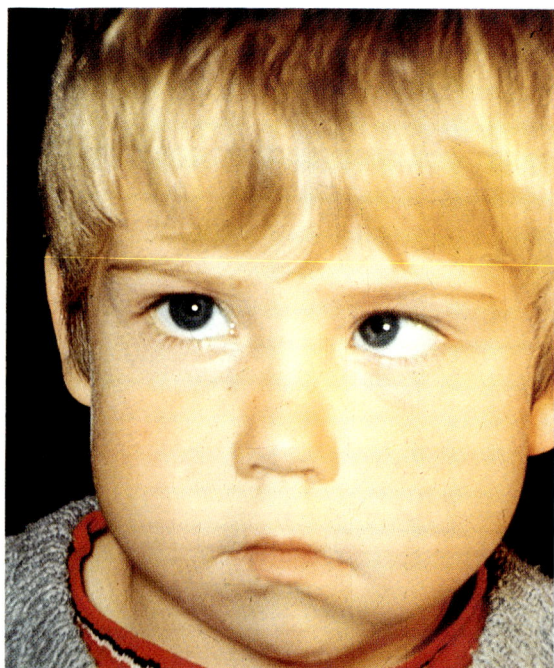

99 Cherubism – a curious type of fibrous dysplasia which presents as swelling of the mandible and later of the maxilla in children between two and four years of age. The deposition of fibrous tissue within the medullary portion of the bone causes marked expansion of the jaw with displacement of the teeth. Distortion of the cheeks causes upward displacement of the globe of the eye. Reaches maximum cosmetic deformity at puberty.

10 The tongue

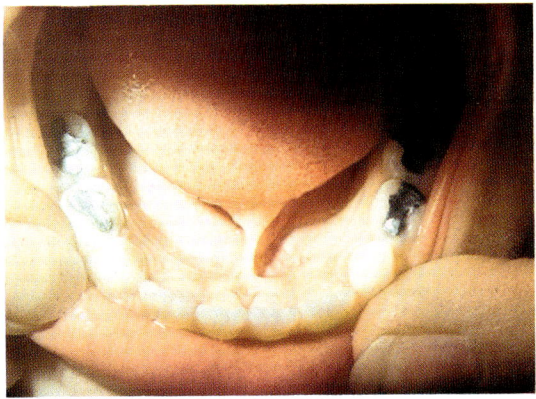

100 Tongue tie (ankyloglossia inferior) – common in infancy but only rarely interferes with normal speech. Surgical release is only required if the tongue cannot protrude beyond the lower gum margin.

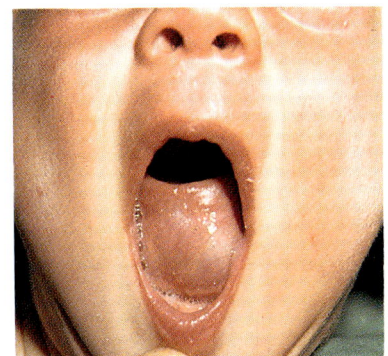

101 Sublingual cyst – usually found in the midline of the inferior surface within the substance of the tongue. May be dermoid cysts, cysts of thyroglossal tract origin or duplication cysts containing ectopic gastrointestinal mucosa. May cause respiratory embarrassment. Treatment is by excision.

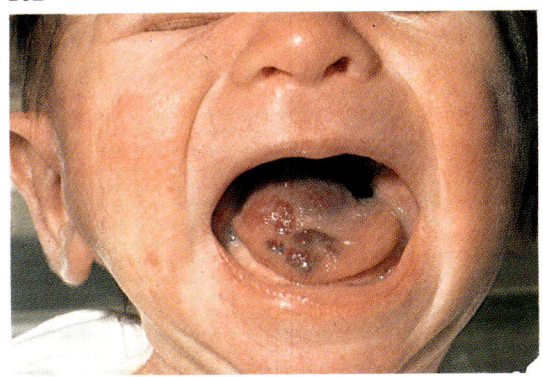

102 Haemangioma of the tongue – localised and projecting from the surface. Bleeds easily from minor trauma. Prevention of infection by sound oral hygiene is important. Local surgical measures (coagulation, sclerosant, excision) are usually sufficient to stop recurrent bleeding.

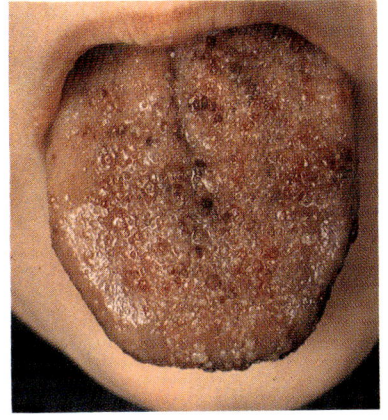

103 Haemangiolymphangioma. Diffuse haemangiolymphangioma of the tongue producing a variegated appearance of the surface. Usually associated with poor oral hygiene, gingivitis and dental caries. Bleeding from the surface caused by minor trauma or from superficial ulcers secondary to chronic infection is common. Treatment is extremely difficult and may involve subtotal glossectomy as a bulk-reducing procedure.

104 Mucus cyst of the tongue presenting as a localised swelling in the midline of the undersurface. It is caused by retention of mucus in a minor salivary gland within the surface of the tongue. Treatment is by local excision.

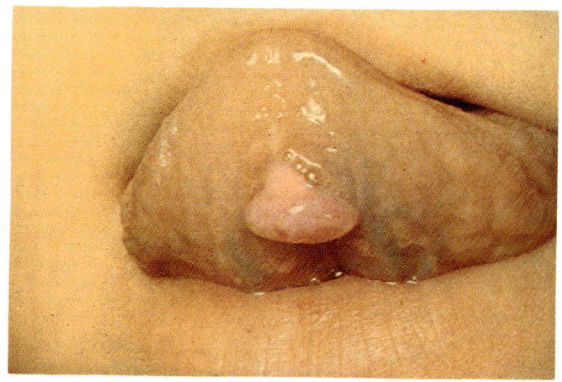

105 Papilloma of the tongue. There is a projecting pedunculated lesion on the surface of the tongue. Commonly an isolated fibrous polyp but occasionally forms part of the orofacial digital syndrome (hypoplastic alae nasi, hypertrophic frenulae of lip and tongue, multilobed tongue, cleft palate, dental defects, deformed hands and, sometimes, polycystic disease of the liver and kidneys).

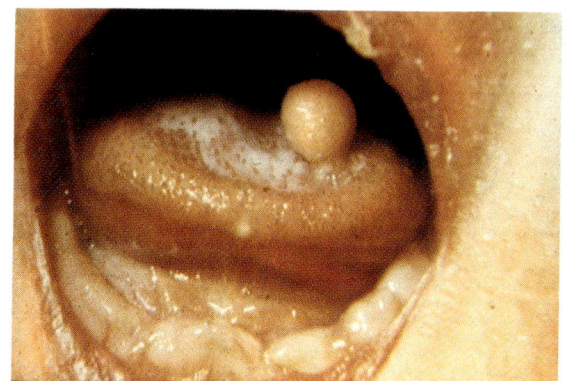

106 Macroglossia is the term given to describe a chronic painless enlargement of the tongue. It may be non-specific with an overgrowth of all tongue tissue or specific when the enlargement is caused by haemangioma, lymphangioma, neurofibroma. In the non-specific form macroglossia may be associated with Down's syndrome (mongolism), as in the child illustrated, mental retardation, cretinism or exomphalos.

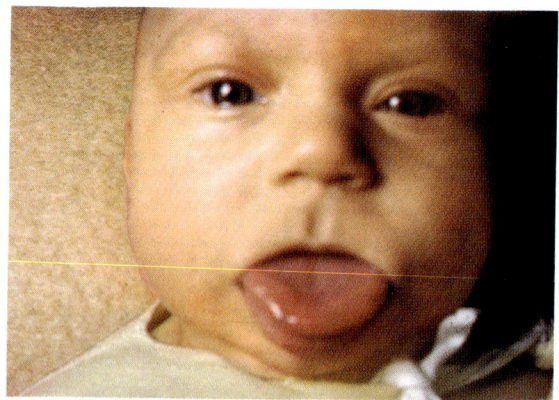

107 Macroglossia. Diffuse non-specific macroglossia associated with Beckwith-Wiedermann syndrome (EMG syndrome). The syndrome consists of the association of exomphalos, macroglossia, macrosomia (occasionally with a cleft palate), facial naevus flammeus, indented ear lobes, hyperplasia of the kidneys and pancreas.

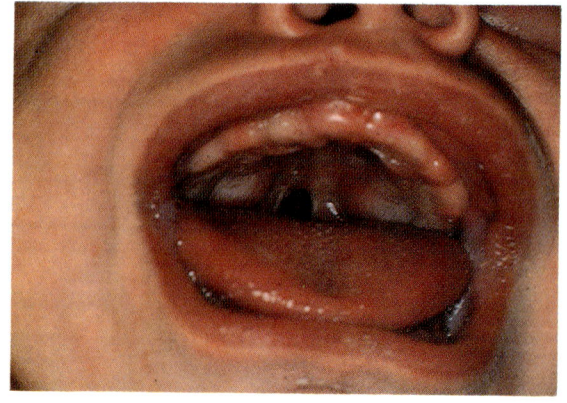

11 The ears

108 Microtia is a congenital abnormality which varies in extent from complete absence of the ear (anotia) to small remnants or to a well-formed miniature ear. Commonly associated with imperforate external auditory canal, absence of tympanic membrane and defects of the middle ear. Unilateral deformity six times more common than bilateral.

109 Preauricular sinus may present as a minute discharging orifice at the anterior border of the helix of the ear or as an acutely inflamed cystic swelling. Treatment consists of excision for the chronically draining sinus or where there has been previous infection. The tract pursues an unpredictable course and may communicate with the external auditory canal, the middle ear, or end blindly in the cartilage of the helix.

110 Preauricular tags vary from a projection of excess skin, for which simple ligation in the neonatal period is all that is required, to lesions containing a combination of cartilage and fibrous tissue. For the complex lesion, formal excision of all ectopic tissue is required.

111 Accessory auricle. Multiple accessory auricles including bilateral pedunculated lesions on the cheeks. These 'tags' are situated on the line of fusion between the maxillary and mandibular processes of the first branchial arch. Treatment is by formal excision.

112 'Bat ears' (protruding auricle) caused by a defect in the normal folding process of the antihelix. The supporting cartilage of the ear holds the ear at right angles to the skull. May be unilateral or bilateral. Cosmetic correction by one of a variety of plastic procedures is often requested by the parents.

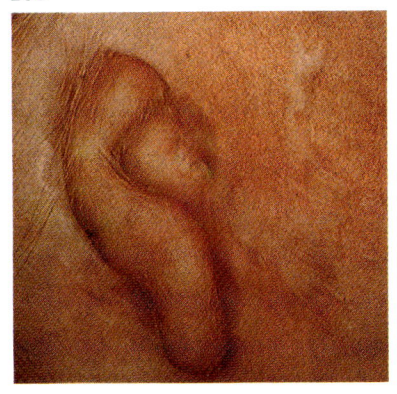

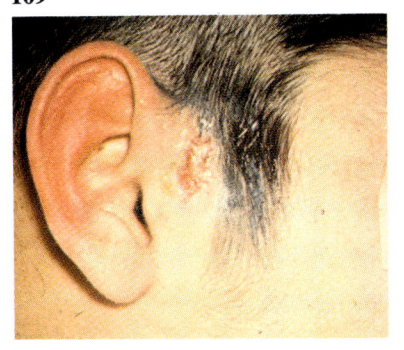

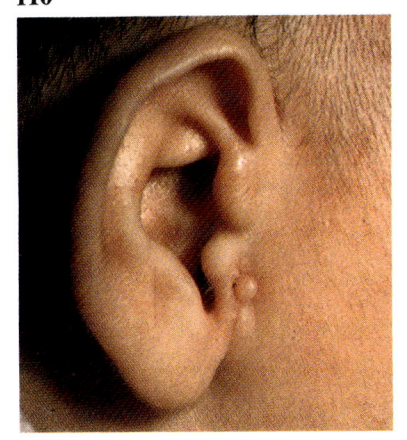

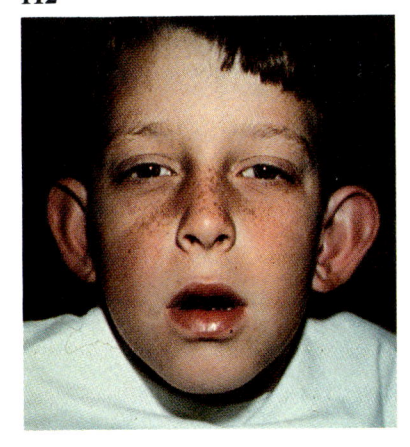

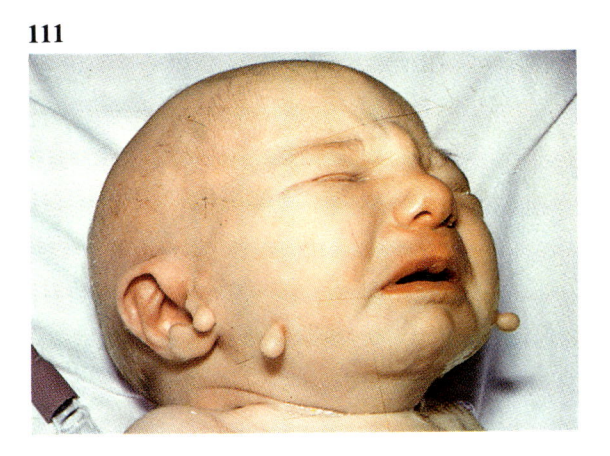

12 Face and skull

113 Crouzon's disease (Apert's disease, craniofacial dysostosis) is caused by premature closure of the suture lines in the vault of the skull with resulting abnormally raised intracranial pressure. The facial deformity consists of proptosis (caused by hypoplasia of the orbits), hypertelorism, depressed bridge of the nose, antimongoloid slant of the eyes, prognathia and a high-arched palate. May have associated syndactylism and mental deficiency. Treatment is by complex combined craniofacial surgery (Tessier).

114 Treacher-Collins syndrome (mandibulofacial dysostosis). The facial component consists of an antimongoloid slant of the eyes, coloboma of the lower lid, facial bone dysostosis, abnormally shaped ears, conductive hearing defect and flame-shaped projection of hair on to the cheeks from the neck. Inheritance is by autosomal dominant trait.

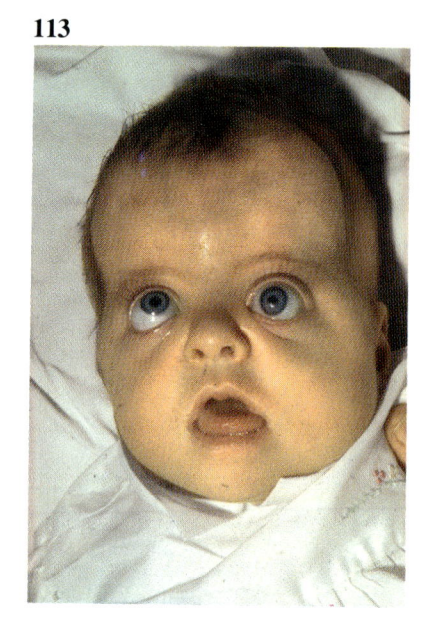

115 Congenital scalp defect. A full-thickness defect in the region overlying the posterior fontanelle. The lesion (if small) may heal spontaneously by the ingrowth of epithelium from the edges of the defect. Large areas require covering with skin-grafts or by rotation flaps.

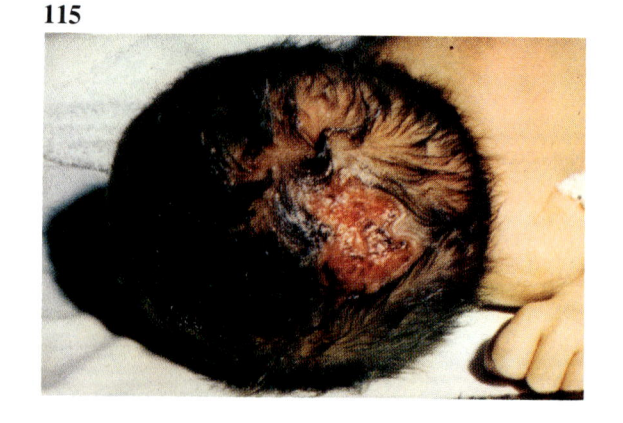

116 Congenital dermal sinus. The peculiar distribution of hair in the midline of the occipital region indicates the orifice of the stratified squamous-epithelium lined tract. The tract may end blindly in the subperiosteal tissue or may extend through a minute bony defect into the extradural or intradural space. Usually diagnosed only after an unexplained episode of meningitis. Treatment is by surgical excision. Probing or sinography are contraindicated because of the risk of introducing intracranial infection.

117 Dermoid cyst in the midline of the scalp. There may be a small dimple on the apex of the lesion through which a tuft of hair may extrude. May be associated with an intracranial element through a defect in the skull. An xray will demonstrate the defect.

118 Haemangiomata of the face pursue a natural history similar to haemangiomata in other situations. They are generally of mixed capillary and cavernous composition and tend to increase rapidly in size to reach a maximum at approximately six to nine months of age. Thereafter, a steady slow regression begins until about seven years, when the lesion may have completely disappeared. This 18-month-old child has bilateral haemangiomata of the parotid regions and a lesion which is completely obliterating the right eye. Regression can be stimulated by systemic steroids or by local sclerosant infiltration.

119 Facial cellulitis. Extensive facial cellulitis after a penetrating injury of the left cheek. This acute spreading infection may also be caused by dental infections. Vigorous antibiotic chemotherapy is indicated to prevent cavernous sinus thrombosis.

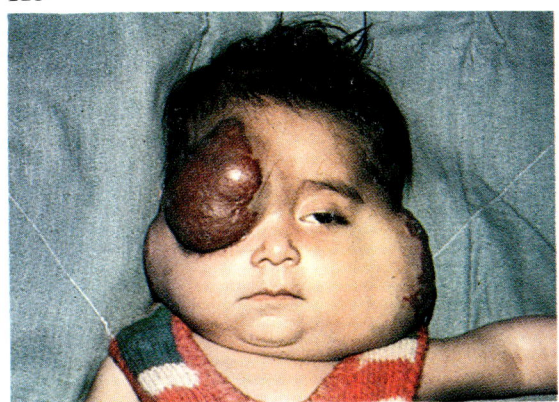

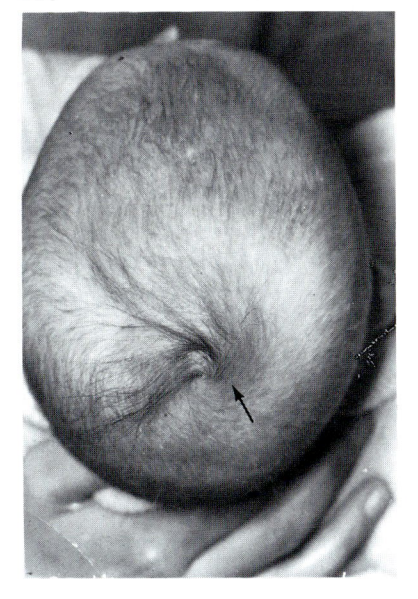

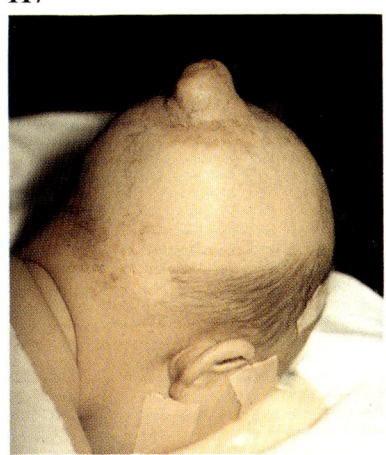

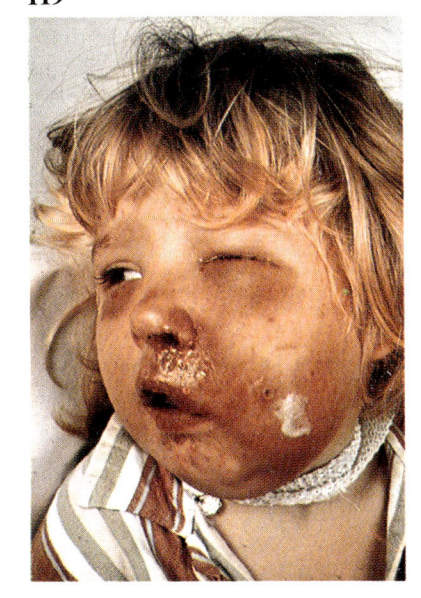

120 Haemangioma of the chin. Occasionally active treatment is required as in this two-month-old child who had a fairly localised ulcerating lesion prone to recurrent episodes of bleeding.

121 Haemangioma. Extensive haemangioma predominantly involving the right side of the face causing obliteration of the eyelids and occlusion of the right nostril. Platelet trapping and development of a bleeding tendency should be suspected in this type of lesion (Kasabach-Merritt syndrome).

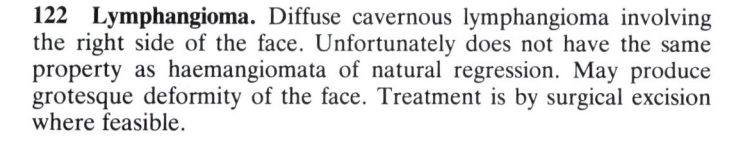

122 Lymphangioma. Diffuse cavernous lymphangioma involving the right side of the face. Unfortunately does not have the same property as haemangiomata of natural regression. May produce grotesque deformity of the face. Treatment is by surgical excision where feasible.

123 Teratoma of the right parotid region producing an enormous pulsating subcutaneous mass. A rare tumour in this region. Treatment is by complete excision.

124 Angiosarcoma of the right parotid producing an ulcerating fungating mass. A rare tumour. Treatment is by radiotherapy and/or chemotherapy with surgery reserved for resection of a residual mass.

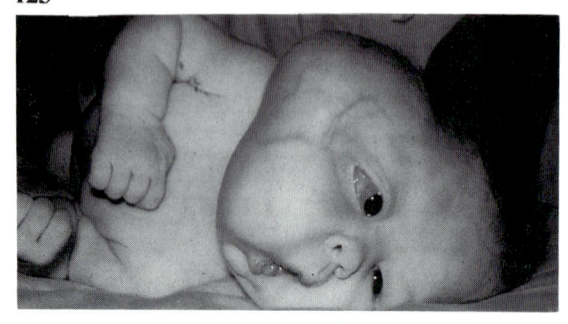

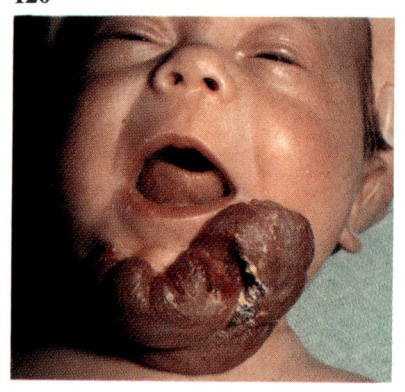

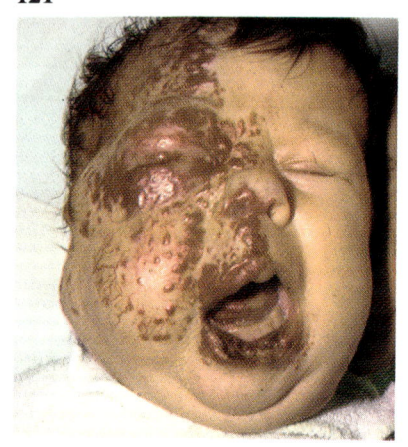

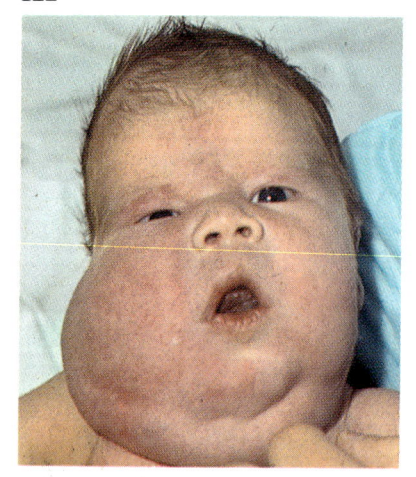

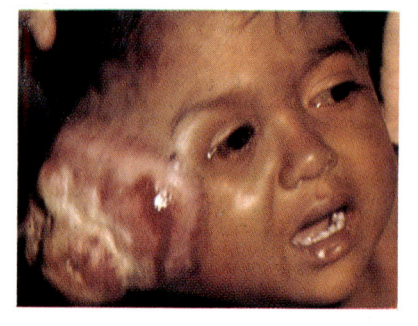

13 Salivary glands

125 Recurrent parotitis is characterised by episodes of acute painful swelling of the parotid glands, accompanied to a greater or lesser extent by a systemic reaction. Beads of pus can be expressed from the parotid duct. Treatment is by broad-spectrum antibiotic therapy and analgesics in the acute phase, together with measures to encourage drainage, e.g. massage, use of acid sweets and chewing gum.

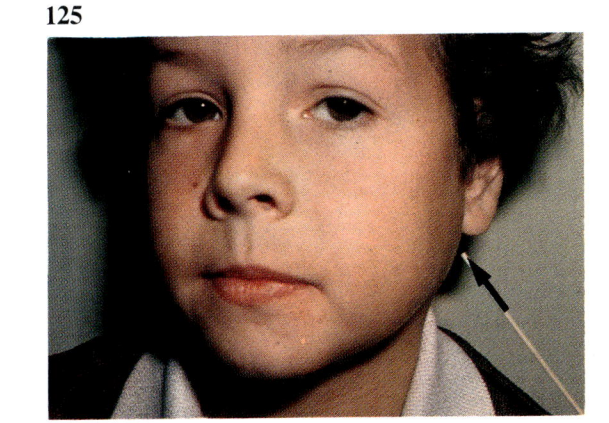

126 Normal parotid sialogram showing the narrow parotid duct branching into finer radicles.

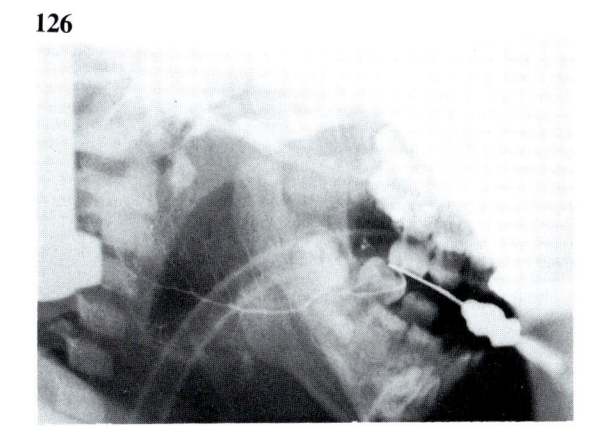

127 Sialectasis. Sialogram in a child with recurrent parotitis. There is diffuse sialectasis consisting of small globules of contrast material associated with the intra-lobular ducts.

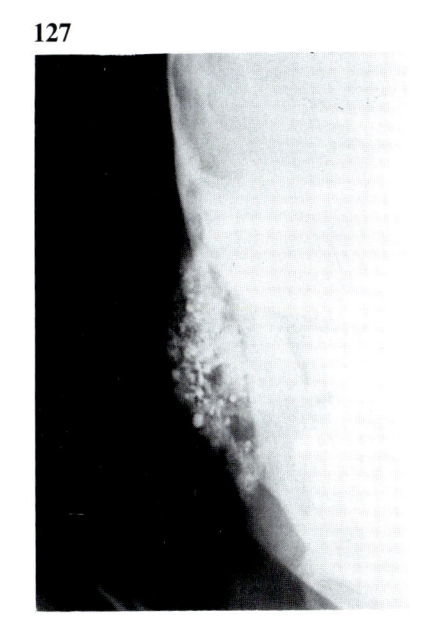

128 Mixed haemangioma of the parotid showing the fine capillary element in the skin overlying the gross cavernous mass. Natural history is towards spontaneous regression but infiltration of sclerosant or use of systemic or local steroids may hasten the process. Surgical extirpation is rarely indicated because of vulnerability of the facial nerve.

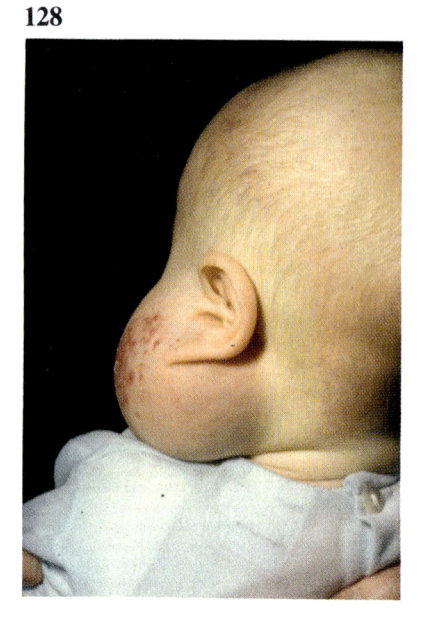

129 Submandibular calculus produces recurrent attacks of submandibular inflammation usually precipitated by eating. The stone can sometimes be felt in the floor of the mouth and is occasionally visible when it impacts near the duct orifice.

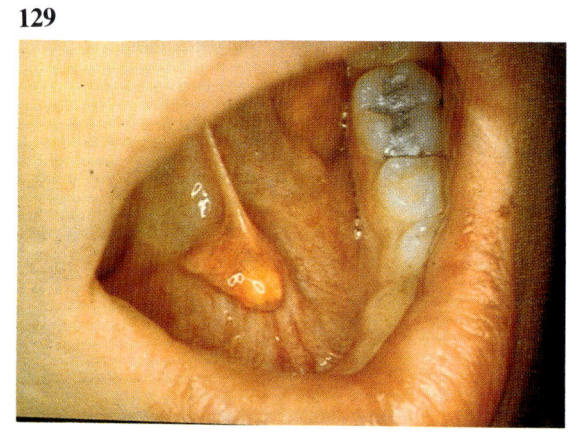

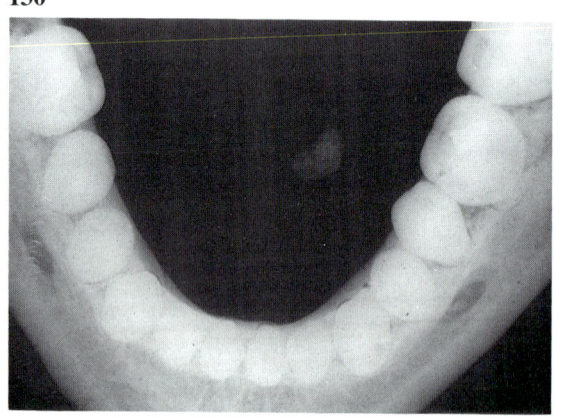

130 Submandibular calculus contains a high proportion of calcium and is often visible on plain xray of the floor of the mouth.

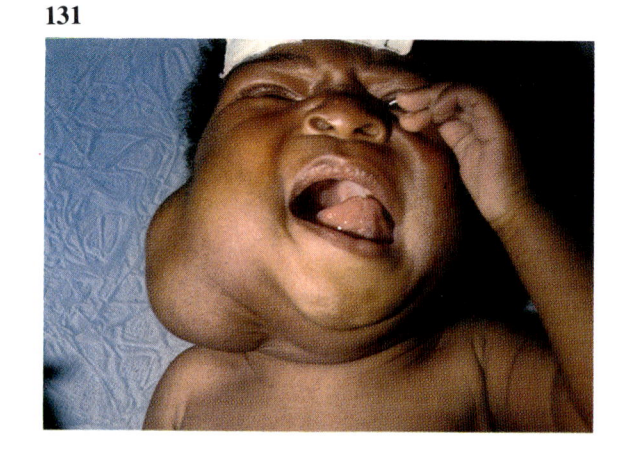

131 Teratoma of the parotid is a rare tumour of infancy. It contains a variety of tissue derived from different germinal layers. Treatment is by complete excision.

14 Pharynx and larynx

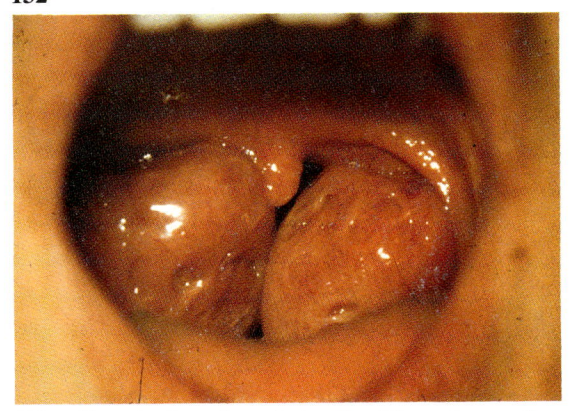

132 Chronically enlarged tonsils. There is usually a history of recurrent attacks of tonsillitis which may be chronically debilitating. Treatment is either by long-term antibiotics or by tonsillectomy.

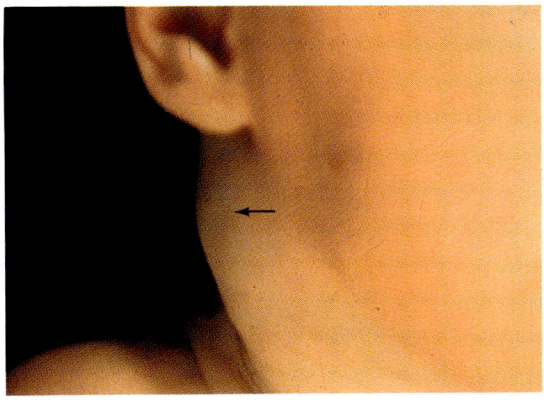

133 Retropharyngeal abscess in an infant. The abscess follows a streptococcal pharyngeal infection and presents with an acutely tender mass in the upper posterior cervical region. A prominent swelling is visible on the ipsilateral side of the posterior pharyngeal wall.

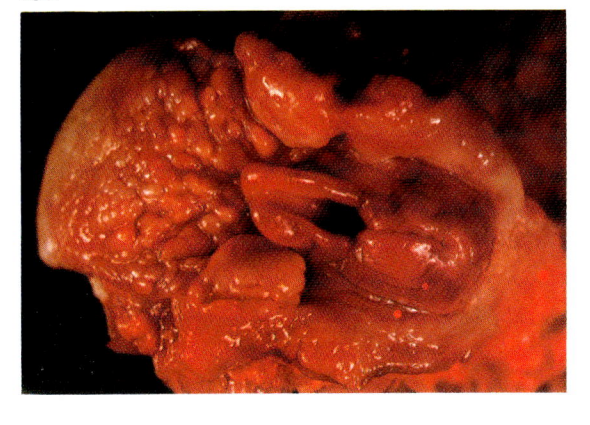

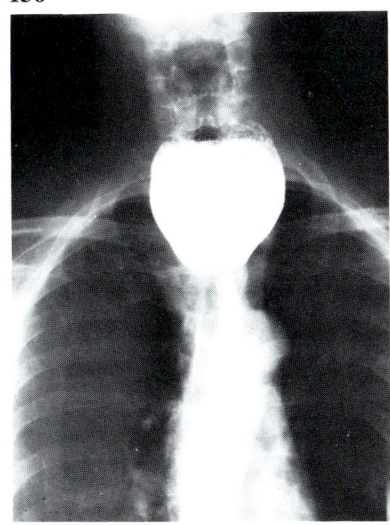

134 Retropharyngeal abscess. Lateral cervical xray in a patient with a retropharyngeal abscess, showing an increased distance between the anterior margin of the second cervical vertebra and the posterior pharyngeal wall.

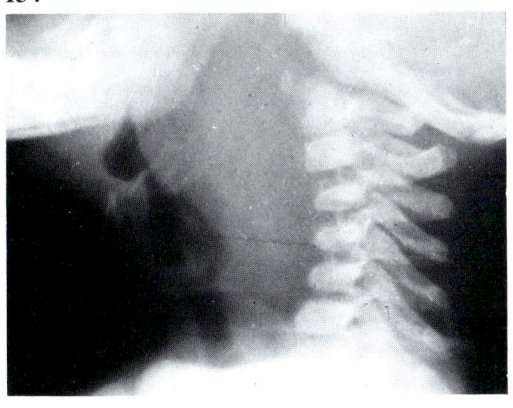

135 Acute epiglottitis. Usually caused by Haemophilus influenza type B infection. There is a rapid onset of dysphagia and dyspnoea which may progress within a short period to respiratory obstruction. The child is usually severely toxic. Treatment is with broad-spectrum antibiotics and humidity. Endotracheal intubation may be necessary for increasing respiratory embarrassment.

136 Pharyngeal pouch diverticulum commonly occurs in elderly males but has been described in the newborn when it presents with swallowing difficulty. Passage of a nasogastric tube may be arrested in the diverticulum. In the immediate neonatal period the condition may be indistinguishable from oesophageal atresia with distal tracheo-oesophageal fistula. Contrast radiography will elucidate the problem.

15 Thyroid gland

137 Thyroglossal cyst may form anywhere along the pathway of the persisting thyroglossal tract which extends from the foramen caecum of the tongue to the pyramidal lobe of the thyroid gland. More commonly located at the level of the hyoid bone and presents as an asymptomatic lump in the midline of the neck. Treatment consists of excision of the entire thyroglossal tract including the central portion of the hyoid bone.

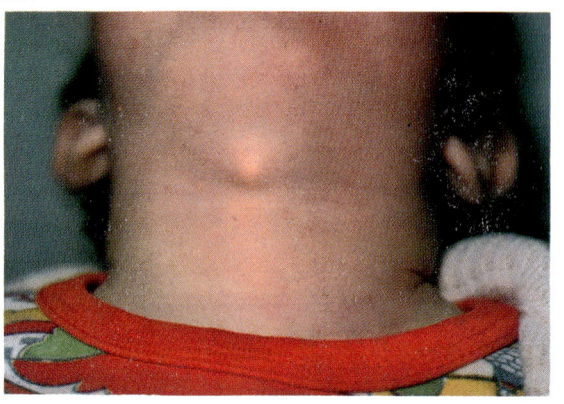

138 Infected thyroglossal cyst. The infection usually responds to antibiotic therapy, but incision and drainage may be required. This may result in sinus formation. Formal excision should follow soon after infection has resolved. Recurrence rate is higher after previous infection.

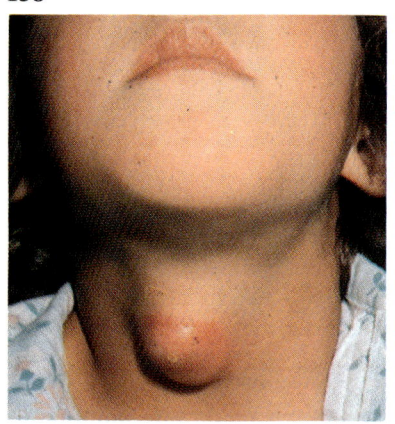

139 Thyroid scintigram after administration of radio-iodine used to demonstrate the position of the thyroid gland in a child with an anterior cervical 'cyst'. The scanogram reveals a superior ectopic position of the thyroid gland at the precise site of the so-called 'cyst'.

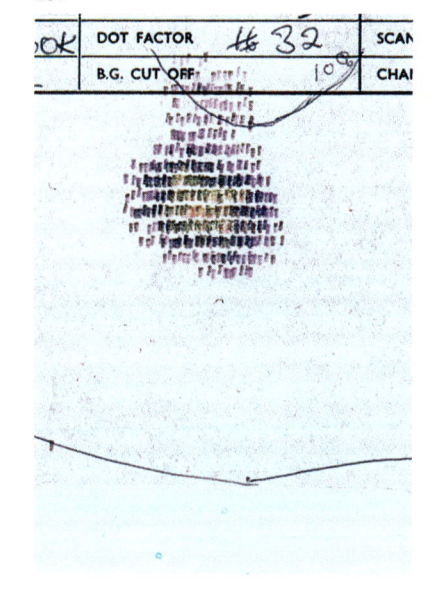

140 Teratoma of the thyroid gland in a four-day-old female infant. Most teratomas of the cervical region are present at birth and are invariably benign. The tumour in this infant arose from the left lobe of the thyroid gland.

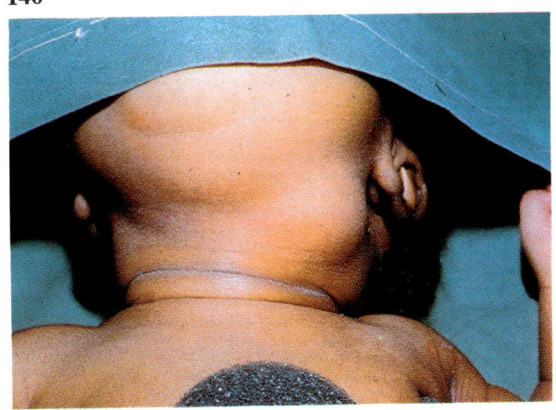

141 Teratoma of the thyroid gland. The resected specimen shows presence of a rudimentary lens structure (A), loops of intestine (B) and solid areas (C). Microscopic examination showed areas of thyroid tissue, intestine, squamous and respiratory epithelium.

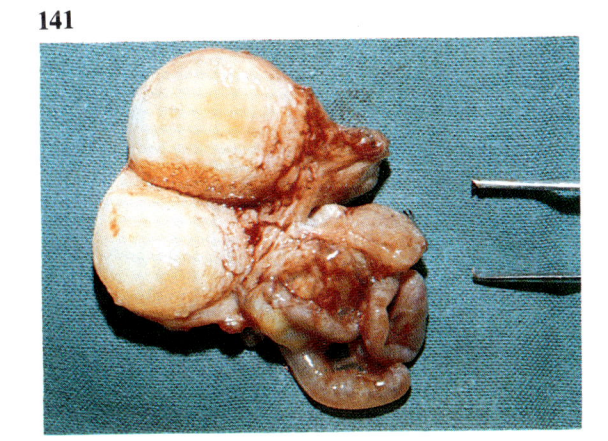

142 Anterior cervical abscess in a young girl. The origin may be from an acute suppurative thyroiditis, from an infected thyroglossal cyst, from an infected branchial cyst. The child presented with stridor and dyspnoea caused by compression and oedema of the trachea. Treatment is by incision and evacuation of pus in conjunction with antibiotic therapy.

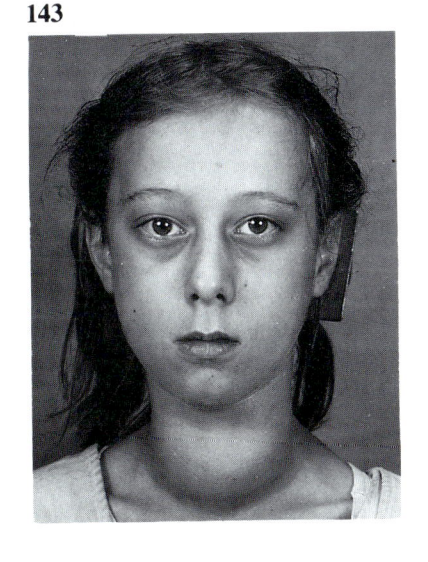

143 Thyrotoxicosis (hyperthyroidism, Graves' disease). Uncommon in children (less than one per cent of cases) but the younger the patient the greater the glandular enlargement. Presenting features in childhood disease are usually emotional instability and motor hyperactivity. Exophthalmos is almost invariably present but only to a modest degree. Medical therapy is usually successful.

144 Hypothyroidism at birth may be caused by endemic disease or by maternal over-treatment with antithyroid drugs. The signs in the early neonatal period are subtle and include prolonged hyperbilirubinaemia, poor feeding and abdominal distension, lethargy and respiratory difficulties.

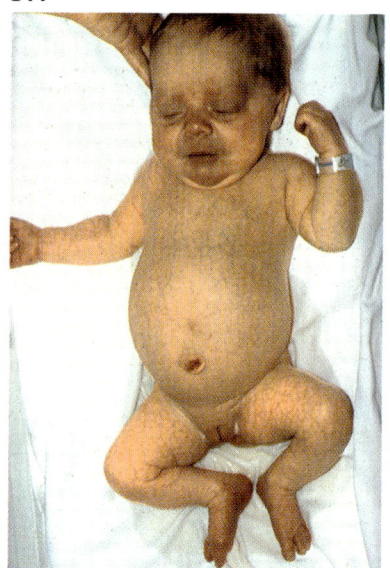

145 Hypothyroidism. The classical features of cretinism include coarse facies with puffy eyelids, flattening of the nasal bridge and an enlarged tongue. Constipation may be a considerable problem and may mimic Hirschsprung's disease. The final outcome is mental deficiency in severe cases. Diagnosis is confirmed by estimation of serum thyroxine levels.

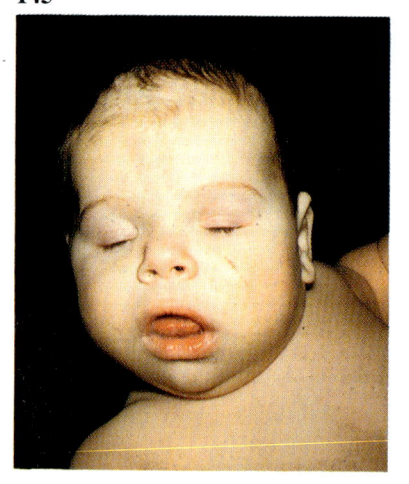

146 Endemic goitre. Puberty goitre (colloid) is frequently seen in children in endemic areas. It is the result of iodine deficiency combined with an increased demand for thyroid secretion at puberty. May be diffuse or nodular. The surface of the thyroid gland is smooth and soft. Rarely associated with pressure symptoms. Generally resolves spontaneously. Surgery is rarely necessary.

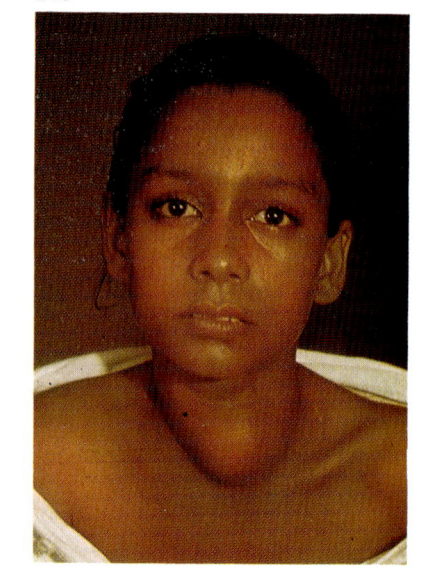

16 The neck

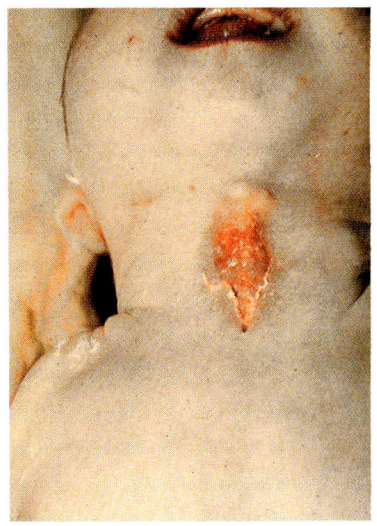

147 Midline cervical cleft. There is a denuded strip of skin 1 to 2 cm wide extending vertically in the midline from the level of the hyoid bone to the suprasternal notch. The exposed subcutaneous tissue is thickened and fibrotic. The defect may heal by ingrowth of epithelium from the periphery. Commonly, excision and Z-plasty is required.

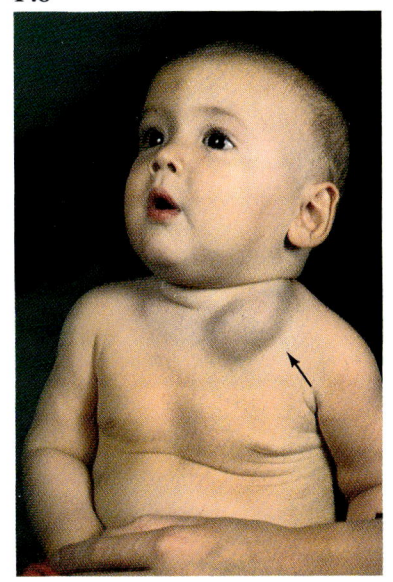

148 Cystic hygroma (lymphangioma) are the commonest lateral cervical masses in the first year of life. The lesion consists of multilocular spaces varying in size from 1 mm to 5 cm in diameter. The locules usually do not communicate. Small unilateral lesions are excised for cosmetic reasons. Spontaneous resolution (c/f haemangioma) is rare.

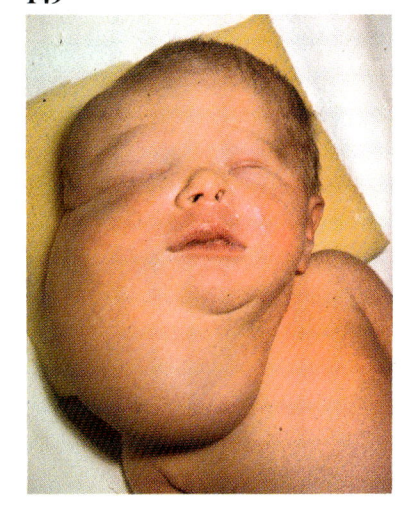

149 Giant cystic hygroma involving the entire right side of the neck with an extension across the midline. There may also be an extension inferiorly into the superior mediastinum. Respiratory embarrassment may be caused by tracheal compression. Surgical excision is the treatment of choice but involves meticulous dissection and may require tracheostomy.

150 Branchial sinus is the central remnant of the second branchial cleft. The external orifice lies in the lower third of the neck on the line of the anterior border of the sternomastoid muscle. Intermittent mucoid discharge is present. The tract ascends into the neck between the external and internal carotid arteries to enter the pharynx on the posterior pillar of the fauces. Treatment consists of complete excision of the sinus and tract.

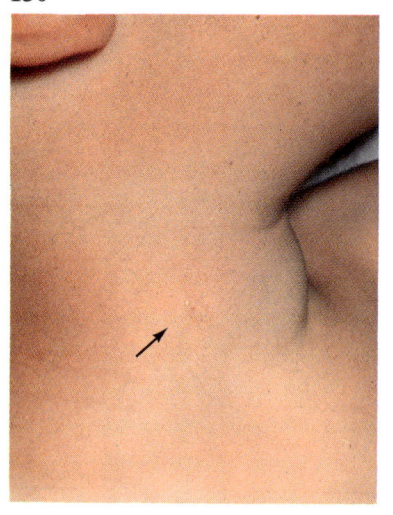

151 Branchial fistula. A contrast study. The contrast was introduced into the orifice in the neck and can be seen tracking up to the pharynx.

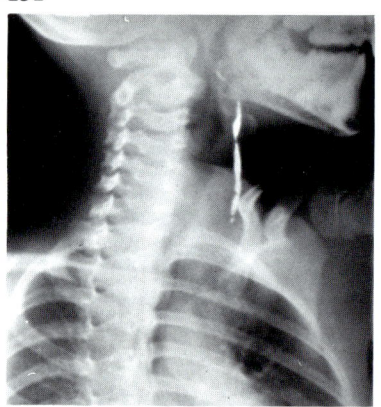

152 Branchial remnant. Cartilaginous remnant of branchial origin presenting as a hard well-defined subcutaneous mass along the anterior border of the left sternomastoid muscle in the lower third of the neck. Treatment is by excision including a tract if present.

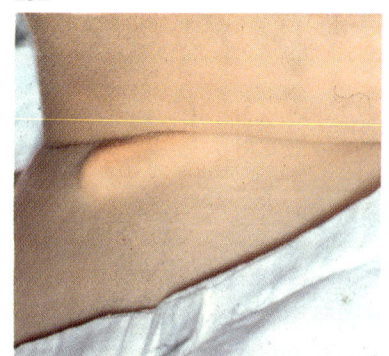

153 Branchial cyst presenting as a small, 2 cm diameter, cystic swelling deep to the sternomastoid muscle. Usually lined with stratified squamous epithelium. Infection and abscess formation may occur. Treatment is by excision of the cyst and tract (when present).

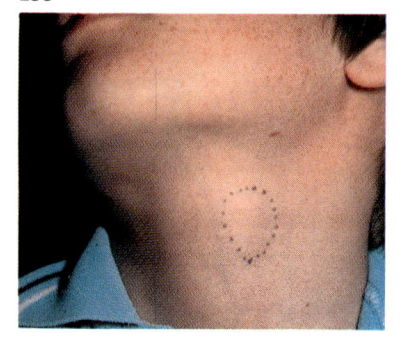

154 Giant left branchial cyst presenting at birth and having the appearance of a cystic hygroma. Microscopic examination revealed a squamous epithelial lined unilocular cyst. May produce respiratory distress caused by compression and displacement of trachea.

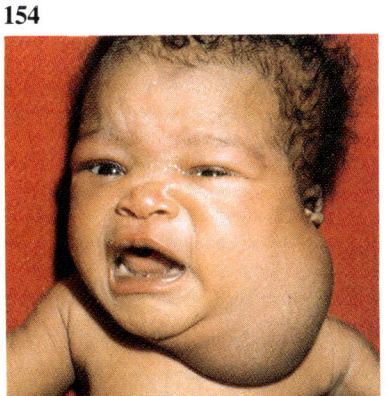

155 Sternomastoid 'tumour'. A firm discrete swelling 1 to 3cm in diameter is palpable in the middle third of the sternomastoid muscle within two to three weeks of birth. The head and face are rotated towards the opposite side. The 'tumour' resolves on conservative treatment with or without passive manipulations.

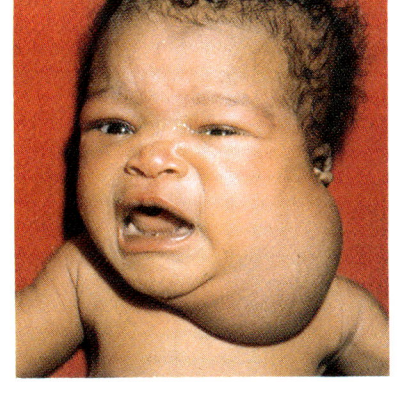

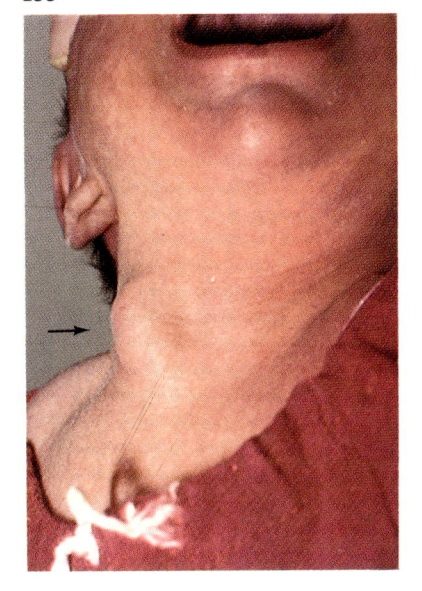

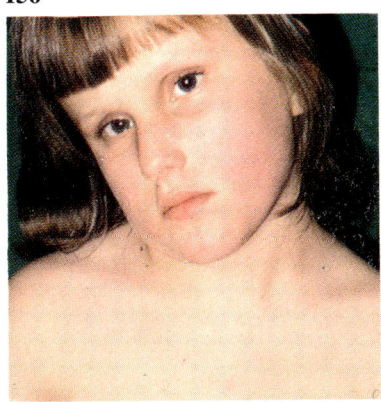

156 Torticollis. Ten per cent of sternomastoid 'tumours' fail to resolve and result in a torticollis with shortening and fibrosis of the sternomastoid muscle. There is usually associated facial hemihypoplasia. Treatment consists of division of the sternomastoid muscle followed by intensive physiotherapy.

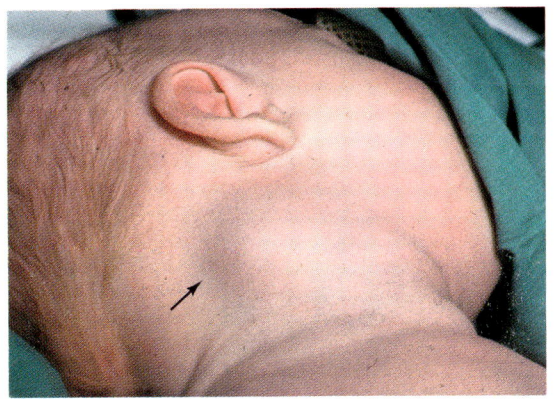

157 Acute cervical lymphadenopathy. This common condition of infancy is caused by a bacterial or viral infection of the nasopharynx. A firm tender swelling of an upper cervical lymph node is present, with or without erythema of the overlying skin which may progress to suppuration requiring incision and drainage.

158 Chronic cervical lymphadenopathy. Unilateral enlargement (greater than 3 cm) or the presence of a single, prominent, firm, non-tender node suggests the possibility of malignancy. Fifty per cent of all malignant neck masses in children are caused by lymphomas. Diagnosis is made on excision biopsy, but only after careful search has been made for a possible primary source.

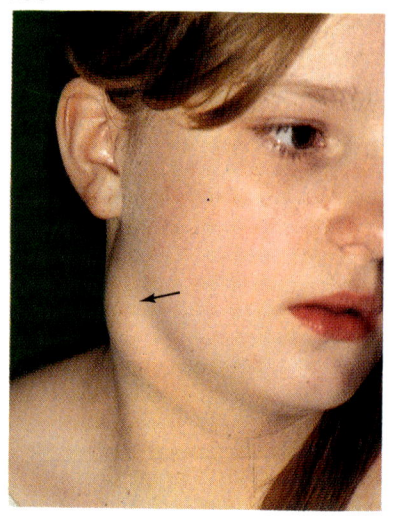

159 Chronic cervical lymphadenopathy caused by tuberculosis is common in certain Third-World countries. The glands are firm, non-tender and matted and may become secondarily infected. Primary site of infection is usually the tonsils.

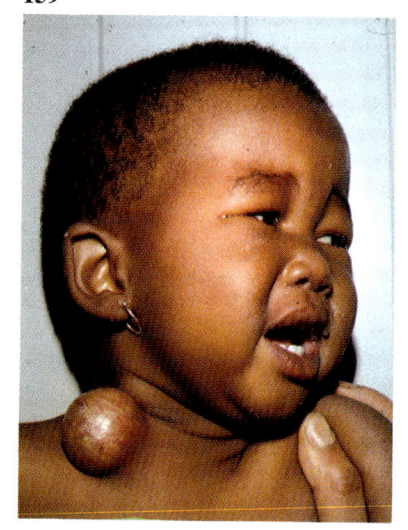

160 Tuberculous ulceration. Involvement of the occipital lymph nodes in association with tuberculosis of the skin with subsequent ulceration. The base of the lesion has become secondarily infected. Heals by secondary intention leaving a scarred contractured area. Treatment is with antituberculous chemotherapy.

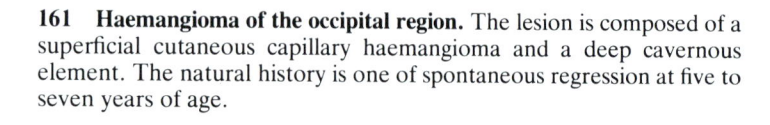

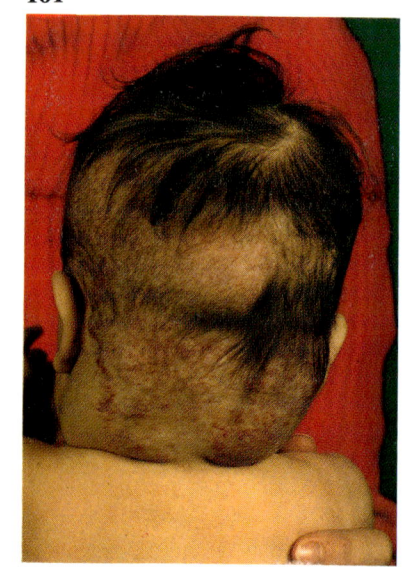

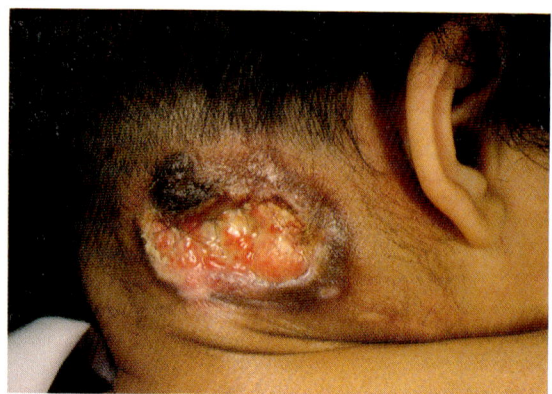

161 Haemangioma of the occipital region. The lesion is composed of a superficial cutaneous capillary haemangioma and a deep cavernous element. The natural history is one of spontaneous regression at five to seven years of age.

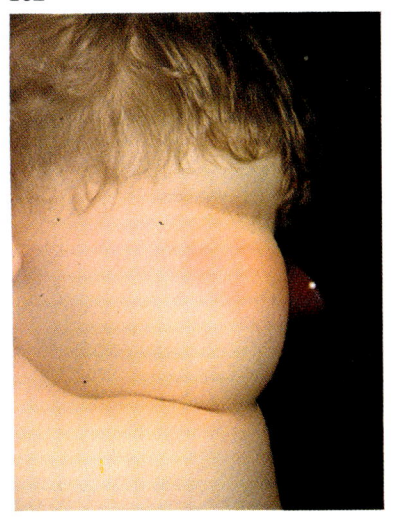

162 Cervical lipoma. There is a large lobulated mass involving the posterior aspect of the neck. Excision of the lesion is the only effective form of treatment.

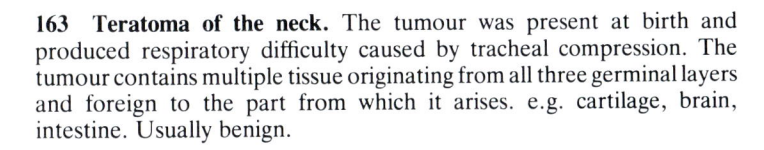

163 Teratoma of the neck. The tumour was present at birth and produced respiratory difficulty caused by tracheal compression. The tumour contains multiple tissue originating from all three germinal layers and foreign to the part from which it arises. e.g. cartilage, brain, intestine. Usually benign.

164 Cervical teratoma. Resected specimen of a benign cervical teratoma revealing cystic and solid areas. The cystic areas were lined by squamous epithelium and the solid areas were composed of lung and brain tissue.

165 Klippel-Feil syndrome caused by failure of vertebral segmentation. There may be a reduced number of cervical vertebrae or multiple hemivertebrae fused into a single osseous mass. The neck is short and movement limited and the hairline low.

166 Turner's syndrome is characterised by short stature, a varying degree of mental retardation and congenital webbed neck. Sex chromosome constitution is XO. The ovaries are streak-like and contain no germ cells. Internal and external genitalia remain infantile but are otherwise normal.

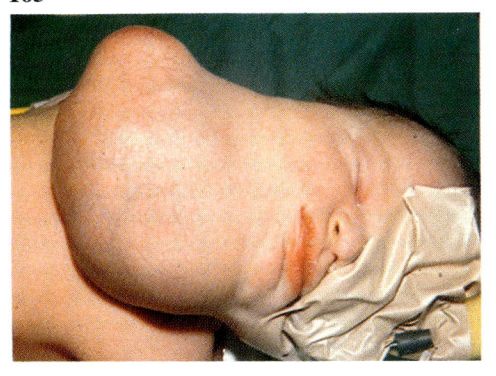

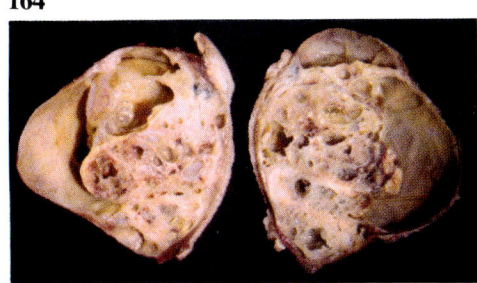

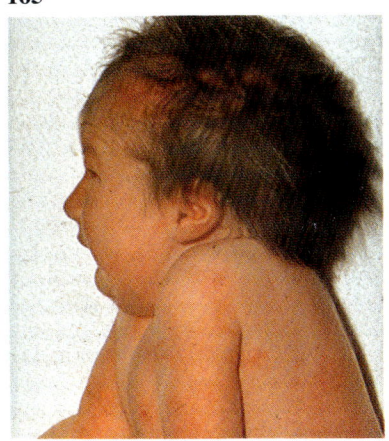

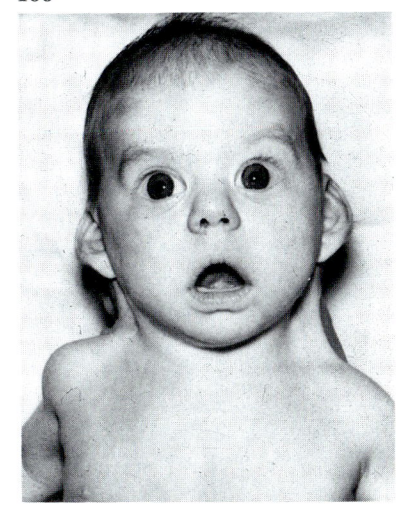

17 The breast

167 Mastitis neonatorum. The enlarged breast of the neonate is particularly prone to infection as a result of stagnation. Staphylococcus aureus is the common organism. Initially diffuse local erythema, tenderness and pyrexia are present. Systemic antibiotics may cure the infection at this stage.

168 Breast abscess is the natural outcome of staphylococcal mastitis neonatorum. There is a well-defined fluctuant swelling of the breast which requires incision and evacuation of the pus.

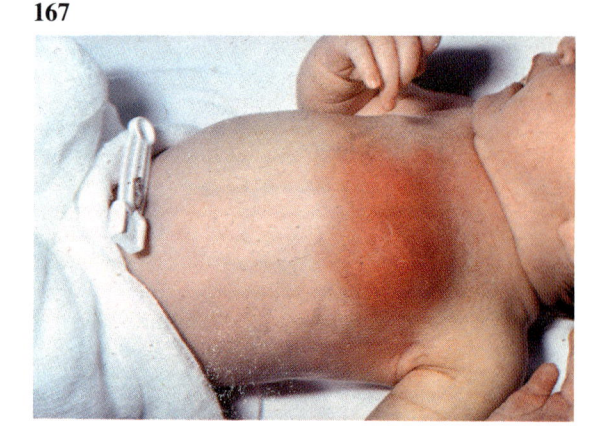

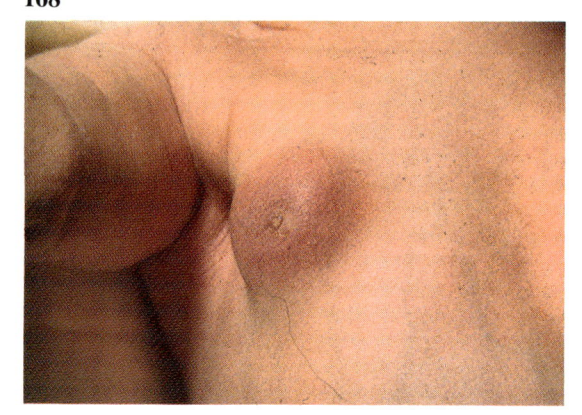

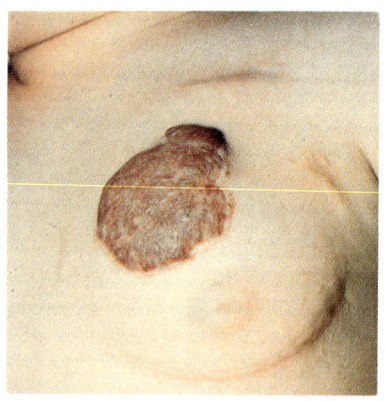

169 Haemangioma of the skin and subcutaneous tissue overlying the left breast. Composed of mixed capillary and cavernous elements it usually regresses spontaneously but may leave a disfiguring scar which requires excision and grafting.

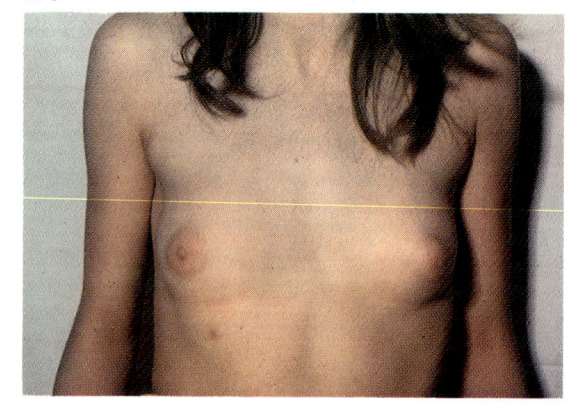

170 Polythelia or accessory nipple is caused by a persistence of breast tissue along the embryonic breast (mammary) line which extends from the axilla to the groin. Treatment is usually unnecessary, but if associated breast tissue (polymastia) is present, excision should be carried out because these accessory breasts undergo all the changes of a normal breast, e.g. hypertrophy, lactation, etc.

171 Pubertal hypertrophy occurs at any time between eight and 15 years of age. It may begin unilaterally and be a source of concern for the child particularly if it occurs in a young girl, and if there is a considerable delay before the opposite breast starts to develop. Biopsy for diagnostic purposes is strictly contraindicated. In precocious development it is important to exclude intracranial, ovarian and adrenocortical tumours.

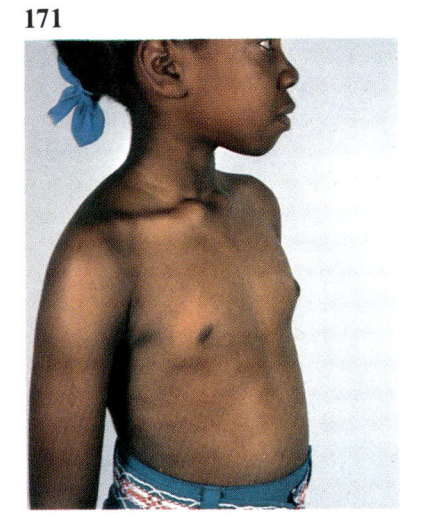

172 Amastia or congenital absence of the breast. Presents as a cosmetic problem and is usually associated with other congenital defects of the chest wall, e.g. pectus excavatum or absent pectoralis major muscle.

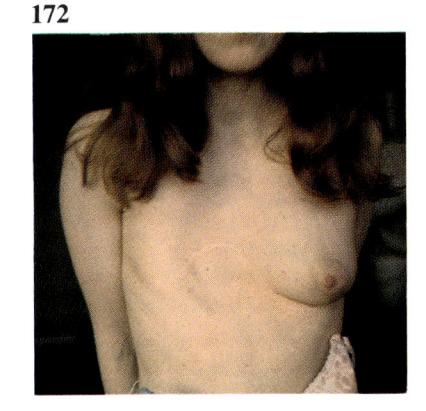

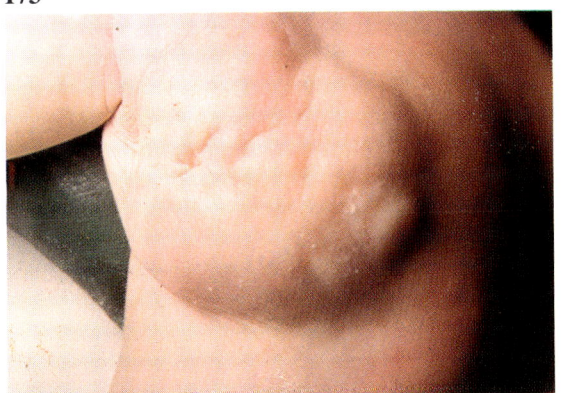

173 Lymphangioma of the right breast region extending into the axilla. No propensity to spontaneous regression. Produces a significant cosmetic deformity and has a tendency to develop rapidly spreading cellulitis and lymphangitis.

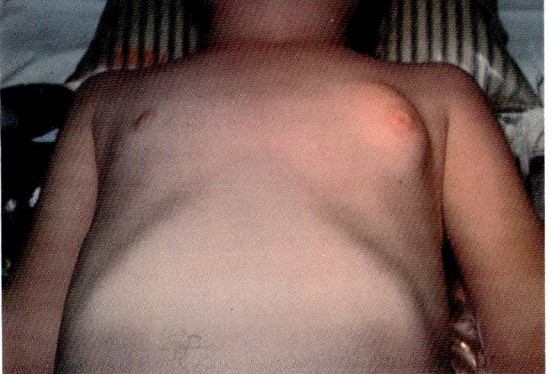

174 Galactocoele of the left breast. Caused by the distension of one of the main lactiferous ducts by unaltered milk or cheese-like material of milk inspissation. The cyst forms a smooth painless subareolar swelling. Usually appears after the end of lactation but has been described at puberty (as in this 13-year-old boy).

18 The chest wall

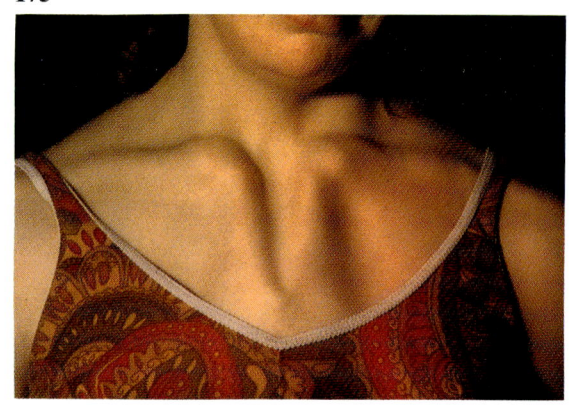

175 Upper sternal cleft. Caused by failure of midline fusion of the paired sternal bands. Produces an obvious cosmetic defect of the upper chest wall into which the heart may bulge. Operative repair should be undertaken in early infancy to obviate the need for multiple chondrotomies or the use of prosthetic material.

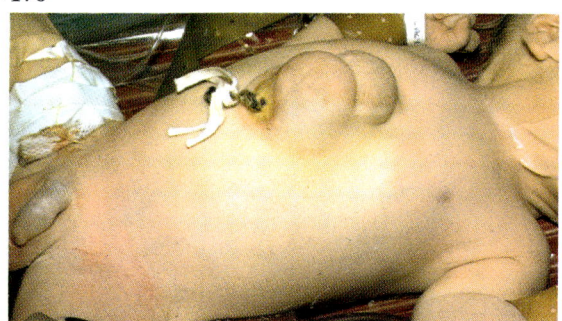

176 Distal sternal cleft. Only seen in association with other defects. Most common association is with a pentalogy of anomalies (thoracoabdominal ectopia cordis). The five anomalies are: 1 midline supraumbilical abdominal wall defect (including exomphalos); 2 split lower sternum; 3 a defect in the anterior part of the pericardial diaphragm; 4 defect in anterior part of the diaphragm; 5 an intracardiac defect (e.g. septal defect, dextrocardia, diverticulum of left ventricle).

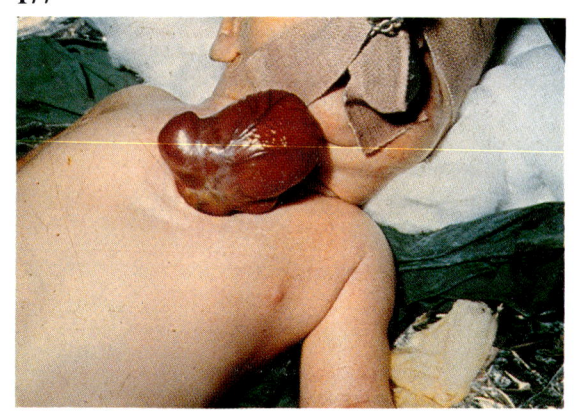

177 Ectopia cordis. The heart is lying exposed on the anterior sternal wall. It is covered by pericardium only. There are usually severe associated intracardiac malformations. Survival is rare.

178 Pectus excavatum. There is a mid-sternal depression of the chest wall which presents in the neonate and infant with paradoxical indrawing of the depression with inspiration. More common in infants with respiratory distress. Usually resolves once respiratory problem has been overcome.

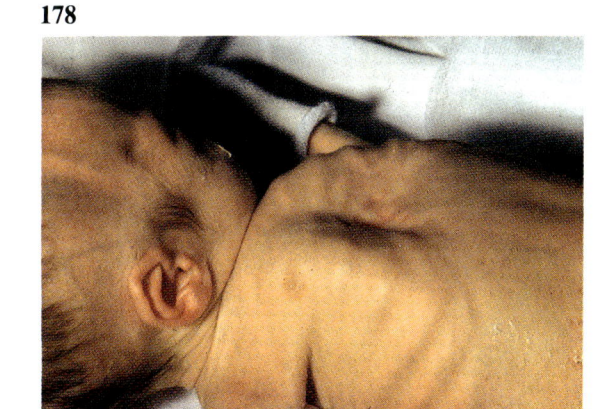

179 Pectus excavatum. Typical deformity in a six-year-old girl with maximum depression involving the lower sternal region. The shoulders are held in the characteristic rounded stooped posture. Operative correction is usually undertaken around five years of age for cosmetic and psychological reasons.

180 Pectus excavatum. Lateral xray of the chest in a child with severe pectus excavatum showing the marked concavity of the lower sternum and the shortened distance between the posterior part of the sternum and the anterior surface of the thoracic vertebrae at the point of maximum depression.

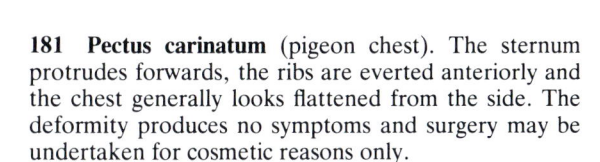

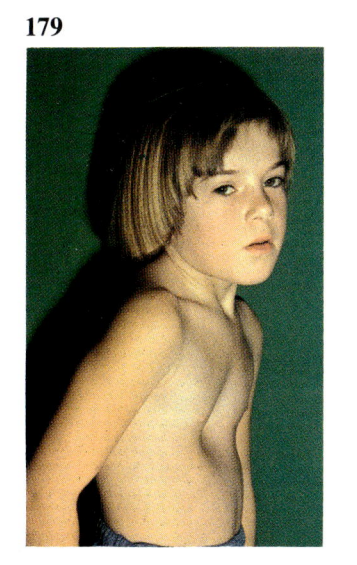

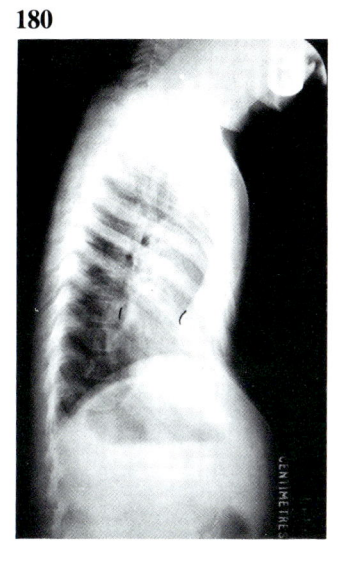

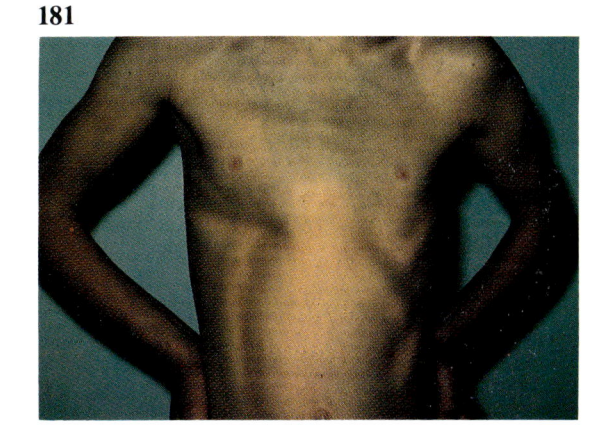

181 Pectus carinatum (pigeon chest). The sternum protrudes forwards, the ribs are everted anteriorly and the chest generally looks flattened from the side. The deformity produces no symptoms and surgery may be undertaken for cosmetic reasons only.

182 Absence of pectoralis major. The muscle is represented by a fibrous strand stretching across the lower border of the anterior axillary fold. A cutaneous haemangioma overlies the absent costal part of the pectoralis muscle. Often associated with rib defects on the same side (Poland's syndrome). In girls, hypoplasia of the breast may necessitate augmentation mammoplasty.

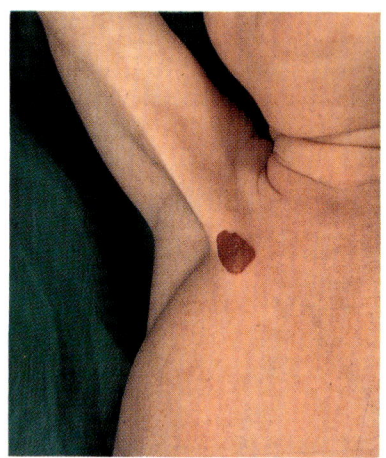

183 Congenital absence of ribs. The left lateral chest wall is deformed and there is associated scoliosis caused by vertebral anomalies. The deformity may be accentuated by soft-tissue deficiency. Surgical correction consists of bridging the gap in the thoracic wall with a bony strut (usually rib).

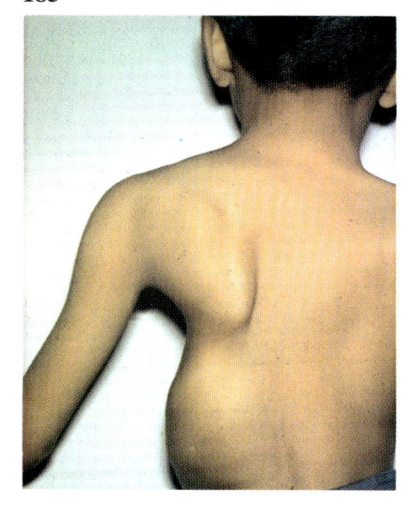

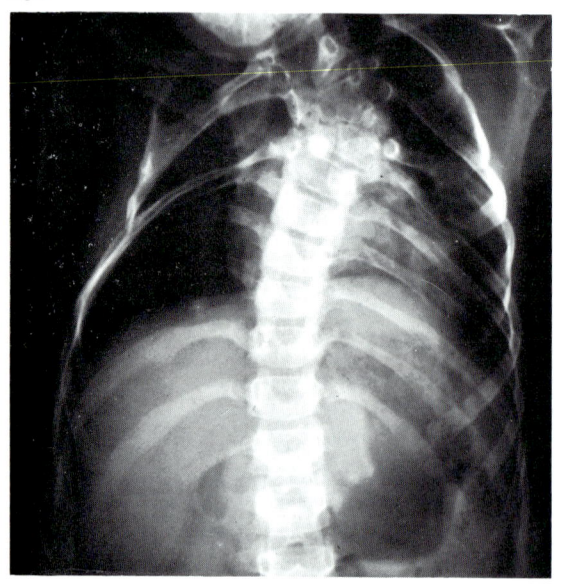

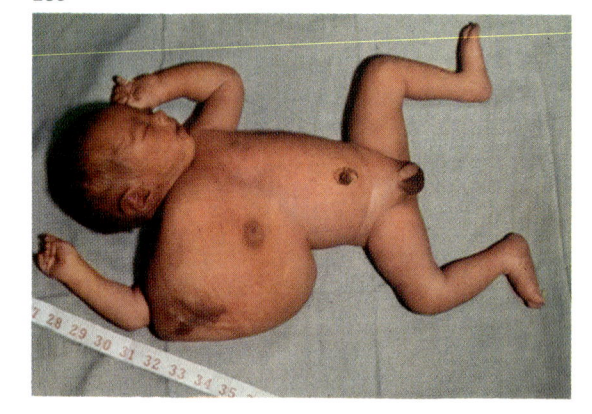

184 Congenital absence of ribs in the right hemithorax of an infant. Note the severe deformity of the upper thoracic vertebra and the associated scoliosis.

185 Lymphangioma of the chest wall. The entire right hemithorax has been replaced by lymphangiomatous tissue. Respiratory distress was evident soon after birth and was irreversible. Note the displacement of the right nipple.

19 The oesophagus

186 Excessively mucusy baby at birth. Requires frequent oropharyngeal suction to clear airway of excess saliva. Oesophageal patency should be examined by passing a large (No 10 French) catheter through the mouth. The diagnosis of oesophageal atresia is suspected if the tube fails to enter the stomach and is arrested approximately 10cm from the lower-gum margin. Coughing and dyspnoea with the first feed is a classical clinical presentation, but represents late diagnosis.

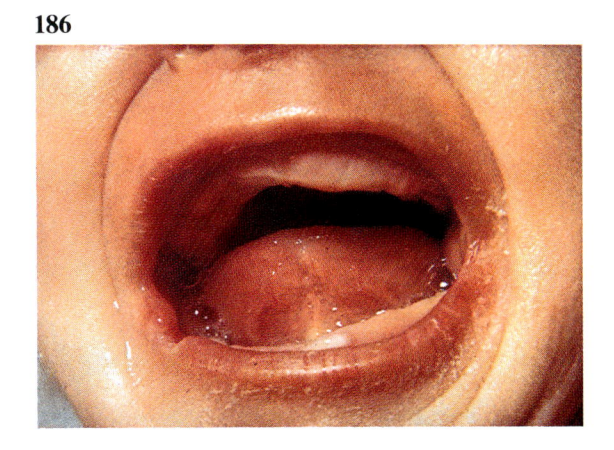

187 Oesophageal atresia. Diagram of the various varieties. The most common type is where there is a proximal blind ending oesophageal pouch and a distal tracheo-oesophageal fistula (90 per cent). Isolated atresia without tracheo-oesophageal fistula occurs in five per cent of cases.

(a) Isolated oesophageal atresia.
(b) Oesophageal atresia with proximal tracheo-oesophageal fistula.
(c) Oesophageal atresia with distal tracheo-oesophageal fistula.
(d) Oesophageal atresia with proximal and distal tracheo-oesophageal fistula.
(e) Tracheo-oesophageal fistula (H-type) without associated atresia.
(f) Distal oesophageal stenosis.

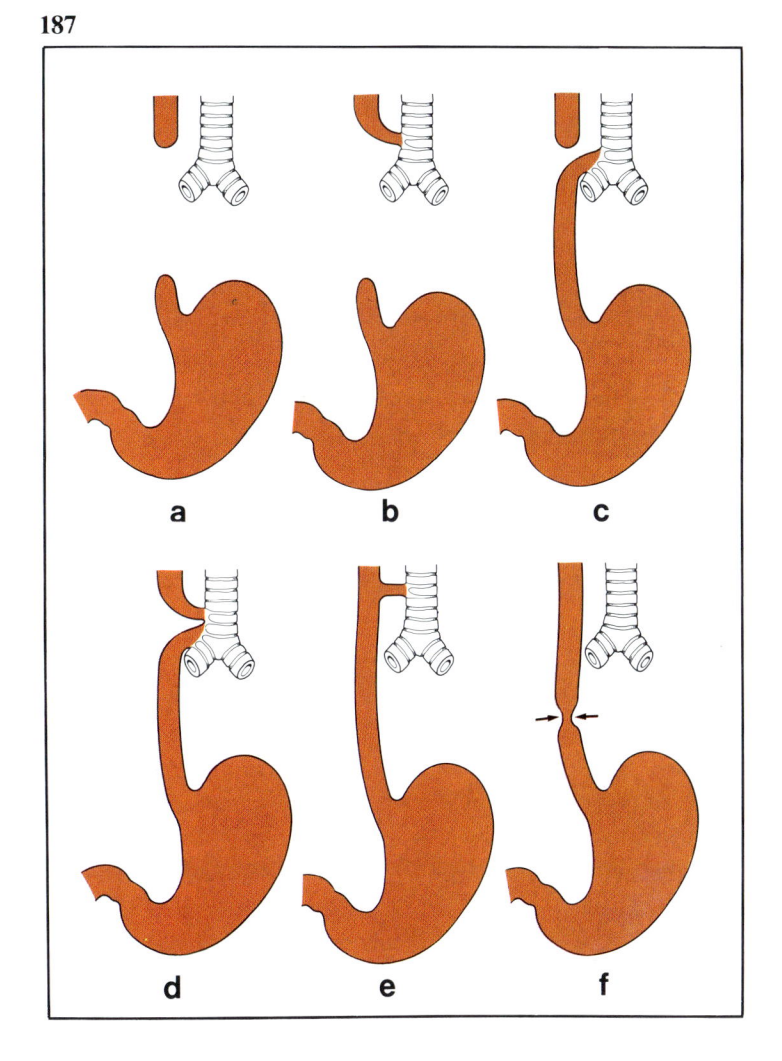

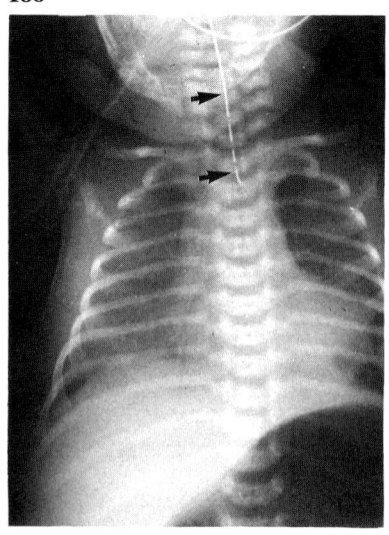

188 Oesophageal atresia. Note the presence of a catheter (with radio-opaque markers) in the blind upper oesophageal pouch. Air has been injected immediately before the xray to outline the upper pouch. The gas in the intestines indicates the presence of a distal tracheo-oesophageal fistula.

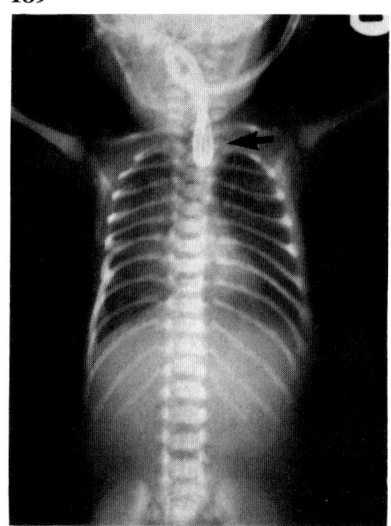

189 Oesophageal atresia in a baby. The radio-opaque catheter is seen curled up in the upper oesophagus. It is mandatory to include the abdomen in the initial radiological assessment. Absence of gastrointestinal gas suggests an isolated atresia without distal tracheo-oesophageal fistula. In these patients the gap between the upper and lower oesophageal ends is usually too large to allow immediate primary anastomosis.

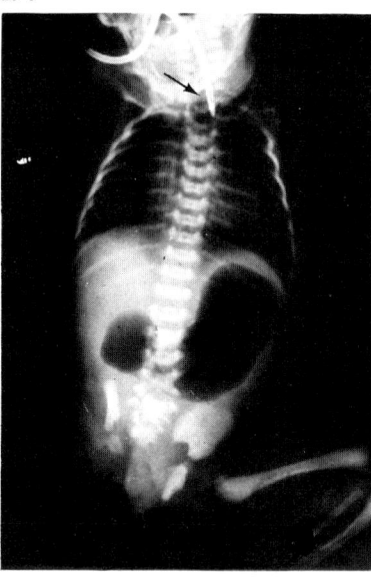

190 Oesophageal atresia in an infant. The abdominal part of the xray shows the 'double bubble' appearance characteristic of duodenal atresia.

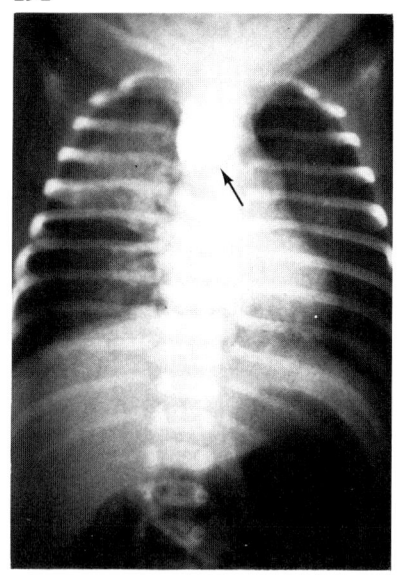

191 Oesophageal atresia. The use of radio-opaque contrast in the diagnosis of this condition may lead to inhalation pneumonia unless rigid precautionary measures are adopted. This xray shows an overfilled upper oesophageal pouch and an upper lobe consolidation indicating prior inhalation.

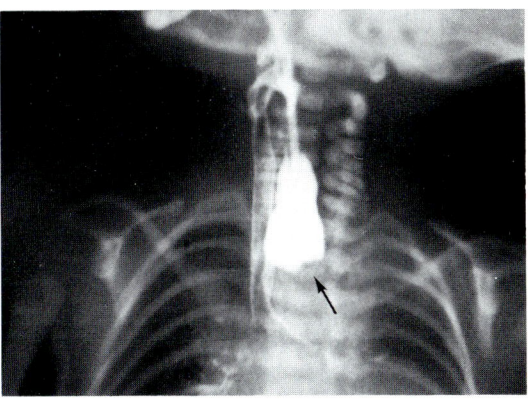

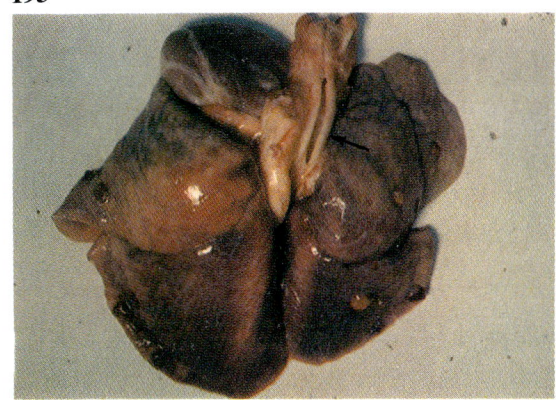

192 Oesophageal atresia. Contrast swallow demonstrating dilated blind upper oesophageal pouch with spillage of contrast over the pharynx into the tracheobronchial tree.

193 Tracheobronchial cleft. A necropsy specimen showing the extensive longitudinal communication between the posterior wall of the trachea and the oesophagus. Clinically presents as a tracheo-oesophageal fistula with cyanosis and choking attacks during feeds. Diagnosis may be made on endoscopy.

194 Tracheo-oesophageal fistula (H or N type). May present in the newborn with paroxysms of coughing during feeds. Abdominal distension is prominent. In later infancy and childhood it causes recurrent respiratory infections. Diagnosis may be extremely difficult to substantiate. Endoscopy with the use of a dye (methylene blue) may be helpful. Cine-radiography in the prone position may outline the oblique upward course of the fistula. Depending on level of the fistula, cervical or thoracic ligation should be performed.

195 Recurrent tracheo-oesophageal fistula. Occurs in 5 to 10 per cent of infants after repair of oesophageal atresia. An early anastomic leak after oesophageal repair is usually the first indication of a developing fistula. Clinical presentation similar to the congenital type of tracheo-oesophageal fistula.

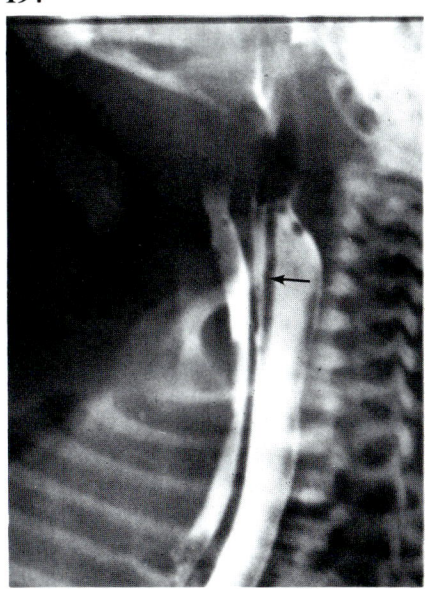

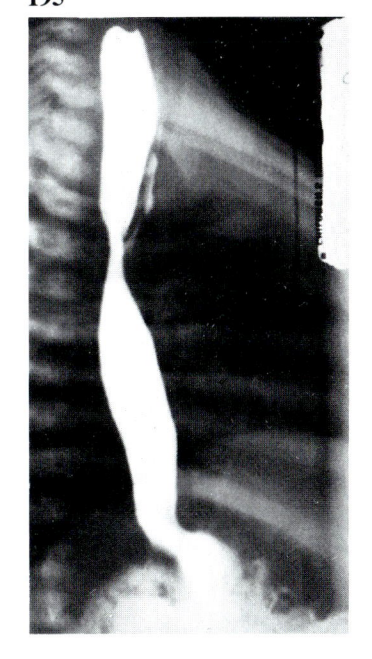

196   Achalasia of the oesophagus. Rare in childhood – only five per cent of patients experience onset of symptoms before 14 years of age. Dysphagia, regurgitation of food and weight loss. Barium oesophagogram shows a dilated incoordinated oesophagus which tapers distally into a narrow oesophago-gastric junction ('rat tail'). Treatment is by cardiomyotomy.

197   Hiatus hernia. Diagram of the (a) normal anatomy of the stomach and the oesophagus with the oblique junction lying well below the diaphragm. In the (b) sliding hernia the junction is displaced above the diaphragm, while in the (c) rolling hernia the junction remains intra-abdominal in position.

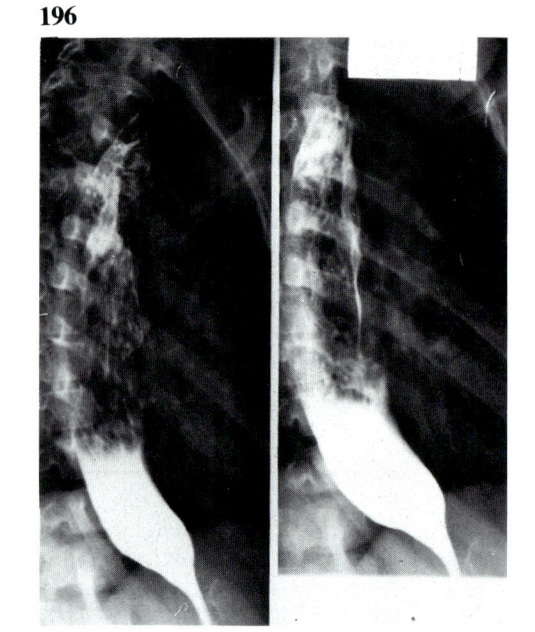

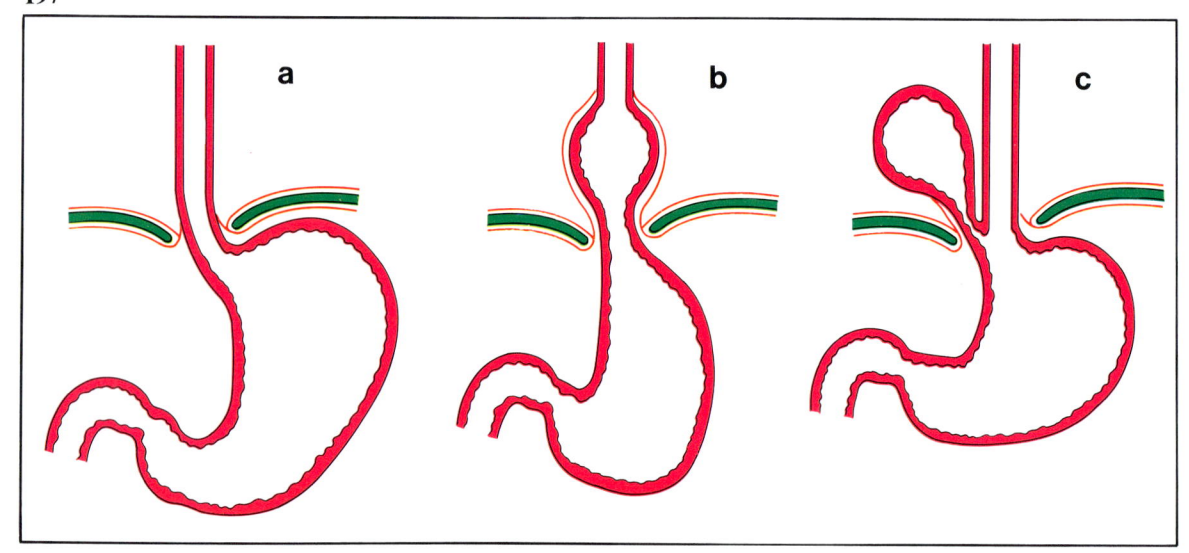

198   Chalasia. There is incompetence of the lower oesophageal sphincter without apparent upward displacement of the gastro-oesophageal junction. Free reflux occurs. Common in infancy but tends to resolve on conservative management (small regular thickened feeds, sitting posture in feeding chair).

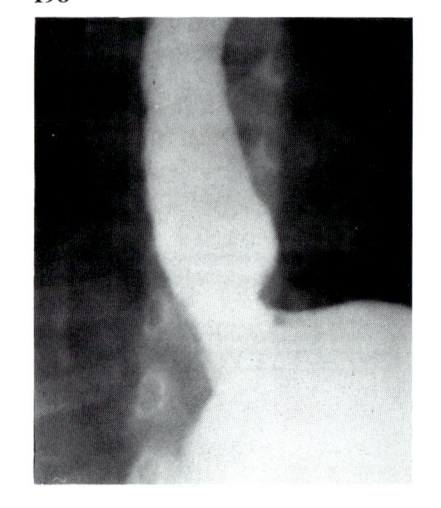

199 Sliding hiatus hernia with reflux oesophagitis. The herniated stomach is shown above the diaphragm and oesophagitis is indicated by the coarse irregular oesophageal mucosa. Symptomatology consists of persistent vomiting which is often blood-stained, dysphagia with or without epigastric pain, failure to thrive, hypochromic microcytic anaemia, recurrent episodes of aspiration pneumonia, episodes of apnoea in the infant and rumination.

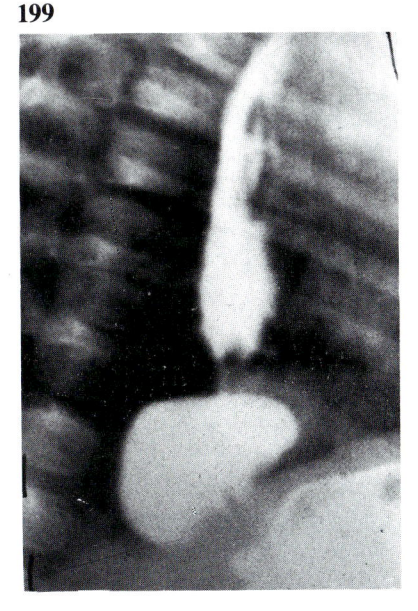

200 Sliding hiatus hernia with stricture of the lower oesophagus. A long tight stricture is seen extending distally from the mid-oesophagus. The parallel gastric mucosal folds are visible, extending above the diaphragm through the hiatus indicating a small hiatus hernia. The child fails to thrive because of inadequate intake of food and suffers recurrent episodes of choking and regurgitation.

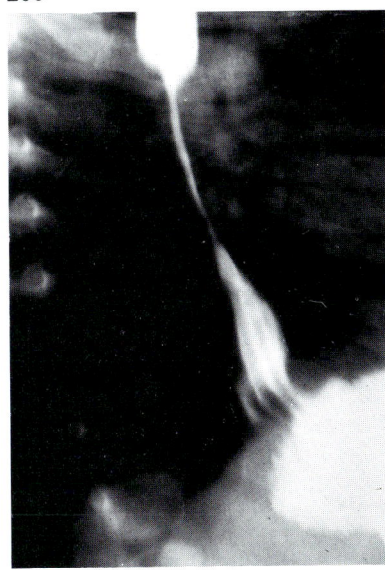

201 Paraoesophageal hiatus hernia (rolling hernia). Oesophagogram showing the entire fundus of the stomach displaced in the chest above the diaphragm. Presents in infancy with dysphagia, respiratory problems and/or chronic anaemia from peptic ulceration within the stagnant fundus of the stomach.

202 Incompetence of the lower oesophageal sphincter. The oesophagogastric junction is widely patent. The oesophageal mucosa shows no evidence of reflux oesophagitis.

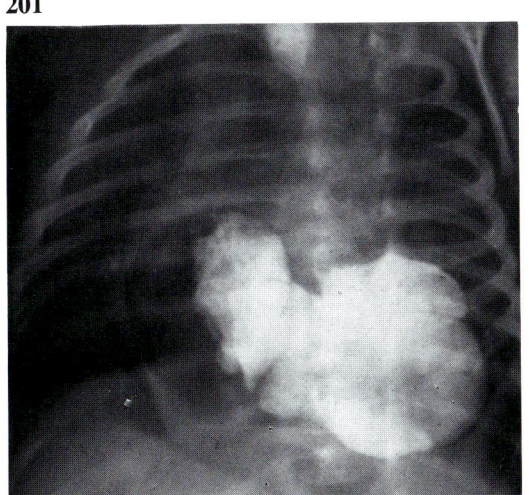

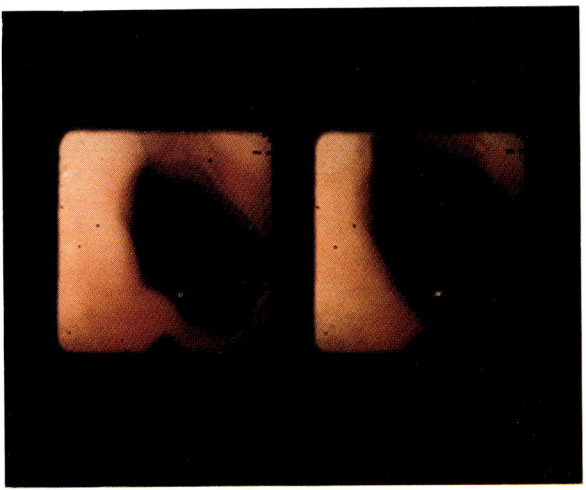

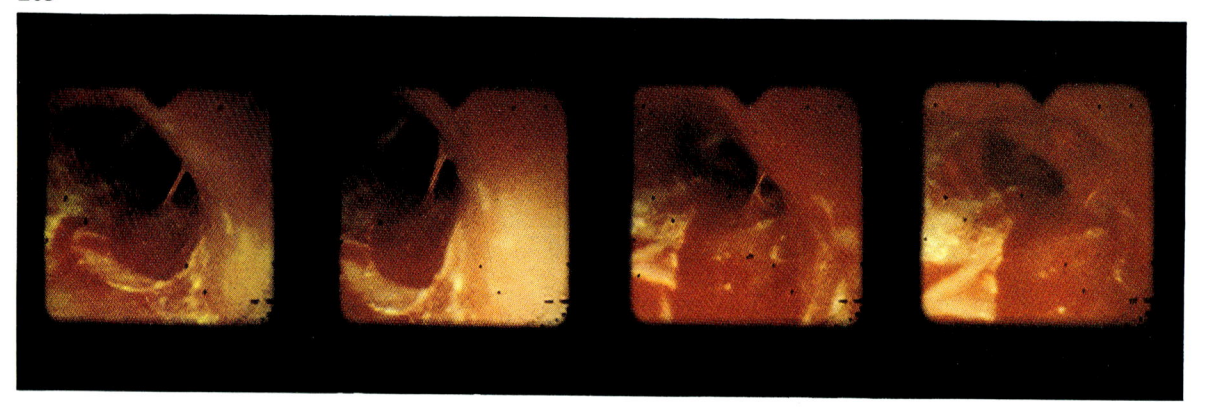

203 Reflux oesophagitis. Endoscopic view showing severe ulcerative oesophagitis with erythema and friability of the mucous membrane of the lower oesophagus.

204 Foreign body in the oesophagus. Ingestion of foreign objects occurs most frequently in first two to three years of life. Impaction common in upper-third at sites of anatomical constriction, e.g. post-cricoid region and at level of aortic arch. Once foreign object enters stomach passage through rest of gastrointestinal tract should proceed uneventfully. Xray shows coin in upper oesophagus.

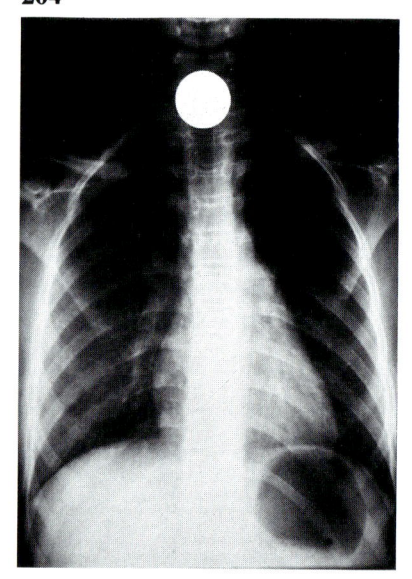

205 Foreign body in the oesophagus. The chest and upper abdomen of a newborn infant showing the endotracheal tube lying in the oesophagus and upper part of the stomach. The endotracheal tube 'disappeared' during resuscitation of the infant at birth. This type of problem arises with emergency intubations attempted by a relatively inexperienced medical attendant.

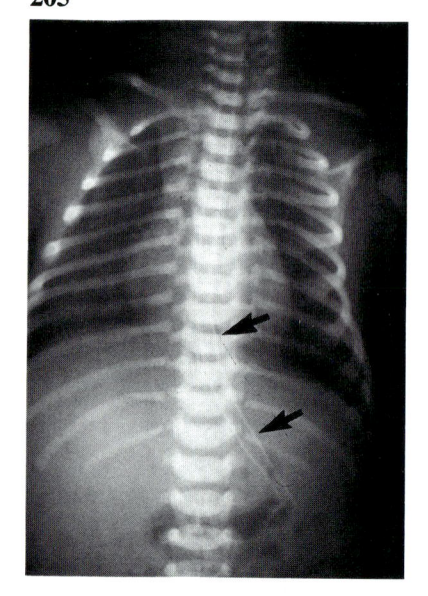

206 Oesophageal web. Most strictures in distal oesophagus are the result of reflux oesophagitis. Occasionally congenital webs occur. Oesophagogram shows shelf-like indentation of the oesophagus well above a normal gastro-oesophageal junction. May be asymptomatic or cause increasing dysphagia.

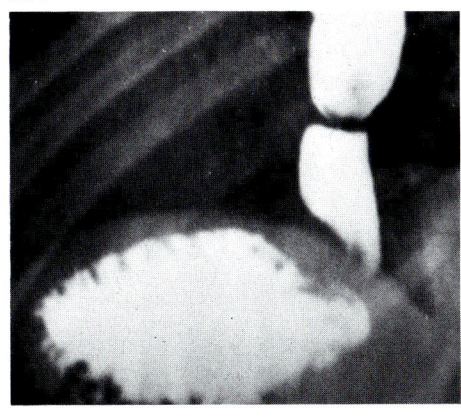

207 Corrosive oesophagitis. Accidental ingestion of caustic soda (lye) results in necrosis of the oesophageal mucosa, the extent varying with the concentration and amount of lye ingested. Mouth burns always present. Active conservative treatment may prevent fibrosis and stricture formation.

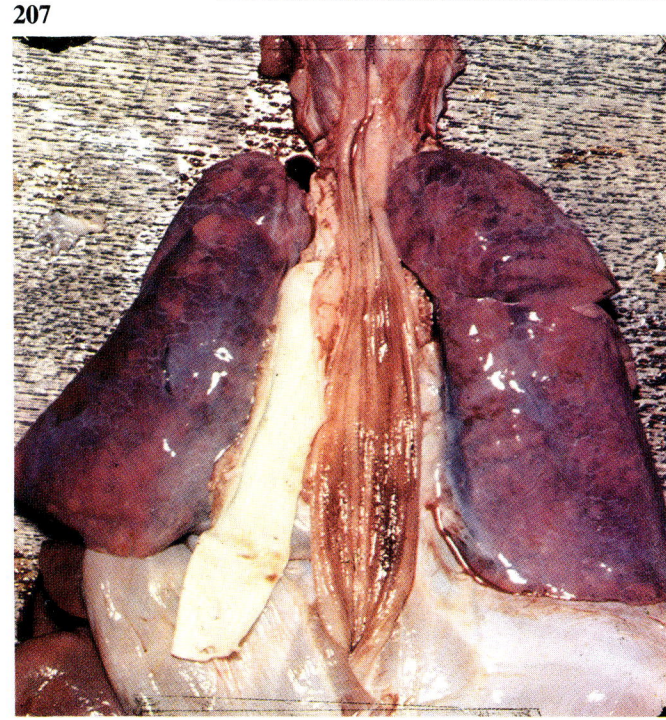

208 Vascular ring. May produce symptoms caused by compression of the trachea (chronic cough, wheeze, dyspnoea) or the oesophagus (dysphagia and vomiting). Barium oesophagogram is the most useful aid to diagnosis and demonstrates posterior indentation of the wall of the oesophagus at the level of the third or fourth thoracic vertebra.

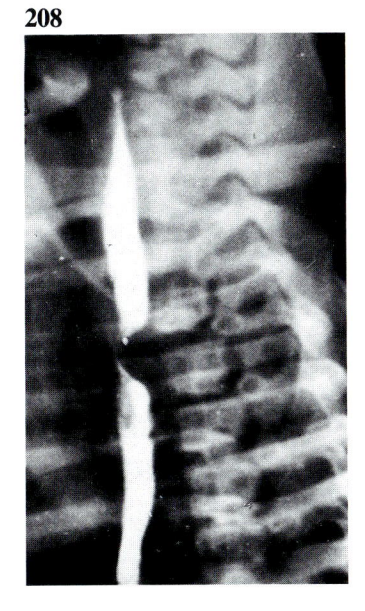

20 The mediastinum

Diagnostic approach to the more common mediastinal masses based on anatomical situation:

Anterior mediastinum: lymphoma (Hodgkin's and non-Hodgkin type), teratoma and dermoid cysts, thymic enlargement and tumours, cystic hygroma, pericardial cysts and diaphragmatic hernia (foramen of Morgagni).

Middle mediastinum: lymphoma, tuberculosis, anomalies of the heart and great vessels.

Posterior mediastinum: duplication cysts of foregut origin, neurogenic tumours, haemangiomas, diaphragmatic hernia (foramen of Bochdalek), anterior meningocoele.

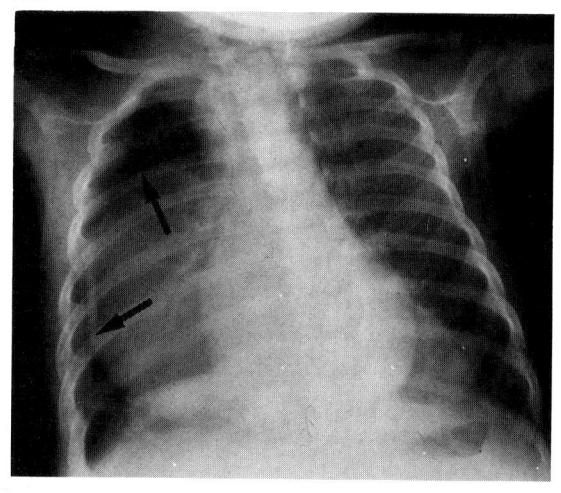

209 Oesophageal duplication cyst. A moderately dense, sharply demarcated, rounded mass is visible in the right hemithorax. May cause symptoms of respiratory embarrassment early in infancy because of a large space-occupying lesion. Symptoms of peptic ulceration with or without penetration into adjacent viscera may occur because the cysts frequently contain ectopic gastric mucosa.

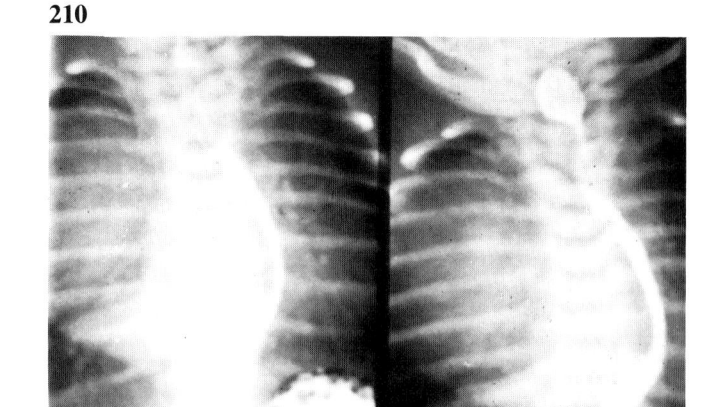

210 Oesophageal duplication cyst. Barium oesophagogram showing displacement of the oesophagus to the left by a well-defined rounded mass in the right hemithorax. Compression of the oesophageal wall produces symptoms of dysphagia in addition to the dyspnoea of the space-occupying lesion. Note also the deformity of the upper thoracic vertebrae, a common association with foregut duplication cysts.

211 Oesophageal duplication cyst. Computerised tomographic scan of the thorax in an infant with a thoraco-enterogenous cyst showing the cystic mass in the right hemithorax containing a fluid level. This indicates a communication with some part of the alimentary tract (oesophagus in the thorax or duodenum or upper jejunum by means of a communication through the diaphragm).

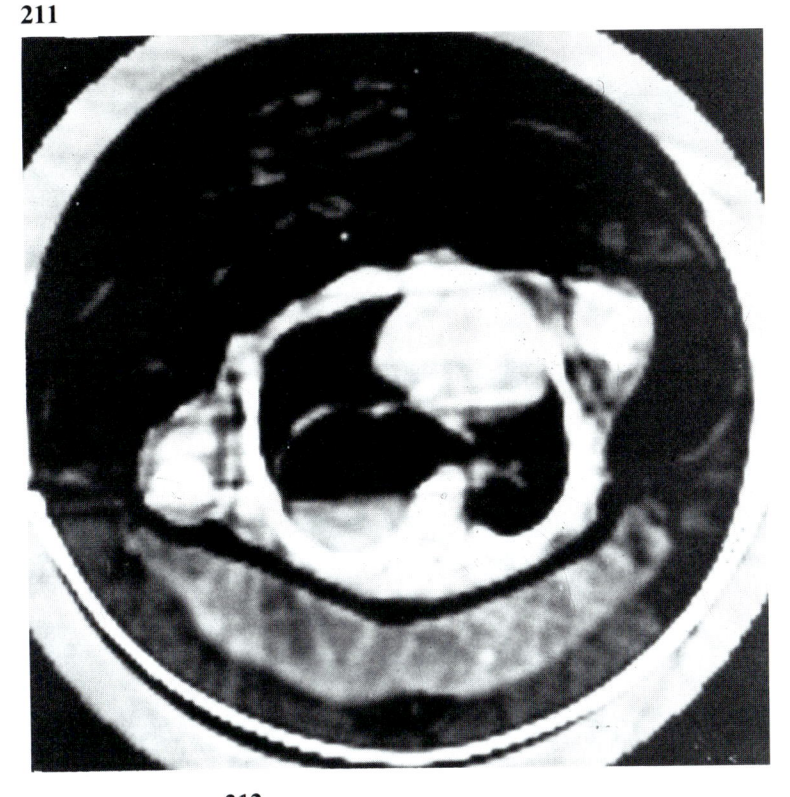

212 Bronchogenic cyst. Resected specimen removed from the posterior mediastinum at the level of the bifurcation of the trachea. Produces symptoms of respiratory obstruction (dyspnoea, wheezing and stridor) caused by compression of adjacent airway. May not be seen on plain xray, but barium oesophagogram reveals a space-occupying lesion between the oesophagus and trachea.

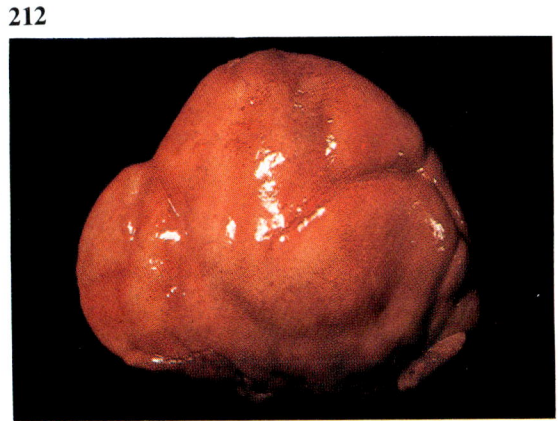

213 Cystic hygroma. The infant presented with a large cystic hygroma of the left side of the neck. Chest xray reveals an extension of the cervical lesion into the left upper mediastinum with displacement and narrowing of the trachea. Treatment is by excision to relieve symptoms of tracheal compression.

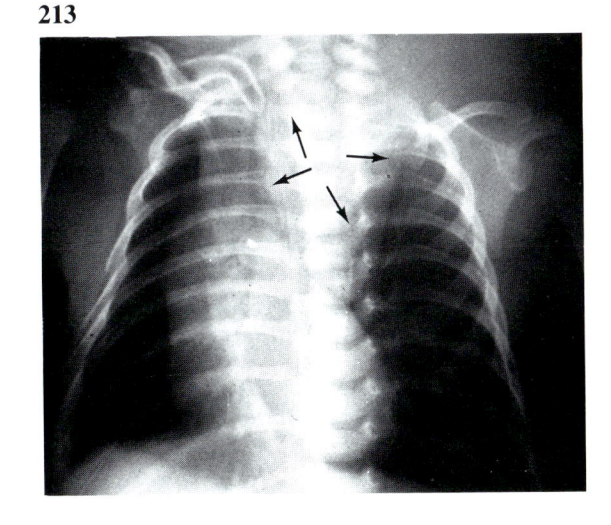

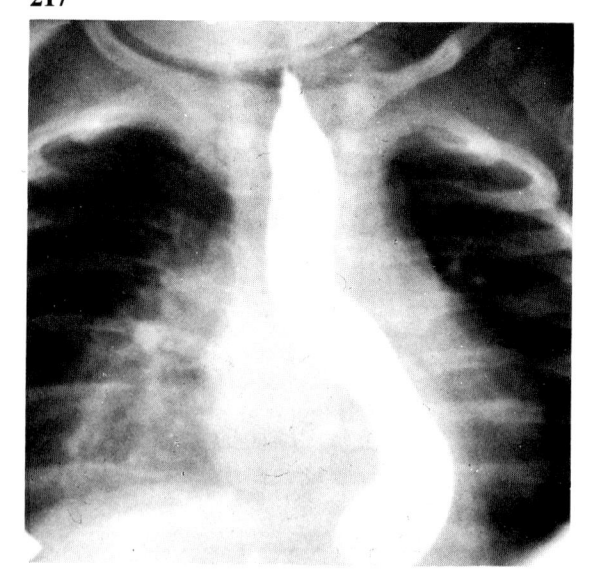

214 Anterior mediastinal teratoma. The superior mediastinal mass was an incidental finding on xray to locate an ingested necklace (seen in the epigastrium). Usually produces symptoms because of displacement and compression of the trachea, oesophagus or heart. Rarely malignant. Treatment is by complete excision.

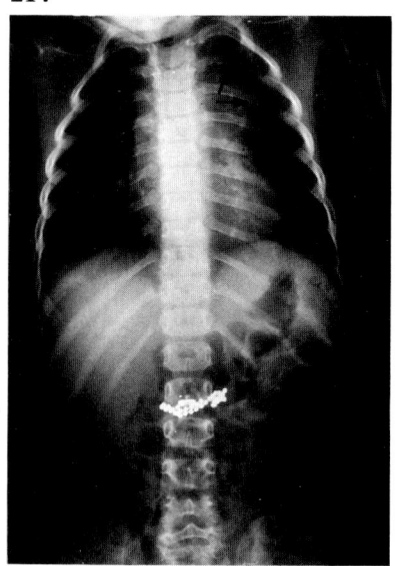

215 Neurofibroma. Arising from neural tissue in posterior mediastinum and is commonly part of von Recklinghausen's syndrome, i.e. generalised neurofibromatosis and skin pigmentation (taches de café-au-lait). Malignant degeneration is not uncommon but occurs mainly in large tumours.

216 Lymphosarcoma. Involvement of the superior mediastinum with dyspnoea and cough or symptoms caused by compression of the superior vena cava is a fairly common mode of presentation of a lymphoma. May present as an emergency with severe airway obstruction. Has marked tendency to progress to acute lymphocytic leukaemia.

217 Neuroblastoma. Malignant tumour arising from neural crest cells in the posterior mediastinum. As the tumour enlarges it causes increasing dyspnoea or recurrent pulmonary infections or dysphagia from displacement of the oesophagus. May also present with symptoms and signs of spinal cord compression caused by extension into intervertebral foramina. Increased catecholamine excretion in urine is diagnostic.

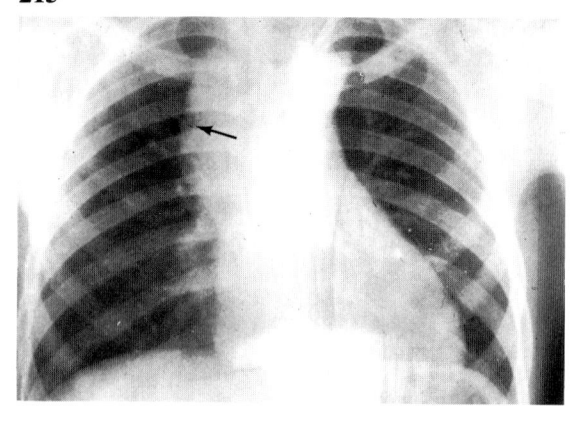

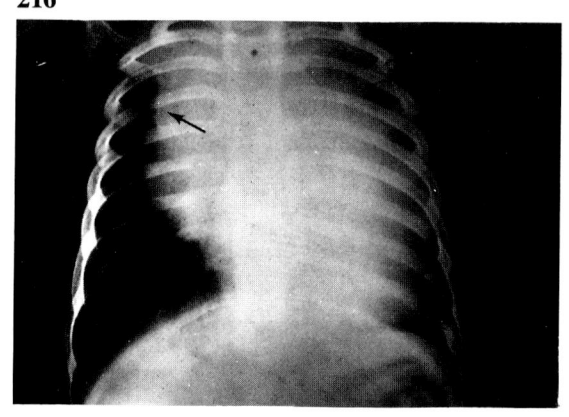

218 Thoracic neuroblastoma arising in the posterior mediastinum and infiltrating the adjacent ribs and soft tissue. Prognosis for mediastinal neuroblastoma is more favourable than for abdominal neuroblastoma.

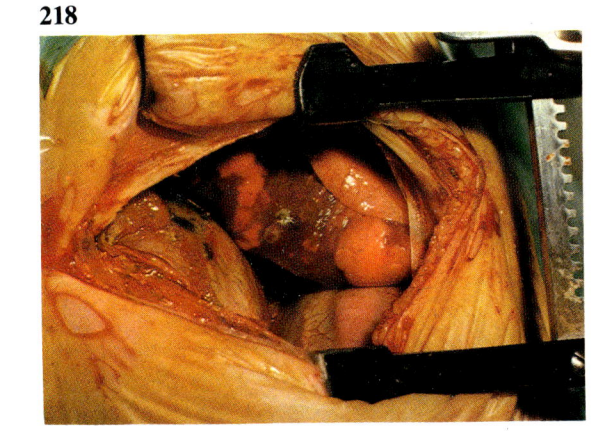

219 Neuroblastoma. Almost total obliteration of the right hemithorax by a space-occupying lesion. Catecholamine excretion raised.

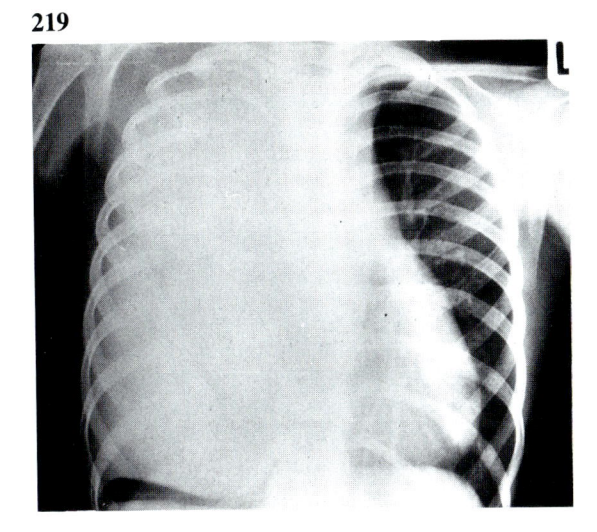

220 Pneumomediastinum. Air in the superior mediastinum is shown outlining the thymus (diagnostic). A lateral xray will confirm the presence of a retrosternal air strip. Usually decompresses itself spontaneously, but large collections may produce circulatory embarrassment and require urgent needle aspiration.

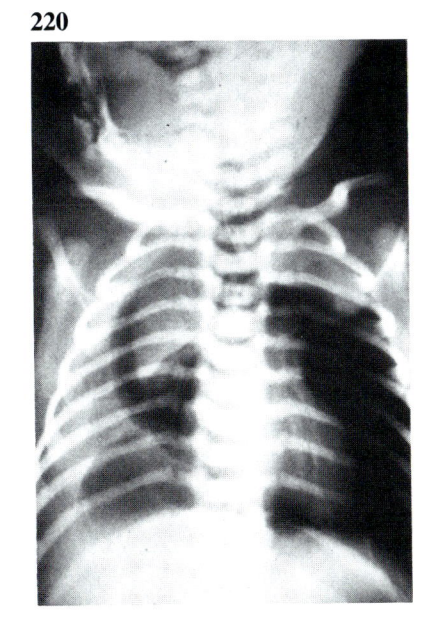

21 The lungs

221 Lobar emphysema is caused by massive overinflation of one lobe, commonly the left upper lobe, of one lung. The overinflated lung compresses the other pulmonary lobes, causes gross displacement of the mediastinum and produces increasing respiratory distress. Because of a structural abnormality (deficient elastic tissue) the involved lobe cannot deflate normally. The xray shows radiolucency of the left hemithorax with the left lower lobe compressed into a triangular shadow at the lower end of the cardiac border and the mediastinum displaced to the opposite side.

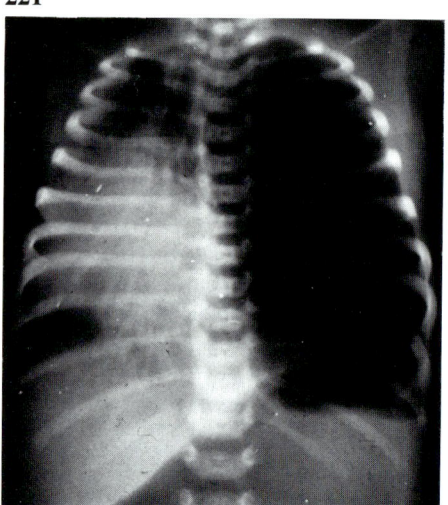

222 Lobar emphysema. Appearance of the affected lobe at thoracotomy. The over-inflated emphysematous lobe bulges out of the wound immediately on opening the parietal pleura.

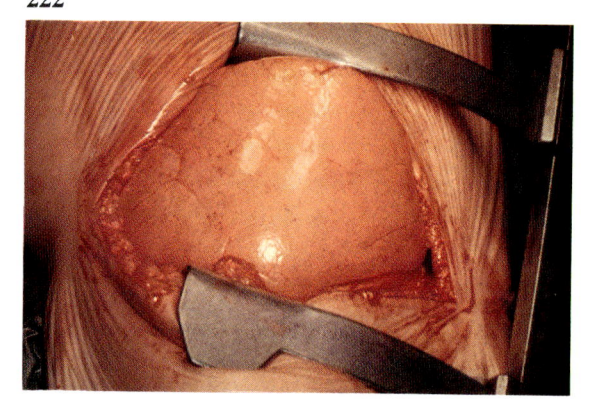

223 Congenital lung cyst. Usually lined with respiratory epithelium and communicates with the bronchial air passages. Often associated with other congenital anomalies, e.g. trilobed left lung, aberrant systemic arteries, etc. Commonly becomes infected because of communication with the airways. The xray shows a large cyst in the mid-zone of the right hemithorax.

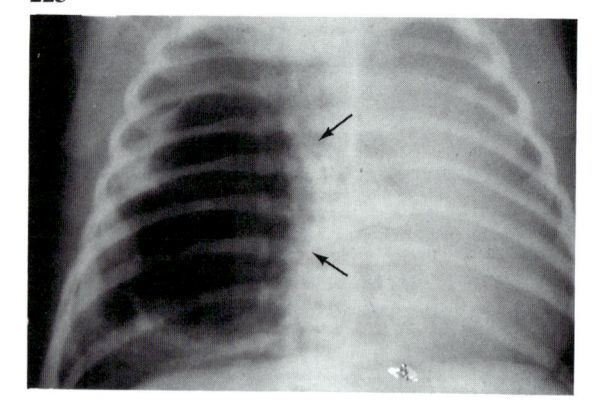

224 Congenital lung cyst. A lateral xray shows the cyst with an air-fluid level. Should be distinguished from acquired lung cysts and from lung abscess. Treatment consists of resection which usually involves lobectomy of the affected lobe.

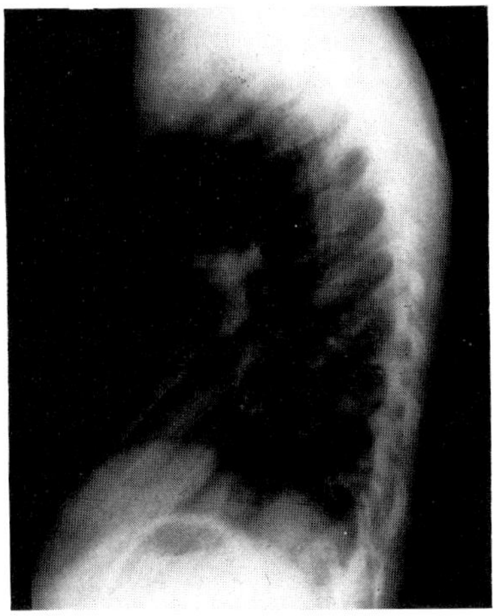

225 Congenital cystic adenomatoid malformation of the left lung. The infant presents soon after birth with respiratory distress. Plain xray of the chest shows multiple large cystic spaces in the left hemithorax with displacement of the mediastinum to the right side. The appearance mimics a left diaphragmatic hernia, but the normal gastrointestinal gas pattern should lead to the correct diagnosis.

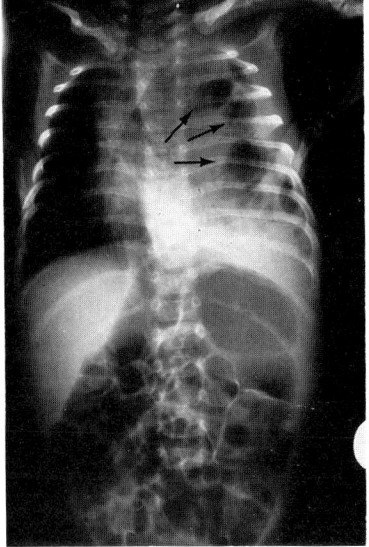

226 Lung abscess. A well-demarcated mass is visible in the right lower lobe. Commonly caused by staphylococcal infection (in this case neonatal osteomyelitis) or secondary to aspiration or foreign-body inhalation. Usually responds to intensive antibiotic therapy.

227 Hydatid cyst of the lung. Caused by infestation with the Echinococcus granulosa. Definitive host is the dog, while man, sheep and cattle are intermediate hosts. The cyst is round, homogeneous with sharp borders. An air-fluid level in the cyst indicates communication with the bronchi. Treatment is by enucleation.

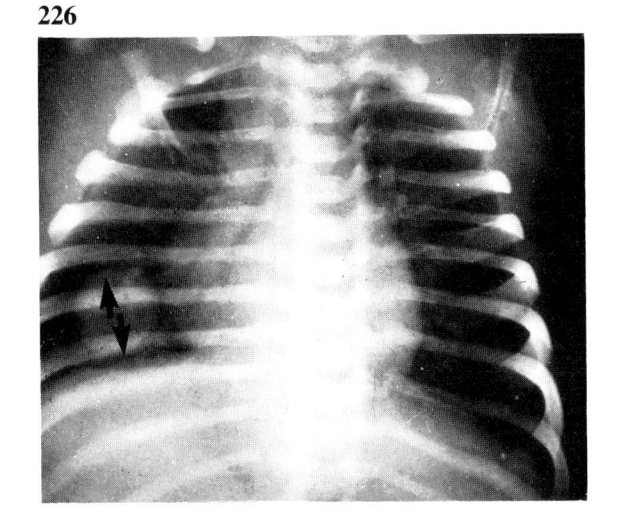

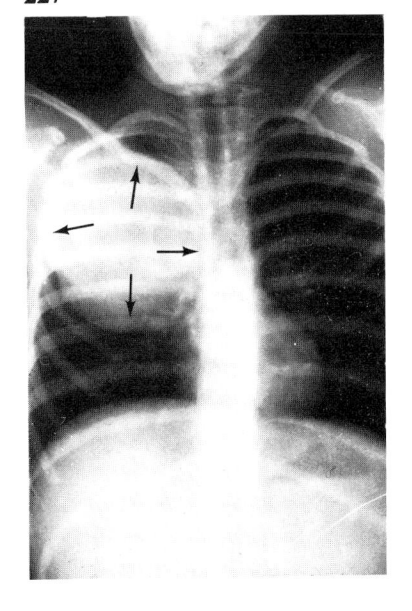

228 Chylothorax. May occur spontaneously in the neonatal period and may be related to a traumatic delivery or after repair of coarctation of the aorta or ligation of patent ductus arteriosus. Produces symptoms of respiratory distress. Xray shows a collection of fluid on the affected side (right more common than left). Diagnosis is confirmed on thoracocentesis. Usually responds to repeated aspiration or tube thoracostomy, with or without the use of medium-chain triglyceride feeds or parenteral nutrition to decrease lymphatic flow (chyle).

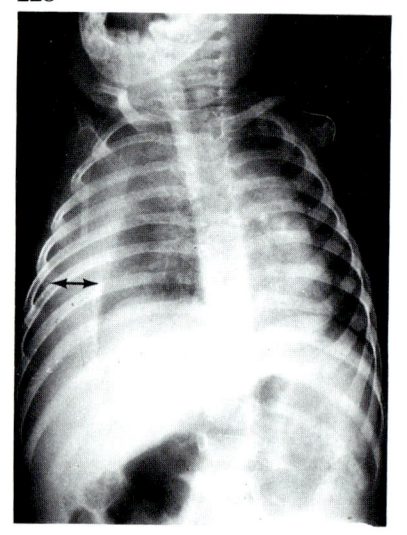

229 Tumours of the lung. Primary tumours of the lung are rare in children. Secondary metastases from Wilms' tumour, osteogenic sarcoma, neuroblastoma are relatively frequent occurrences in oncological services. The chest xray shows a large 'cannon-ball' secondary in the right lung in a child with a nephroblastoma. A number of other metastases can be seen in the left lung.

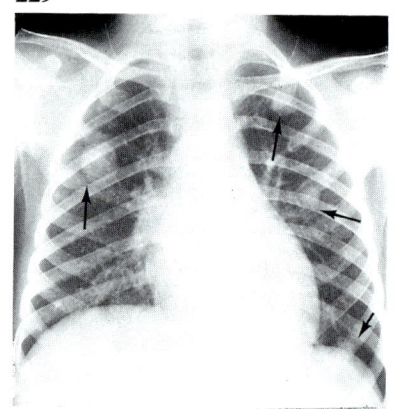

230 Lung metastasis. A resected specimen of the right lower lobe in a 14-year-old girl with osteogenic sarcoma of the right leg for which an ablation had been carried out a few years previously.

231 Inhaled foreign body. Chest xray including contrast material in the oesophagus shows the foreign object lodged in the left main bronchus. Endoscopic extraction is usually possible. Inhalation of a peanut is particularly hazardous because of swelling of the peanut and fragmentation on attempting extraction.

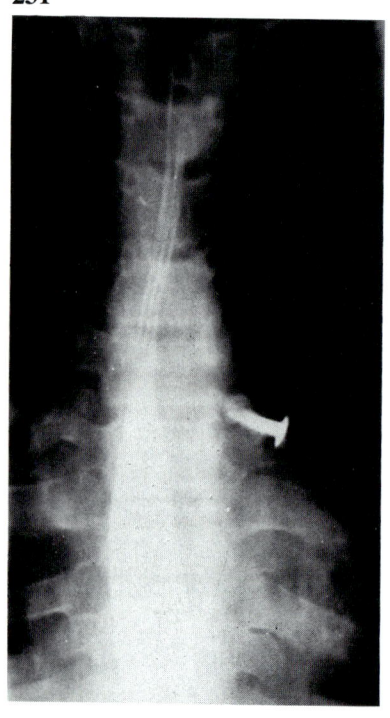

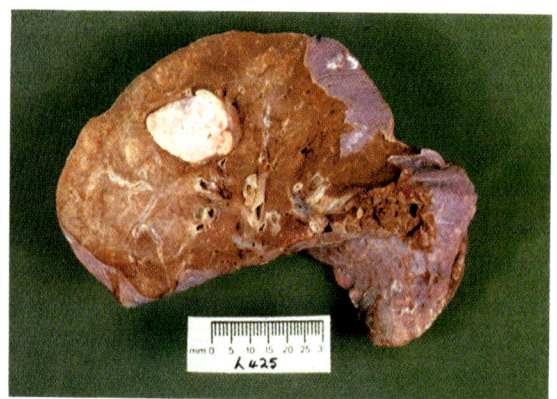

22 The diaphragm

232 Congenital posterolateral diaphragmatic hernia (hernia through the foramen of Bochdalek or pleuroperitoneal canal) usually presents early in the neonatal period with progressively increasing respiratory distress. The infant commonly has a scaphoid abdomen and an apparent dextrocardia. Borborygmi may be ausculated in the chest.

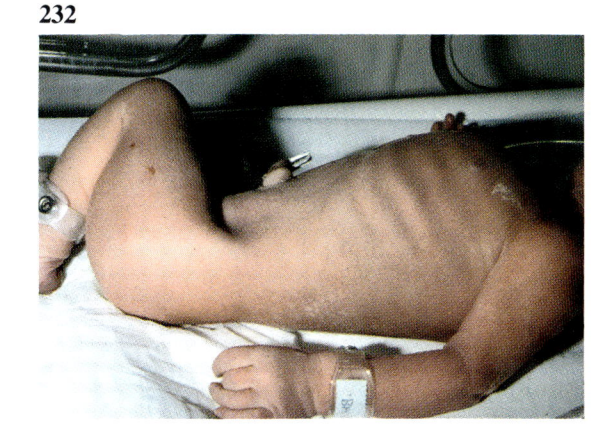

233 Diaphragmatic hernia. There is a defect in the left diaphragm through which stomach, small intestine and spleen have herniated into the left hemithorax. The left lung is compressed and the heart and mediastinum are displaced to the opposite side.

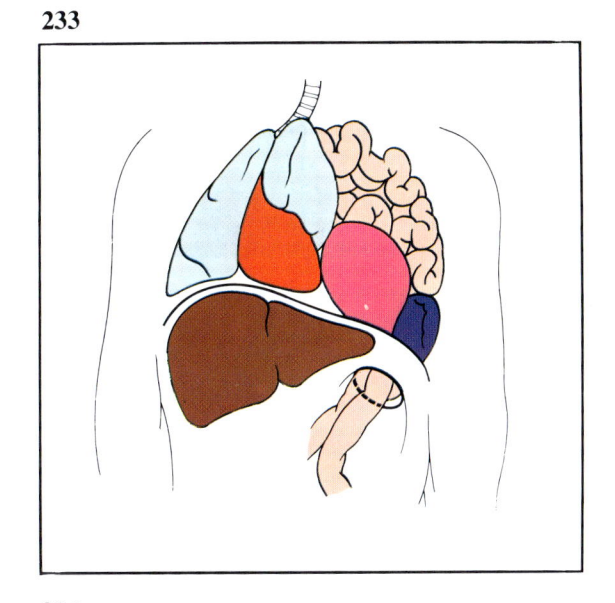

234 Diaphragmatic hernia. The chest xray (which should include the abdomen) shows the presence of loops of intestine in the left hemithorax in continuity with the bowel of the abdomen. The heart is displaced into the right hemithorax. The left side is affected in 90 per cent of cases.

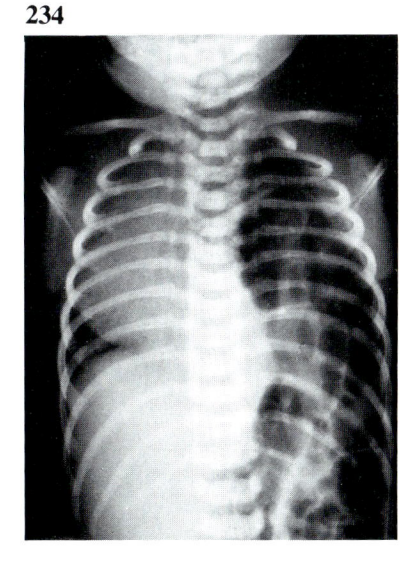

235 Diaphragmatic hernia. A barium meal (not recommended) shows almost the entire small bowel in the left hemithorax. Associated mid-gut malrotation is an almost invariable accompaniment.

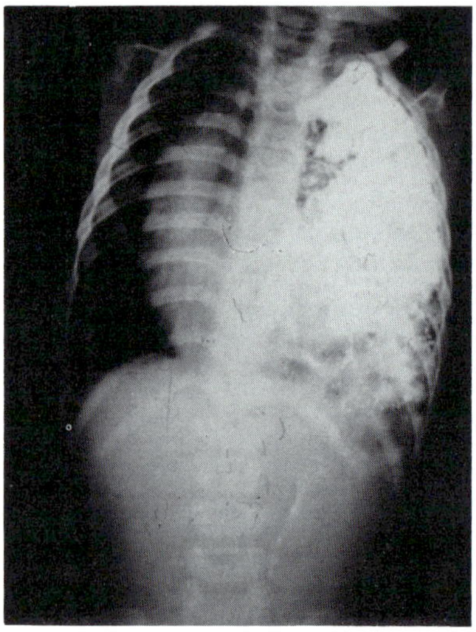

236 Diaphragmatic hernia. A necropsy demonstration of a left side diaphragmatic hernia containing the fundus of the stomach, necrotic small intestine and an infarcted spleen in the left chest.

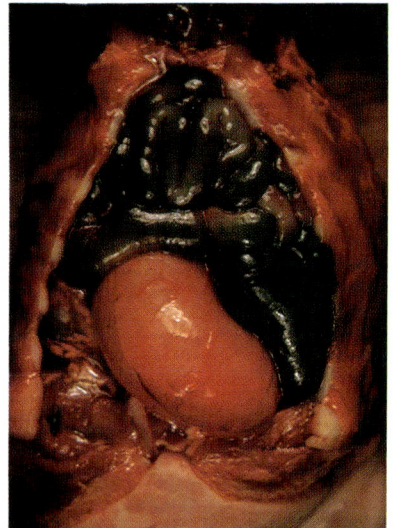

237 Diaphragmatic hernia. An operative view of the defect in the posterolateral aspect of the left diaphragm (after reduction of the contents). The well-developed anterior diaphragm can usually be approximated to the thinner posterior leaflet and closed by direct suture.

238 Right diaphragmatic hernia. May present with respiratory distress in the newborn period, but more commonly the defect in the diaphragm is occluded by the right lobe of the liver and may escape detection for some time.

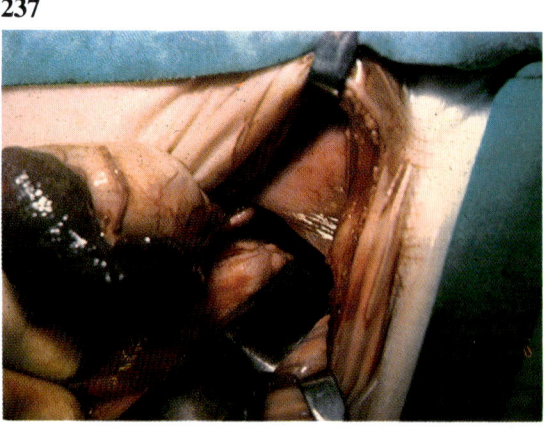

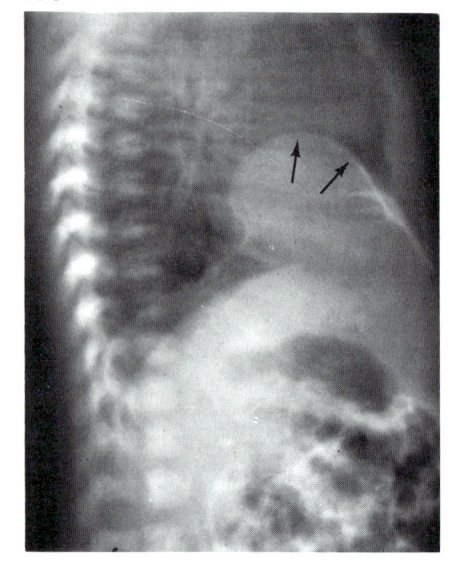

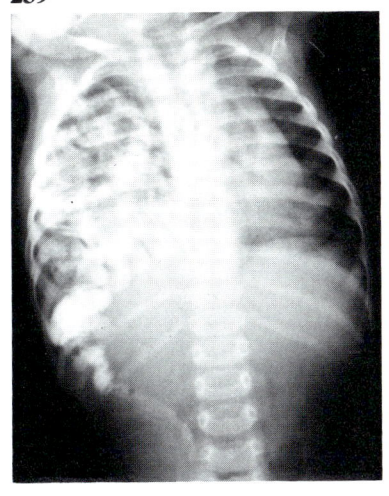

239 Right diaphragmatic hernia. The barium follow-through study shows the presence of intestine in the right chest.

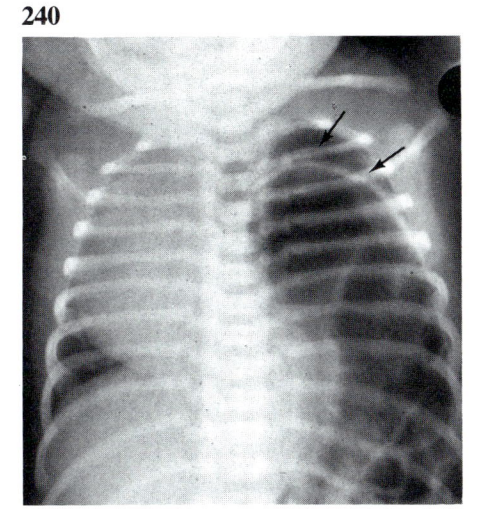

240 Eventration of the diaphragm. May be congenital as a result of muscular hypoplasia or acquired after injury to the phrenic nerve, e.g. during a difficult delivery or acquired during surgery in the thorax. The infant may present with respiratory embarrassment in the neonatal period or with recurrent respiratory tract infections. Xray shows an elevated leaf of the diaphragm with paradoxical movement on respiration. The mediastinum is displaced to the right.

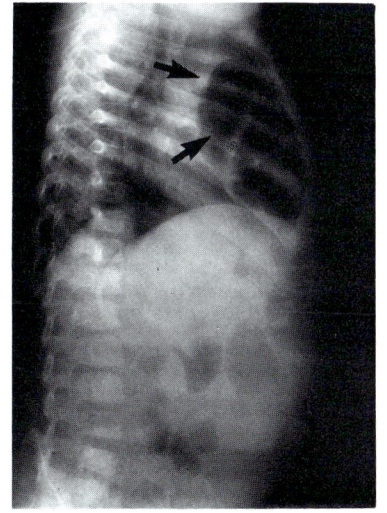

241 Morgagni hernia. The defect is in the retrosternal portion of the septum transversum and the content is most commonly large intestine or omentum. Clinical presentation varies from respiratory distress to symptoms of intestinal obstruction. The lateral chest xray shows the presence of bowel retrosternally in the anterior mediastinum.

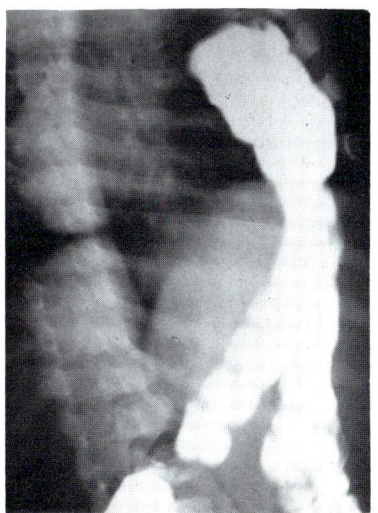

242 Morgagni hernia. A barium enema examination shows transverse colon in the retrosternal area anterior to the cardiac shadow.

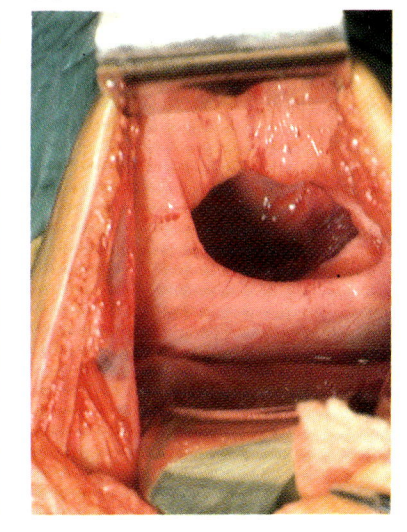

243 Morgagni hernia. An operative view (from the abdomen) showing the defect in the anterior part of the diaphragm. The liver is displaced inferiorly and the heart can be seen anteriorly and to the left in the chest.

23 The abdominal wall

244 Abnormalities of the omphalomesenteric duct (vitelline duct). (See also Section 28.) The vitelline duct is the stalk of communication between the embryonic intestine and the yolk sac which normally becomes atretic between the fifth and sixth week of intrauterine life. A wide variety of anomalies result from the persistence of all or only parts of that structure:
a) omphaloileal fistula
b) Meckel's diverticulum attached to umbilicus by fibrous cord
c) umbilical polyp associated with attached Meckel's diverticulum
d) fibrous connection between umbilicus and ileum
e) cystic remnant of omphalomesenteric duct attached to ileum and umbilicus
f) umbilical polyp with fibrous connection to ileum
g) isolated Meckel's diverticulum

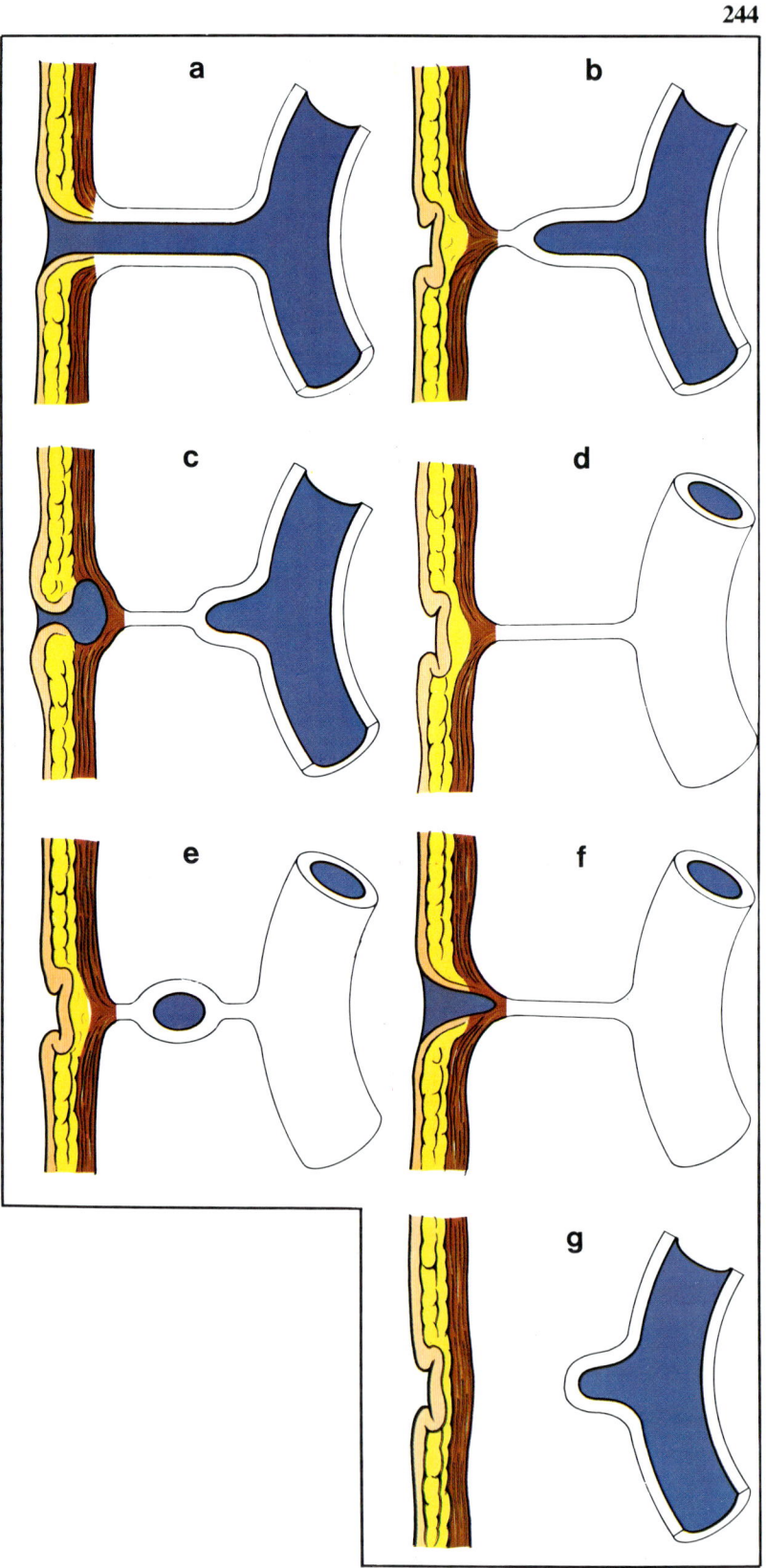

245 Umbilical granuloma is simply an overgrowth of granulation tissue at the site of attachment of the normal umbilical cord. Produces a blood-stained discharge. Responds to cauterisation with silver nitrate or to simple ligation of the stalk at its base.

246 Umbilical polyp. Represents persistence of the distal remnant of vitello-intestinal epithelium at the umbilicus. Has the appearance of a mucosa-covered polyp. Does not respond to cauterisation and should be completely excised.

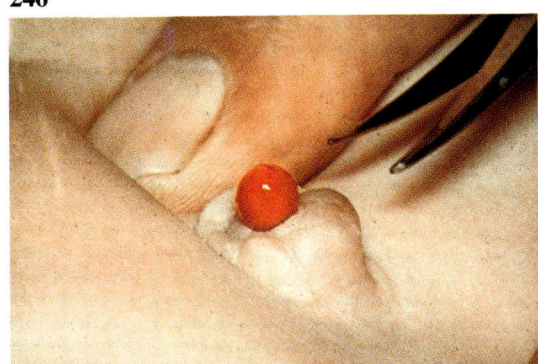

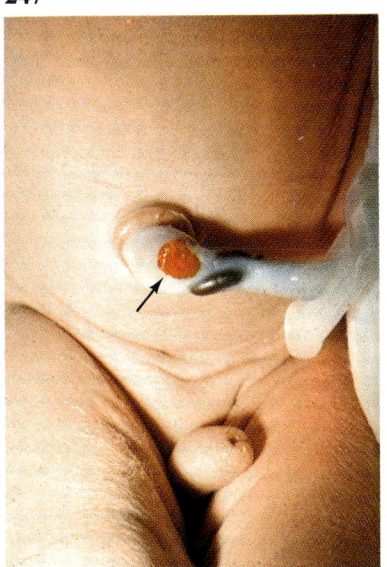

247 Patent omphalomesenteric duct is a fistulous communication between the ileum and the umbilicus. Discharges meconium and/or flatus. The orifice is covered with intestinal mucosa. Prolapse of the duct or the ileum through the orifice occurs in about one-third of cases. Treatment requires total excision with or without the attached ileum.

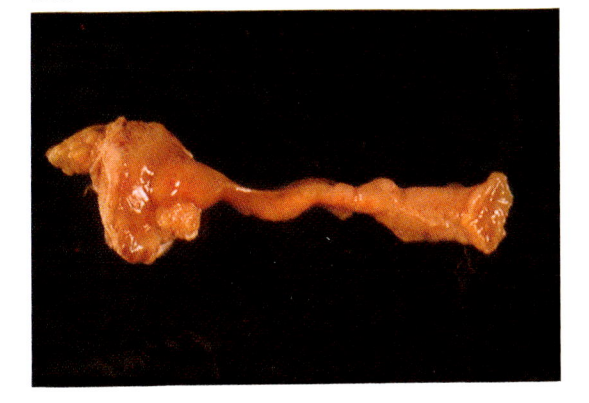

248 Omphalomesenteric duct. Resected specimen with the disc of skin including the umbilicus. A short segment of ileum has been removed with the duct.

249 Meckel's diverticulum is the persistent proximal portion of the vitelline duct. It contains all layers of the intestinal wall and typically projects from the antimesenteric surface of the ileum approximately 25 cm from the ileocaecal junction.

250 Perforated Meckel's diverticulum. Forty per cent of Meckel's diverticula contain ectopic gastric mucosa. Peptic ulceration may develop in the ileal mucosa adjacent to the diverticulum. The ulceration may be complicated by haemorrhage or ileal perforation.

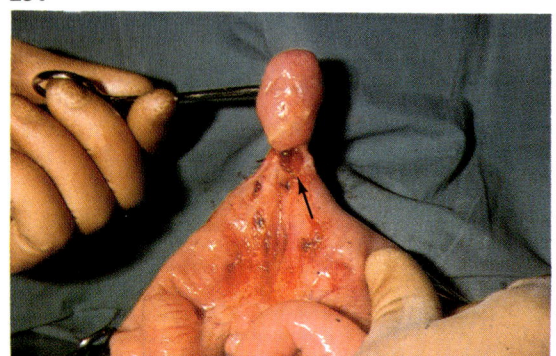

251 Intestinal obstruction secondary to Meckel's diverticulum. Obstruction of the ileum by fibrous bands, volvulus or intussusception. The straight erect abdominal xray showing dilated loops of intestine with air-fluid levels is non-specific.

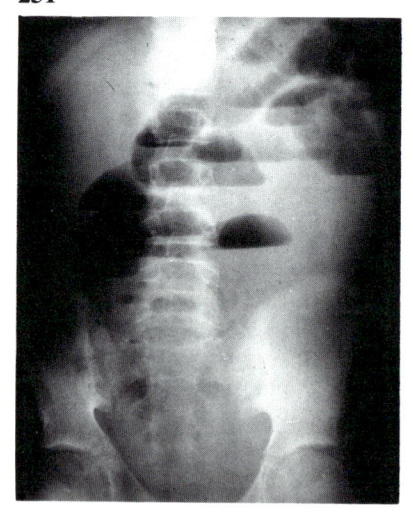

252 Patent urachus is a persistence of the communication between the allantois stalk and the primitive cloaca. It may present as a fistula with the discharge of urine through an orifice at the umbilicus. Important to exclude bladder outlet obstruction (posturethral valves).

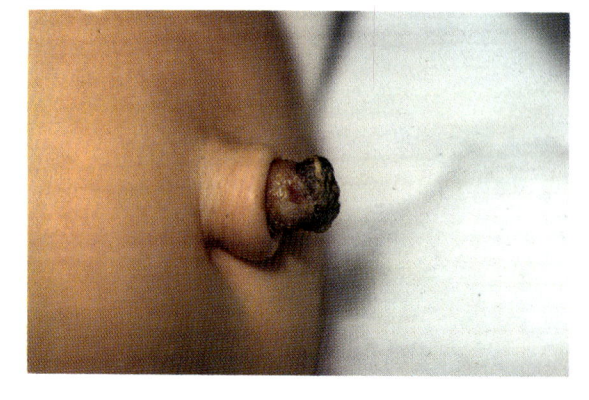

253 Urachal cyst. Persistence of the mid-portion of the urachus with obliteration of both ends leads to the development of a cystic lesion. Presents as an infra-umbilical mass. Cystogram shows deformity of the dome of the bladder. Treatment is by extraperitoneal resection.

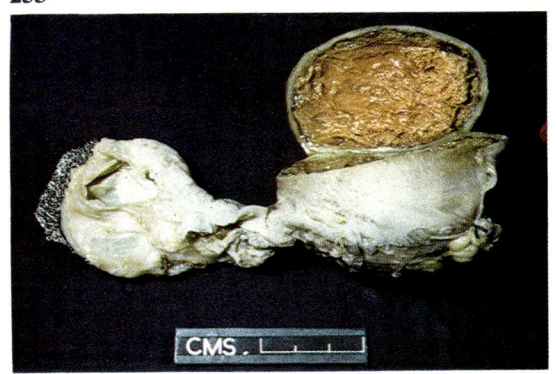

254 Umbilical hernia. Caused by failure of cicatrisation of the umbilical ring. Common in Negroid races. Reduces very easily and complications are rare in childhood. Spontaneous regression is common – 90 per cent. Umbilical herniorrhaphy is required if the hernia persists beyond the fifth year.

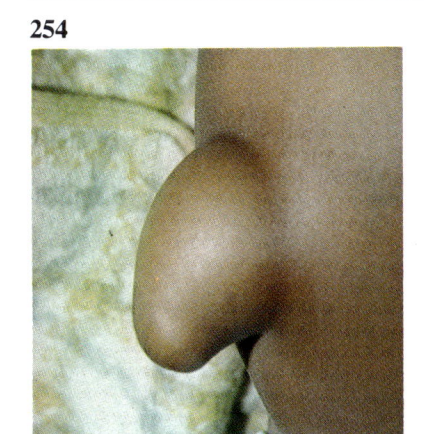

255 Perforation of an umbilical hernia by a safety pin when applying a napkin in a writhing crying infant.

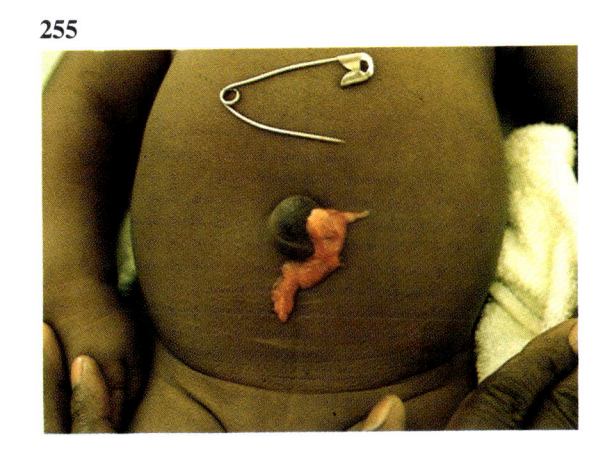

256 Supraumbilical hernia. The hernia is periumbilical in location and occurs through a defect in the linea alba above (or below) a normal umbilicus. Spontaneous regression does not occur and surgical repair is required.

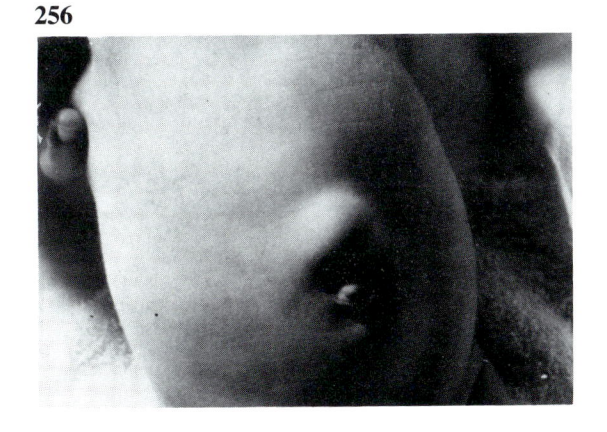

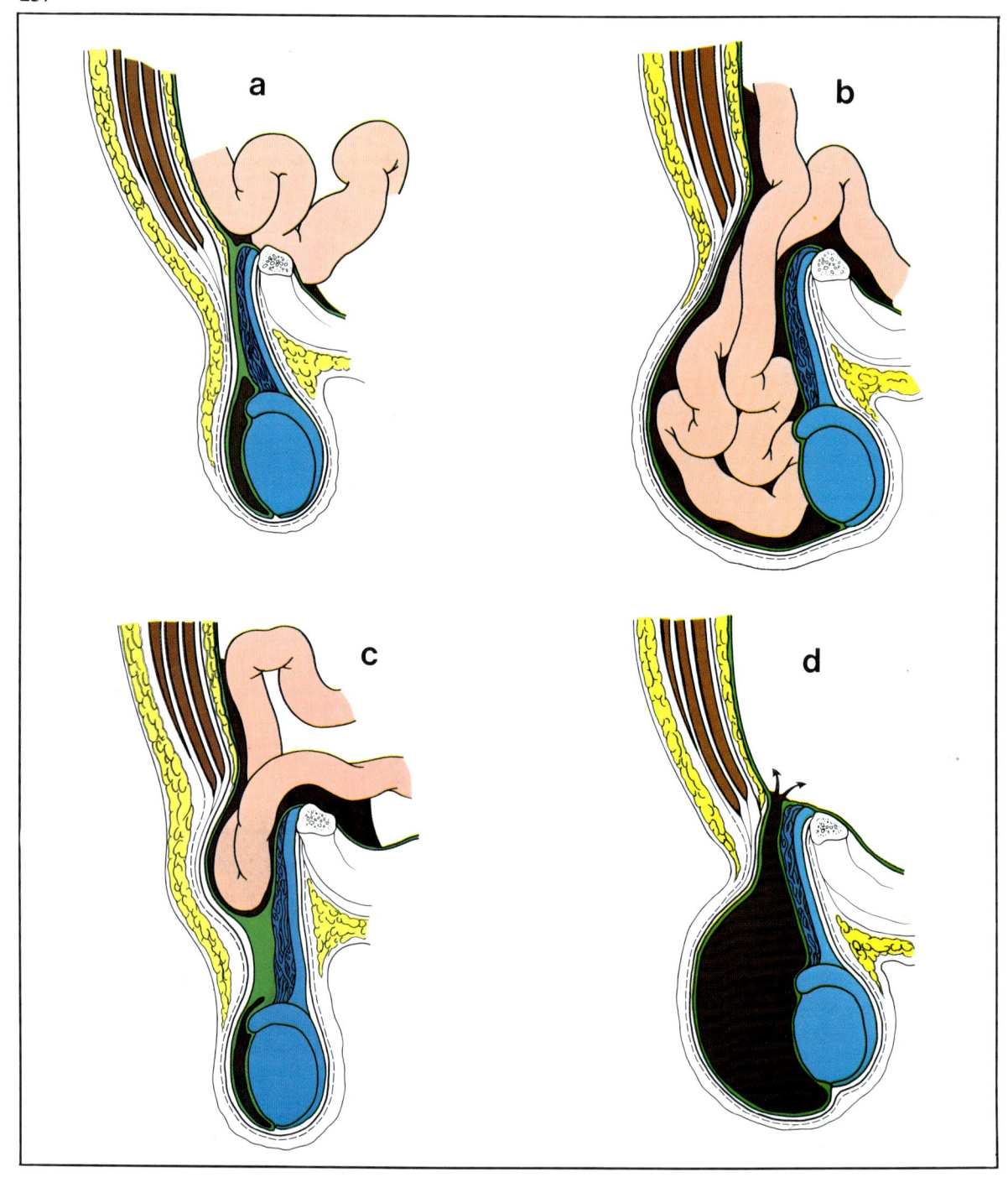

257 Development of inguinal hernias and hydrocoeles
a) Normal anatomy of the inguinal region showing complete obliteration of the processus vaginalis between the peritoneum at the internal inguinal ring and the tunica vaginalis of the testis.
b) Complete indirect inguinal hernia. The processus vaginalis has failed to obliterate and a loop of intestine is shown descending to the scrotum.
c) Incomplete indirect inguinal hernia. The proximal part only of the processus vaginalis has failed to obliterate.
d) Communicating hydrocoele. The process of obliteration of the processus vaginalis is incomplete. There is a narrow communication between the peritoneal cavity and the scrotum where fluid collects. The narrow communication prevents intestine from entering the sac.

258 Bilateral inguinal hernia. Complete hernia is evident on both sides. In infancy there is a significant risk of irreducibility and strangulation of the hernial content. Surgery (herniotomy) should be undertaken on a semi-urgent basis.

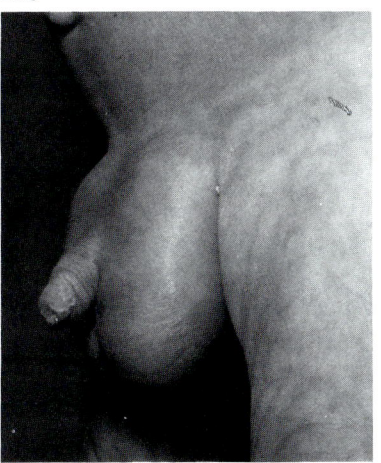

259 Left incomplete indirect inguinal hernia in a male infant. The bulge in the groin does not extend down into the scrotum. This type of hernia is commonly seen by the parents or family practitioner and frequently cannot be demonstrated during consultation. Surgery should be undertaken on the strength of a good history as the incidence of irreducibility approaches 50 per cent in the first three months of life.

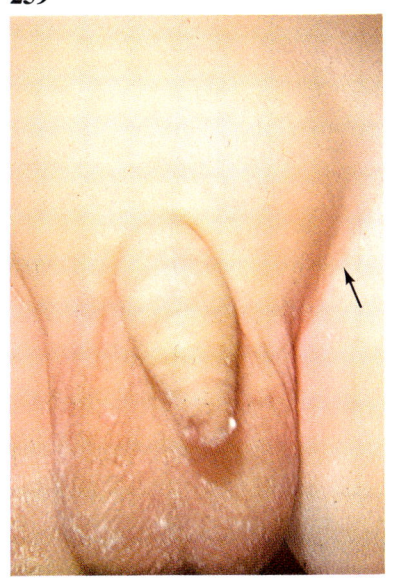

260 Irreducible right indirect inguinal hernia. Incarceration of an inguinal hernia may be the first indication of a defect at the site and is commonest in the first three months of life. The infant presents with screaming attacks and vomiting. The hernial contents can be frequently reduced into the peritoneal cavity by taxis at the neck of the sac. The infant may have to be sedated before successful manipulation. Occasionally urgent surgery is required, particularly if the contents of the hernia have become gangrenous. The viability of the testis may also be threatened.

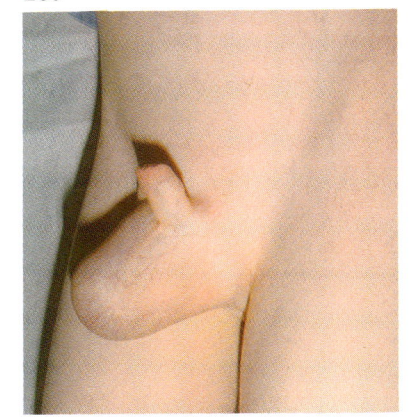

261 Communicating hydrocoele. Most hydrocoeles in childhood are of the communicating type and represent failure of complete obliteration of the processus vaginalis. May be quite tense. Upper extent of hydrocoele easily definable. Most infantile hydrocoeles resolve spontaneously by the age of 18 to 24 months. Surgical treatment is by ligation of the patent processus vaginalis.

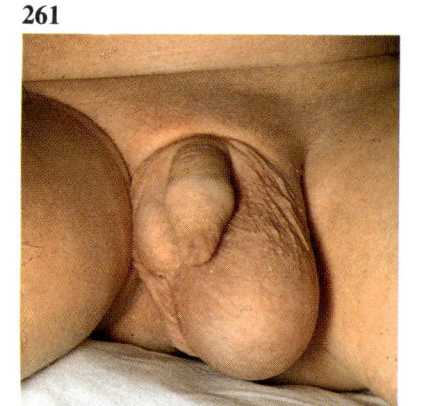

262 Communicating hydrocoele. The swelling is brilliantly transilluminable indicating the fluid content.

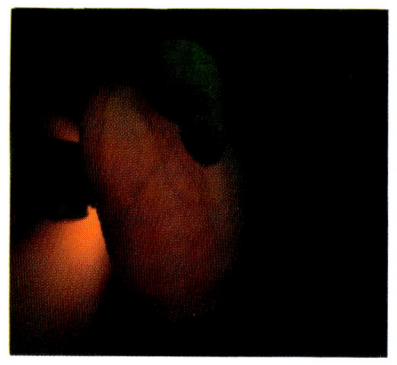

263 Femoral hernia. Rare in childhood. Presents as a rounded reducible swelling below the medial end of the inguinal ligament. May have a palpable impulse on straining. Treatment consists of femoral herniorrhaphy.

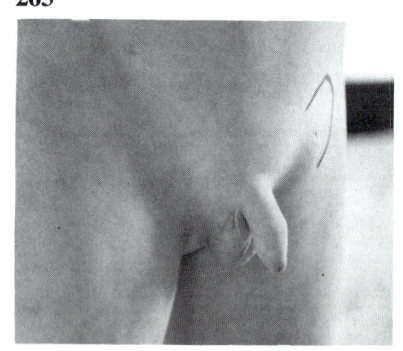

264 Inguinal hernia in a girl. Less common than male inguinal hernia. May contain adnexa such as ovary and/or fallopian tube. One per cent of girls with inguinal hernia (more common in bilateral than unilateral hernia) have 'testicular feminisation syndrome'. The external genitalia are entirely female and the vagina is normal. The cervix, uterus and fallopian tubes are absent and the gonad is macroscopically and microscopically a testis.

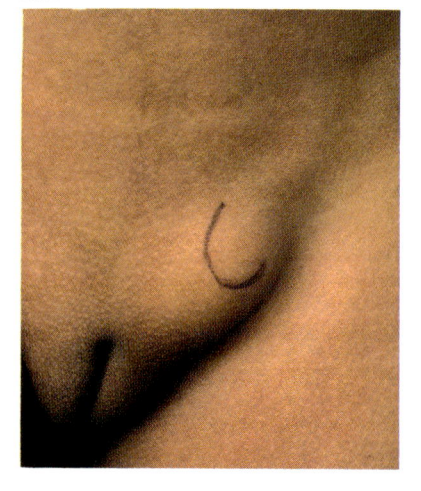

24 Exomphalos (omphalocoele)

265 Skin-covered umbilical defect. The defect is skin covered and is therefore technically an umbilical hernia. Note the caudad insertion of the umbilical cord. This lesion formed part of a pentalogy of anomalies consisting of a midline supraumbilical abdominal wall defect, split lower sternum, deficiency of the anterior diaphragm, a defect in the diaphragmatic pericardium and a congenital intracardiac defect.

266 Exomphalos minor or hernia into the umbilical cord. The herniated intestine is visible through the thin transparent amniotic membrane. May be treated by simply twisting the umbilical cord and reducing the hernial content or by direct surgical repair.

267 Exomphalos minor. The size of the defect in the anterior abdominal wall measures less than 5 cm in diameter. The coverings of the exomphalos are intact. Malrotation of midgut is almost invariable. Treatment is by primary surgical repair of the defect.

268 Exomphalos major. The size of the defect at the umbilicus is greater than 5 cm in diameter. The contents of the sac consist of intestine and liver. Primary repair may result in respiratory embarrassment caused by upward displacement of the diaphragm. Conservative treatment with the application of an antiseptic solution to the sac results in an eschar formation and subsequent rupture is prevented.

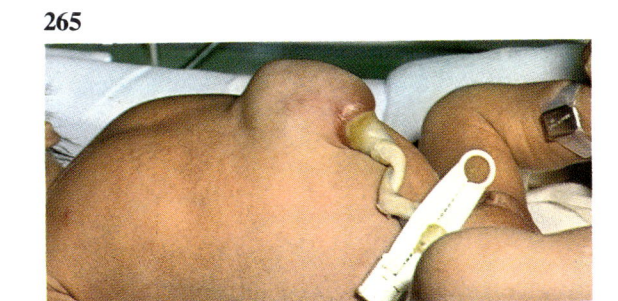

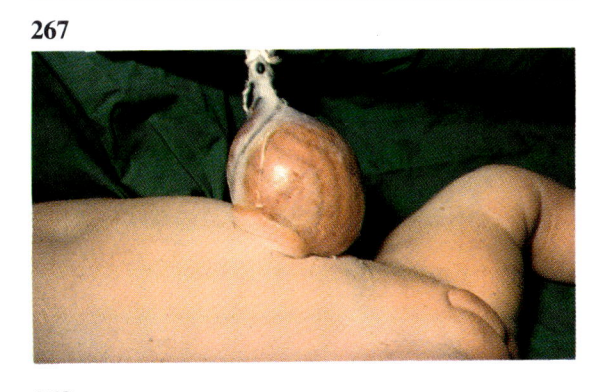

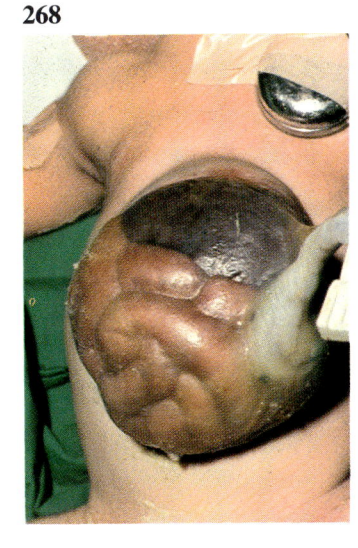

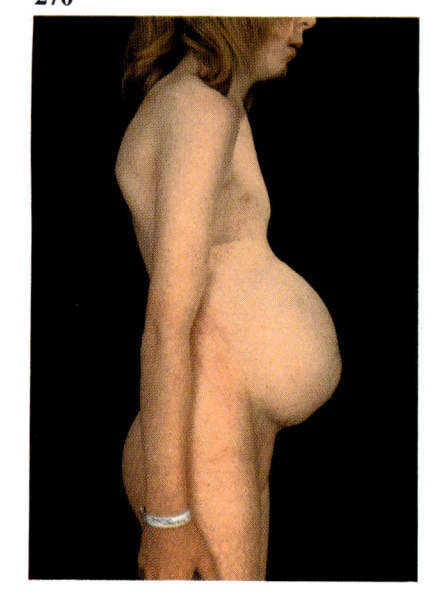

269 Exomphalos major. Treated by application of mercurochrome to the sac. The resulting eschar is subsequently replaced by epithelial ingrowth from the periphery of the lesion. The final result is a large umbilical hernia which usually requires surgical closure at 18 to 24 months of age.

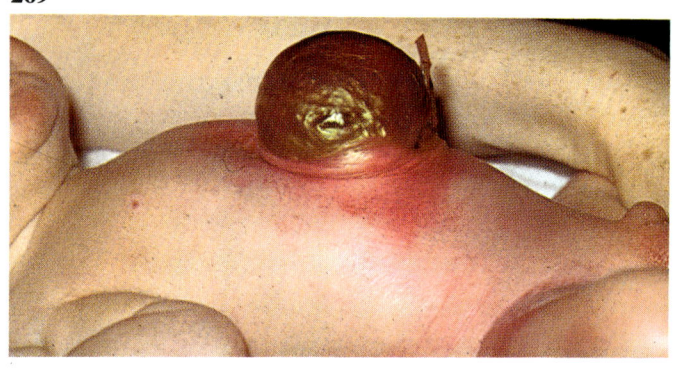

270 Abdominal wall herniation. A major exomphalos was initially treated by skin-flap closure (gross). The resulting anterior abdominal wall defect remained unrepaired until the child was nine years old. Treatment consisted of staged closure using prolene mesh.

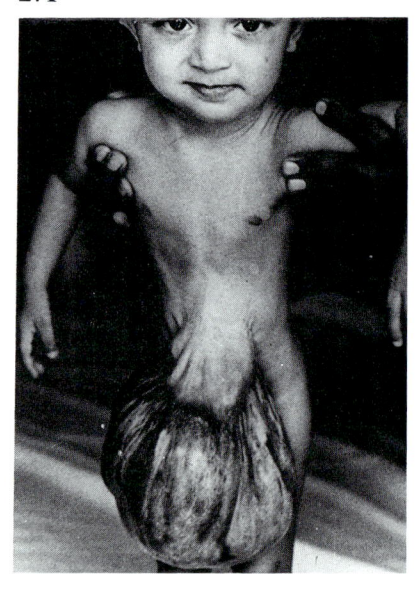

271 Exomphalos major. Failure to repair the resulting umbilical hernia in a conservatively treated major exomphalos has resulted in a massive umbilical hernia which descends almost to the knees of the child.

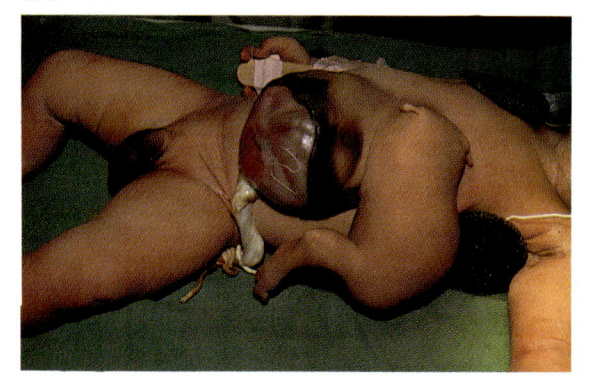

272 Complex exomphalos. In addition to the major exomphalos there is an attached accessory lower limb on the cranial aspect of the defect.

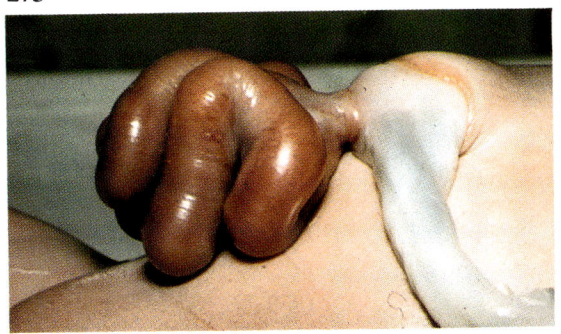

273 Gastroschisis (ruptured exomphalos). There is a defect in the umbilical cord on the right, through which a loop of thickened and oedematous intestine has prolapsed. An atresia was found at the site of protrusion at both ends of the extruded bowel.

274 Gastroschisis. A large amount of small intestine has eviscerated through a defect to the right of a normal appearing umbilical cord. No sac is visible and the intestine is thickened, matted and oedematous. Vascular compression has resulted in ischaemic necrosis.

275 Ruptured exomphalos. The extruded intestine is covered by remnants of the exomphalos sac indicating perinatal rupture. Primary repair is usually feasible in these cases.

276 Ectopia cloaca (vesicointestinal fissure). A defect in the formation of the lower abdominal wall. The combination of anomalies includes an exomphalos major, prolapsed ileum, everted caecum in the midline separating the two hemibladders which form the lateral wall of the defect.

277 Beckwith-Wiedermann syndrome (exomphalos-macroglossia-gigantism (EMG). There is a large tongue and macrosomia in addition to hyperplastic kidneys and pancreas. Neonatal hypoglycaemia commonly occurs in response to the hyperinsulinism and may cause retardation. Monitoring of the serum glucose levels for at least 48 hours is essential if brain damage is to be avoided.

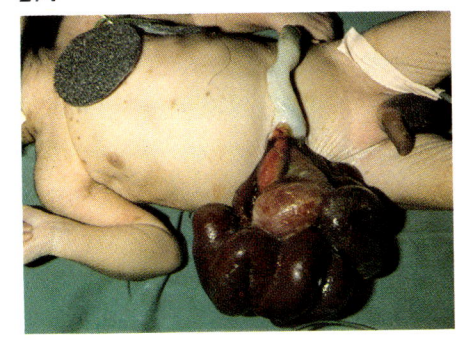

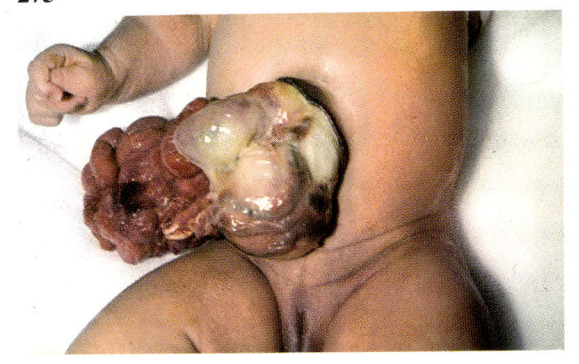

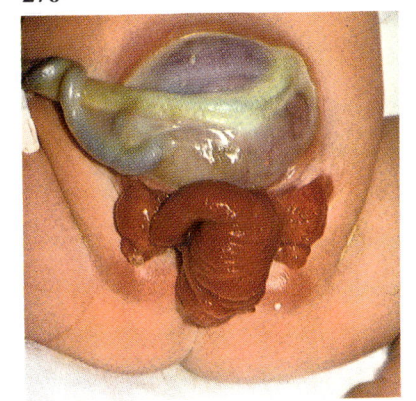

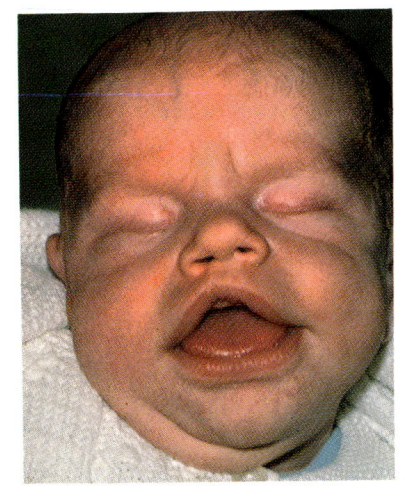

25 The peritoneal cavity

278 Periumbilical erythema. If, in addition to the clinical features of an intestinal obstruction, there is red discoloration of the skin around the umbilicus, complications such as peritonitis or intestinal gangrene should be considered.

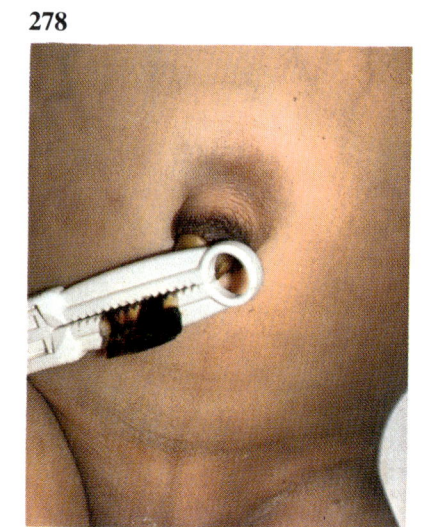

279 Oedema of the abdominal wall. Oedema of the anterior abdominal wall frequently accompanies periumbilical erythema in cases of peritonitis or intestinal gangrene. The abdomen appears shiny and is tensely distended.

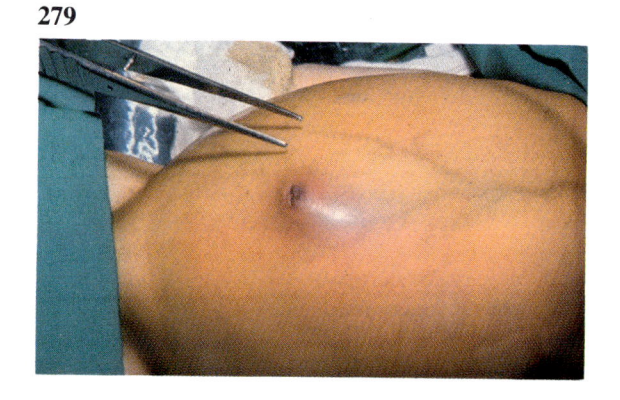

280 Oedema of the abdominal wall. The 'pitting' oedema is shown by the impression left on the abdominal wall by the bell of the stethoscope after auscultation for borborygmi.

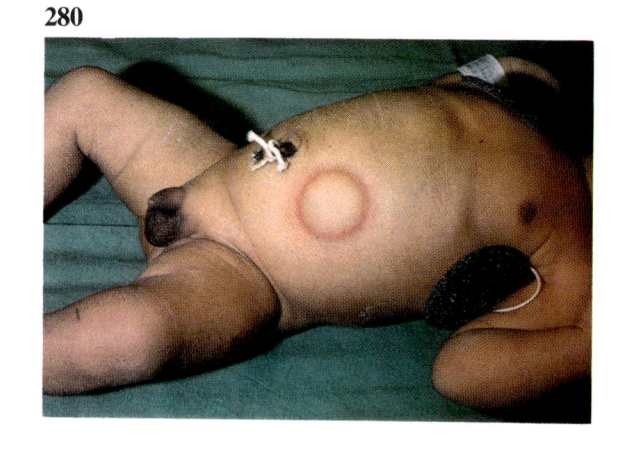

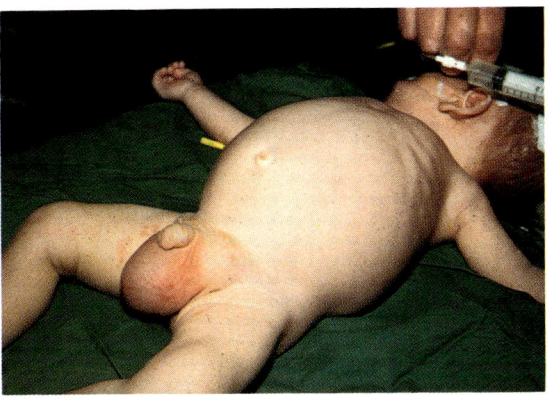

281 Urinary ascites. The peritoneal cavity is filled with urine after extravasation. The commonest cause is posterior urethral valves. Other conditions which predispose to urinary ascites include urethrocoeles, neuropathic bladder and supravesical and infravesical obstructive lesions (e.g. urethral stenosis). Occurs almost exclusively in boys. May occur in the absence of any demonstrable obstructive lesion.

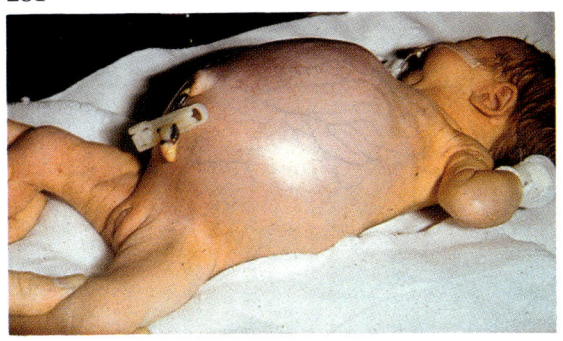

282 Chylous ascites. Results from the leak or effusion of mesenteric, cisternal or lower thoracic ductal lymphatic fluid into the peritoneal cavity. May occur secondary to mechanical intestinal obstruction, malrotation, rupture of a mesenteric cyst, lymphangioma or after trauma.

283 Chylous ascites. Fluid aspirated from the peritoneal cavity is 'milky' in appearance.

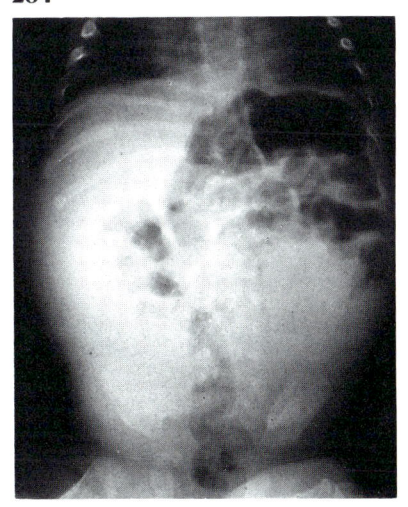

284 Ascites. X ray appearance of fluid (effusion, urinary, chyle, blood) in the peritoneal cavity. The bowel shadows are centrally located and displaced cranially ('flower pot' sign).

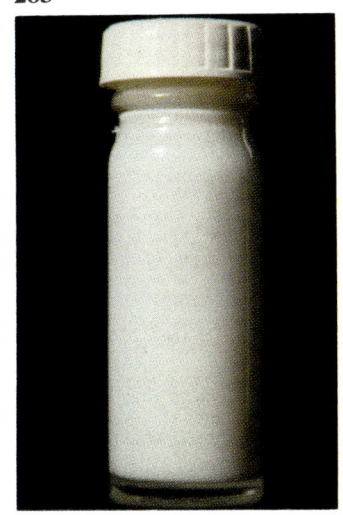

285 Mesenteric cyst. Rare in childhood. Probably develops from embryonic lymphoid centres. Clinical presentation is with abdominal distension and a palpable mass or with intestinal obstruction.

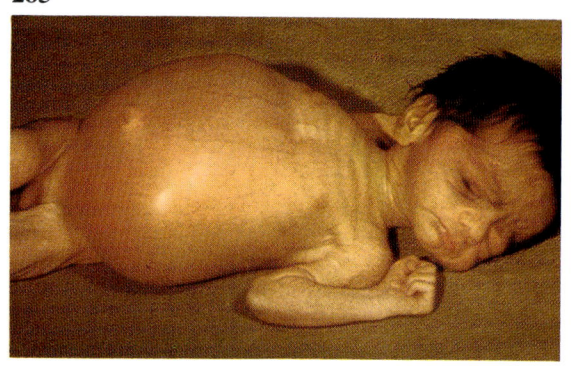

286 Mesenteric cyst. Develops in the mesentery of the small intestine (occasionally transverse mesocolon). Unilocular or multilocular and thin walled. The cyst is not attached to the adjacent intestine and can be 'shelled out' without damage to the blood supply. Absence of a muscular wall differentiates it from duplication cysts.

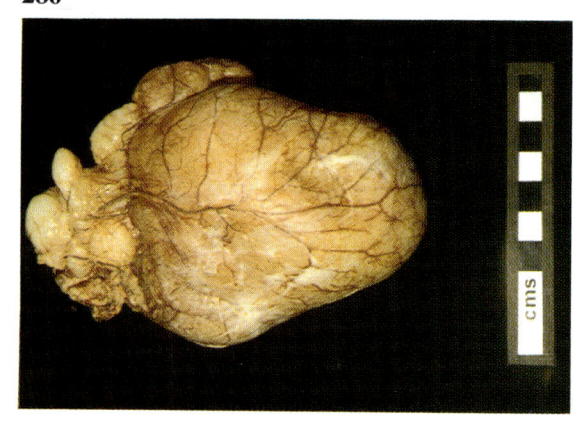

287 Omental cyst. Situated in the greater omentum. Unilocular or multilocular and contains thin watery fluid. Clinical presentation may be with increasing abdominal distension or with acute symptoms caused by haemorrhage or torsion. Treatment is by excision.

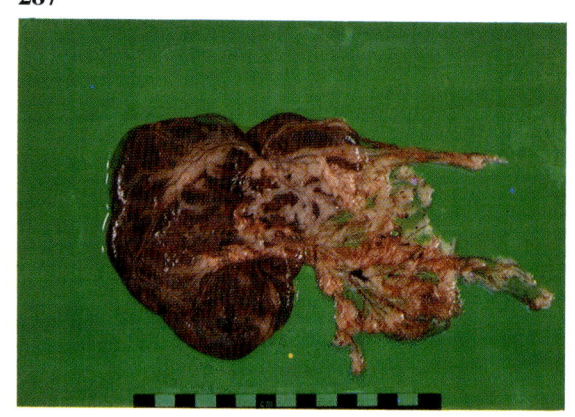

26 The stomach

288 Neonatal gastric perforation. 'Spontaneous' perforation of the stomach presents with sudden massive abdominal distension sufficient to cause respiratory embarrassment.

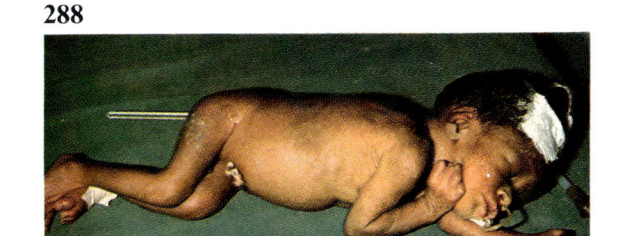

289 Neonatal gastric perforation. Erect abdominal xray shows gross pneumoperitoneum with or without an abdominal air-fluid level and an absence of gas in the stomach. Needle aspiration of the air from the peritoneal cavity may be lifesaving.

290 Neonatal gastric perforation. Supine xray shows gaseous distension of the peritoneal cavity with air outlining the ligamentum teres (falciform ligament) ('football' sign).

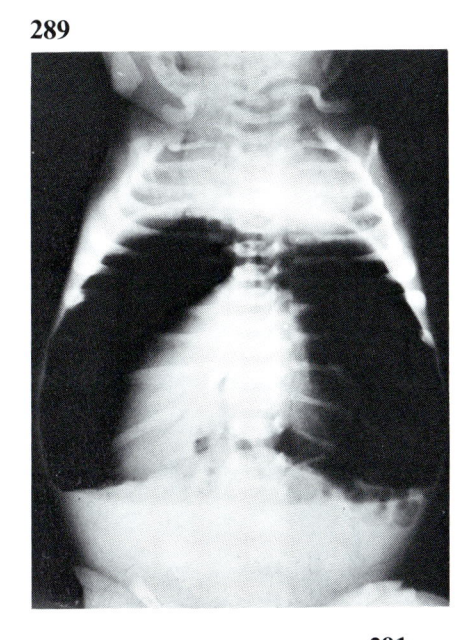

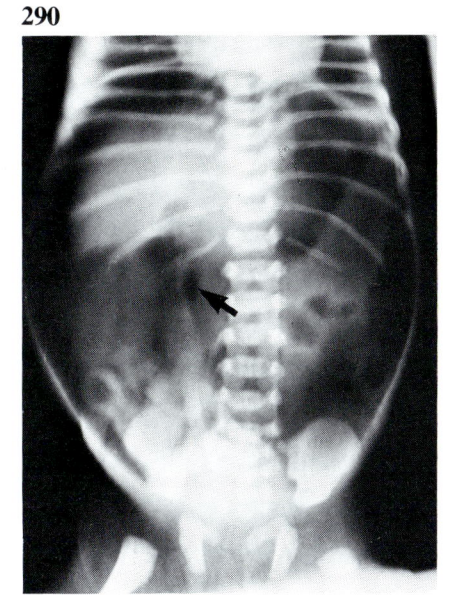

291 'Spontaneous' gastric perforation. At laparotomy there is a ragged tear in the wall of the stomach most commonly situated along the greater curvature, but occasionally involving the anterior wall or lesser curvature. The nasogastric tube can be seen extruding through a defect on the lesser curvature of the stomach.

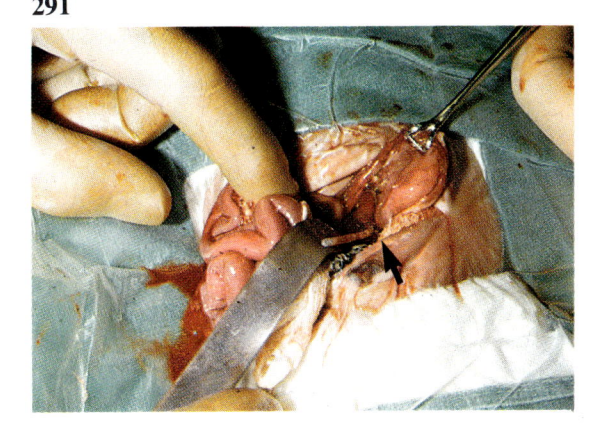

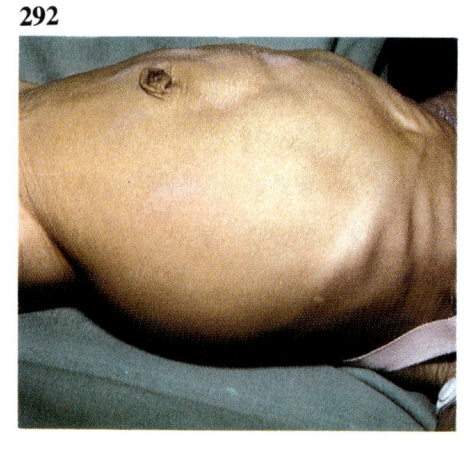

292 Pyloric stenosis. Classical symptoms are projectile non-bile-stained vomiting, constipation and failure to thrive in a two to six week old male (M:F::4:1) infant. Forceful gastric peristalsis may be visible on the abdominal wall. Diagnosis is confirmed by palpating the pyloric tumour in the right hypochondrium.

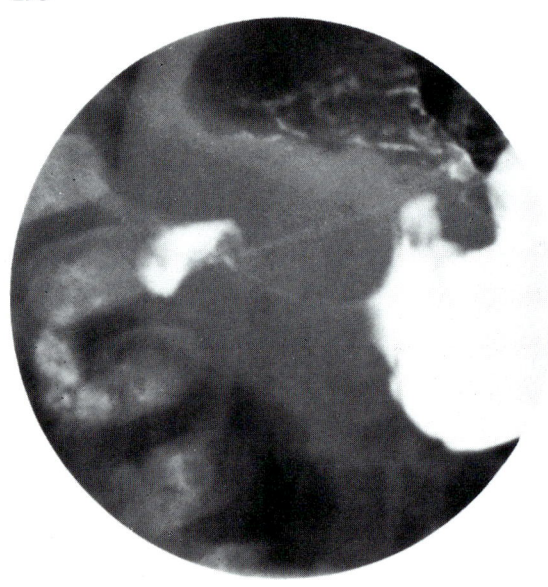

293 Pyloric stenosis. In 10 to 20 per cent of cases the tumour is impalpable. Barium meal reveals an elongated narrow pyloric canal which extends convex upwards to the duodenal cap. Gastric hyperperistalsis and delayed evacuation are also present.

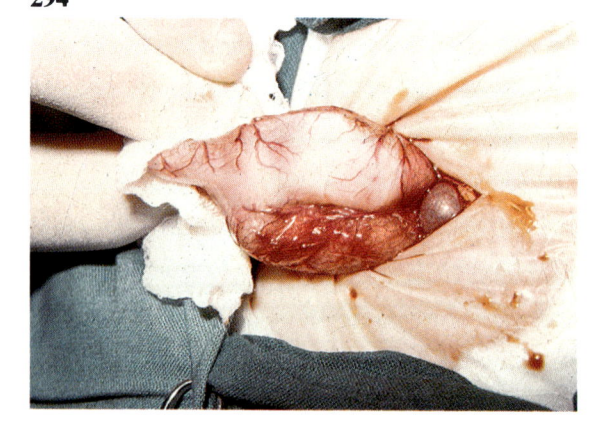

294 Pyloric stenosis. Treatment is by pyloromyotomy. The 'tumour' as seen at operation is about 2 cm long, glistening white in appearance and firm to palpation. The muscular hypertrophy is confined to the pyloric antrum. The incision for the pyloromyotomy is made in the avascular anterior wall of the pylorus.

295 Acute gastric erosions. Usually multiple and associated with stress, e.g. uraemia, burns, septicaemia. Widely and irregularly distributed throughout the stomach, they vary in size from pinpoint to large ulcers. Specimen shows multiple shallow ulcers scattered throughout the stomach.

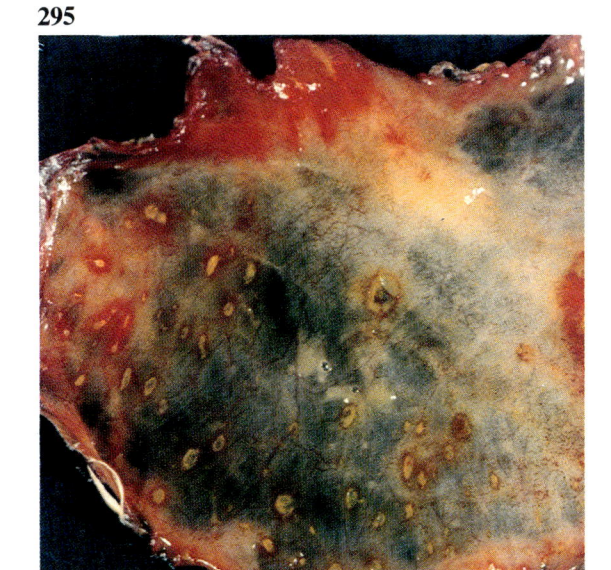

296 Acute gastric ulcer. The entire wall of the stomach is erythematous and a number of deep necrotic ulcers are evident in the antrum and body. Full-thickness penetration of the ulcer on the greater curvature has occurred.

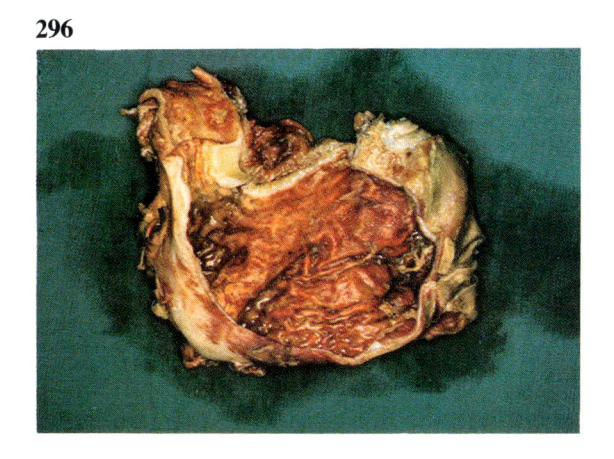

297 Gastric ulcer. Endoscopy photograph shows a superficial lesser curve gastric ulcer. The base of the ulcer appears whitish in contrast to the normal gastric mucosa. The aperture of the pylorus can be seen in the distal part of the stomach.

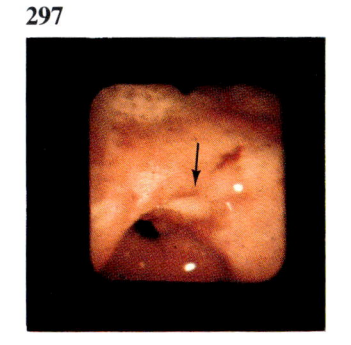

298 Trichobezoar. Space-occupying lesion within the lumen of the stomach composed chiefly of swallowed hair which compacts to form a cast of the stomach and extends by means of a 'tail' into the duodenum and occasionally into the jejunum. A firm non-tender mobile mass is found on abdominal examination. Xray shows the intragastric mass coated with a small amount of barium.

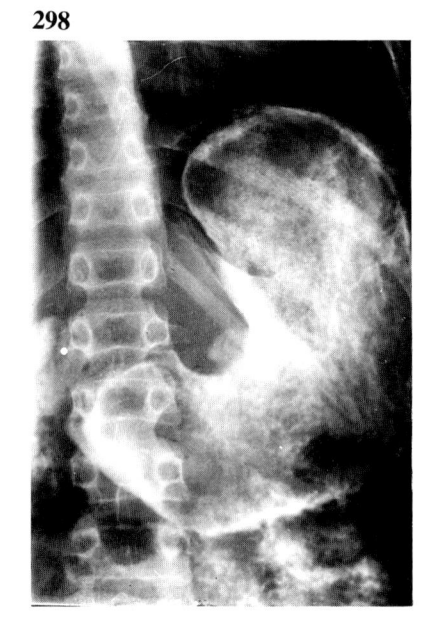

299 Trichobezoar. Excised specimen showing the 'hairy' nature of the mass which is moulded into a cast of the stomach. Note the projecting 'tail' which extended through the duodenum into the proximal small bowel.

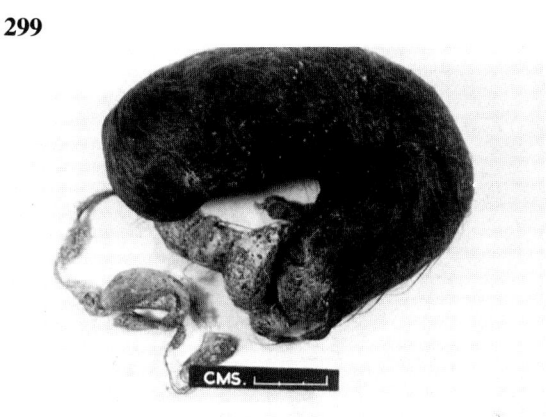

300 Gastric foreign body. Over 90 per cent of swallowed foreign objects which enter the stomach will pass uninterrupted through the gastrointestinal tract. Indications for operative removal included prolonged hold-up (greater than two to three weeks) at one area in the gastrointestinal tract or the presence of a long slender object (e.g. hair grip) in the stomach of a child younger than two years old.

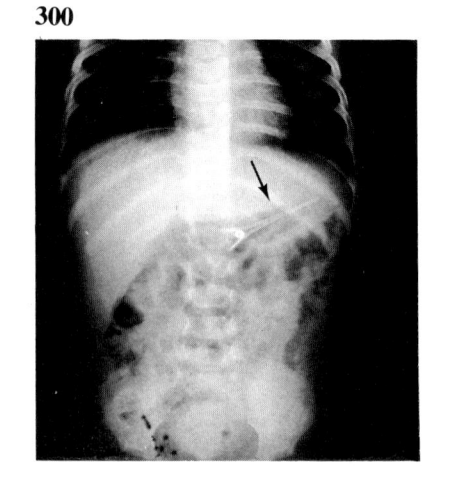

27 The duodenum

301 Bile-stained vomit. Green vomit in an infant indicates mechanical intestinal obstruction until an alternative diagnosis has been established. A diagnostic approach to the infant with bile-stained vomiting is shown in the diagram below.

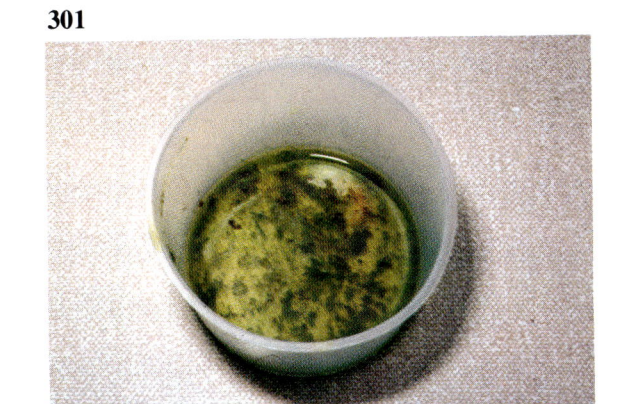

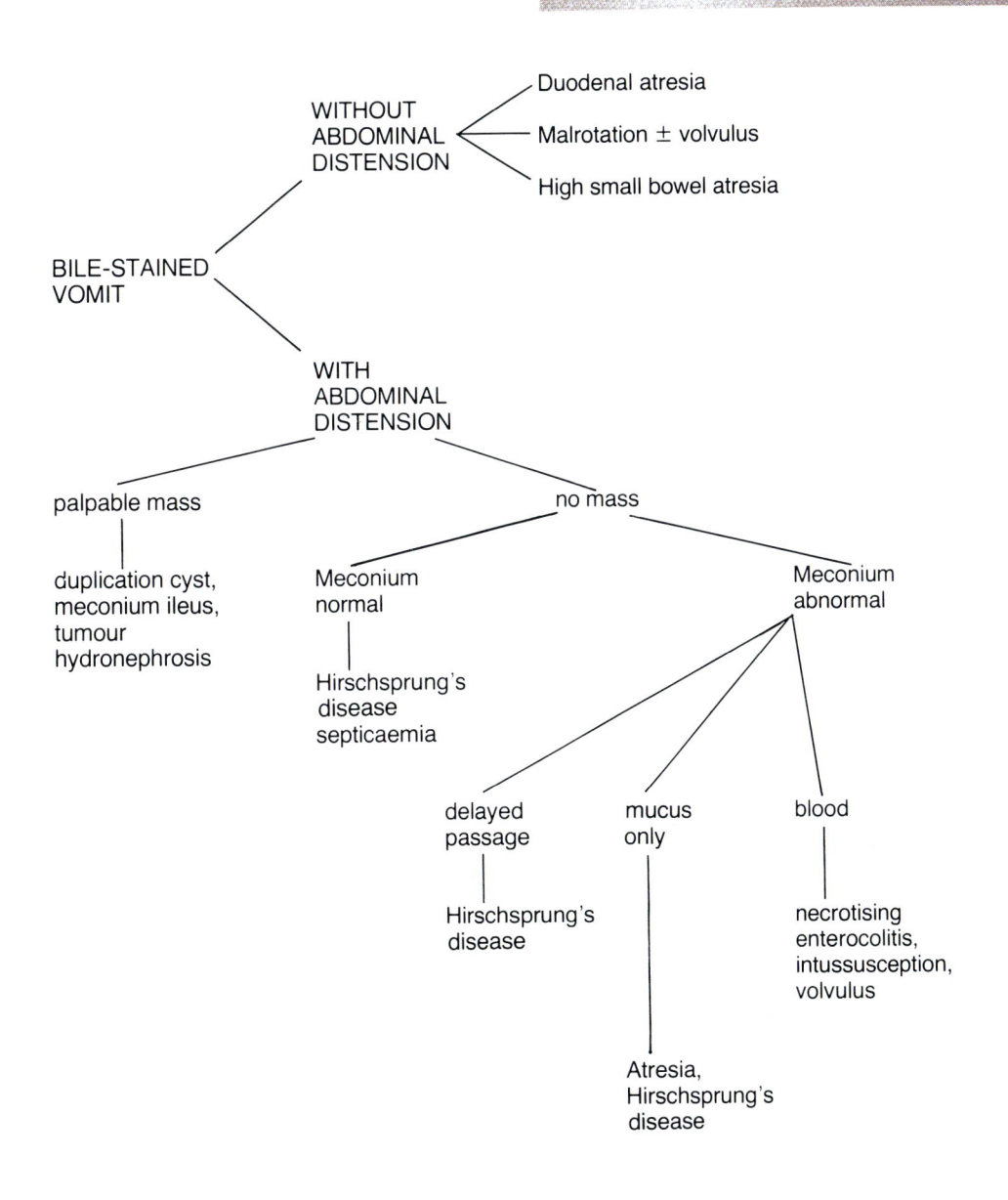

```
                              ┌─ Duodenal atresia
              WITHOUT         │
              ABDOMINAL ──────┼─ Malrotation ± volvulus
              DISTENSION      │
                              └─ High small bowel atresia
BILE-STAINED
VOMIT
              WITH
              ABDOMINAL
              DISTENSION

  palpable mass              no mass

  duplication cyst,     Meconium            Meconium
  meconium ileus,       normal              abnormal
  tumour                   │
  hydronephrosis        Hirschsprung's
                        disease
                        septicaemia

                    delayed        mucus         blood
                    passage        only            │
                       │             │         necrotising
                  Hirschsprung's     │         enterocolitis,
                  disease            │         intussusception,
                                     │         volvulus
                                  Atresia,
                                  Hirschsprung's
                                  disease
```

93

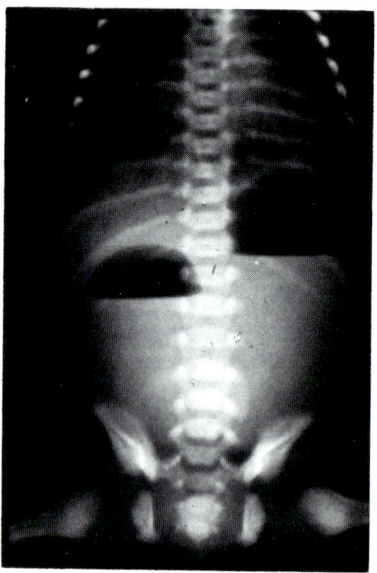

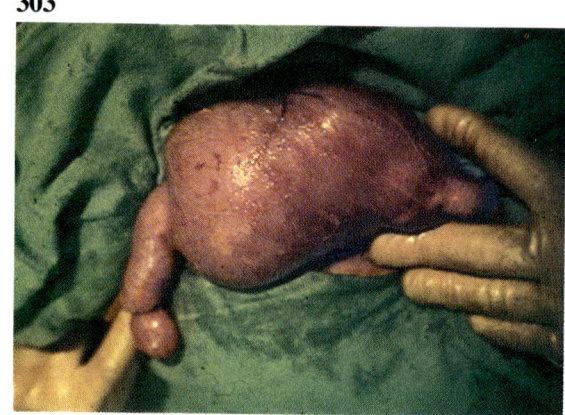

302 Duodenal atresia. In two-thirds of the cases the obstruction is in the second part of the duodenum. The infant presents with bile-stained vomiting with slight upper abdominal distension. Straight erect abdominal xray reveals the classical 'double-bubble' appearance of dilated air-fluid levels in the stomach and duodenum in an otherwise radio-opaque abdomen.

303 Duodenal atresia. The obstruction is in the second part of the duodenum. The proximal duodenum is grossly dilated and hypertrophied. The distal duodenum is narrow and collapsed. High association with Down's syndrome. Treatment is by duodenoduodenostomy.

304 Duodenal diaphragm. The infant presents with bile-tinged vomit, and an abdominal xray reveals a 'double-bubble' but frequently with associated distal intestinal gas shadows. The operative view shows the 'wind sock' diaphragm with a centrally placed aperture in the second part of the duodenum.

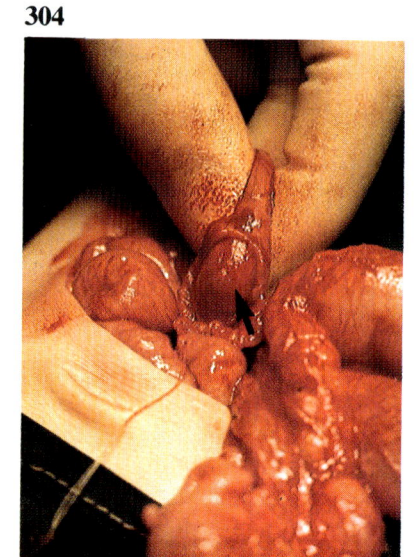

305 Annular pancreas. Almost always associated with an underlying duodenal obstruction anomaly and presents with similar symptoms. The operative photograph shows pancreatic tissue overlying the anterior surface of the second part of the duodenum. Treatment is by duodenoduodenostomy bypassing the area of obstruction.

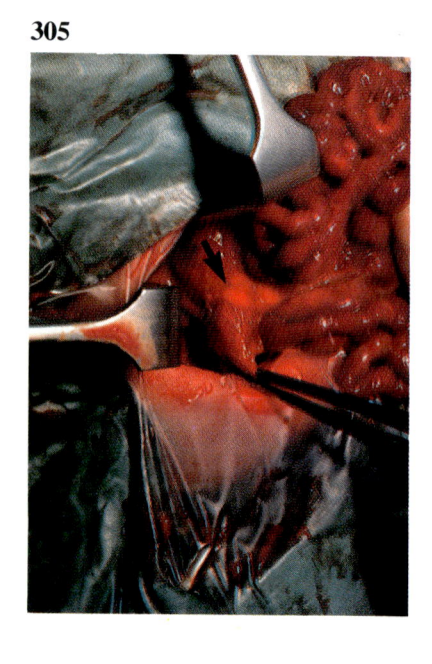

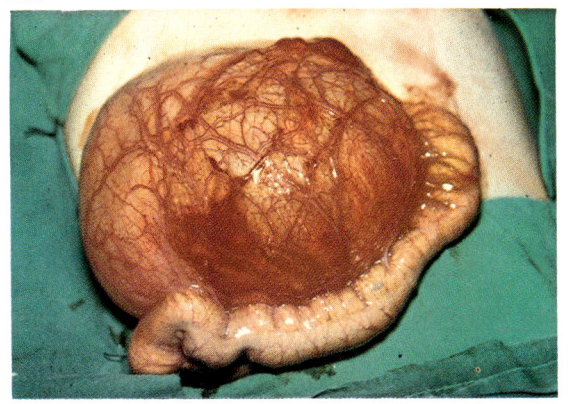

306 Duodenal duplication. The cyst lies in the concavity of the C-loop of the duodenum and produces obstructive symptoms. A mass may be palpable in the epigastric region. The cyst does not communicate with the lumen of the duodenum. Treatment is by cystoduodenostomy because excision is hazardous.

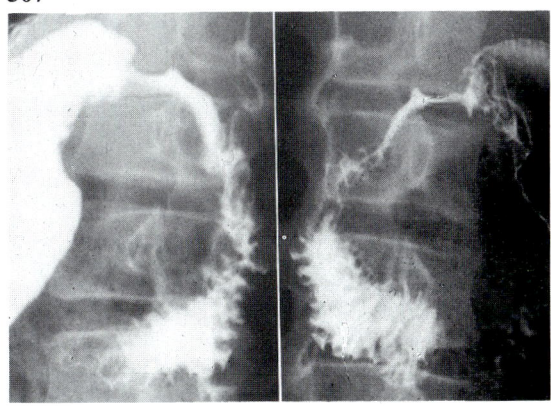

307 Duodenal duplication cyst. Barium meal examination showing a space-occupying lesion in the concavity of the duodenum loop. The duodenal loop is stretched out and widened by the cyst.

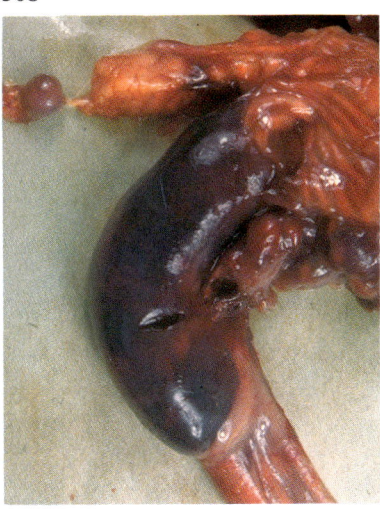

308 Duodenal haematoma. Occasionally develops after blunt abdominal trauma (usually associated with trauma to the pancreas and/or right kidney). Isolated duodenal haematoma presents with bilious vomiting. If other injuries can be excluded conservative treatment is usually successful and the haematoma resolves in 7–10 days.

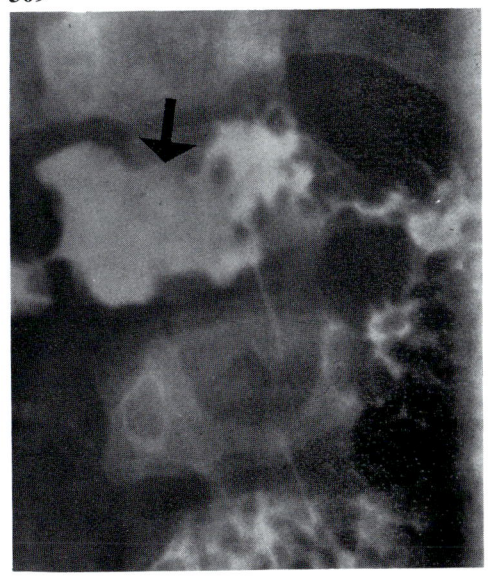

309 Peptic ulceration. Relatively uncommon in childhood. In infancy presents with acute complications, e.g. haemorrhage or perforation. In young children vague abdominal pain and recurrent vomiting may occur. Classical symptom, i.e. postprandial epigastric pain relieved by food and awakening the child at night is confined to the older age-group. Barium meal shows ulcer in the superior fornix of the first part of the duodenum. Note the surrounding 'halo' indicating mucosal oedema.

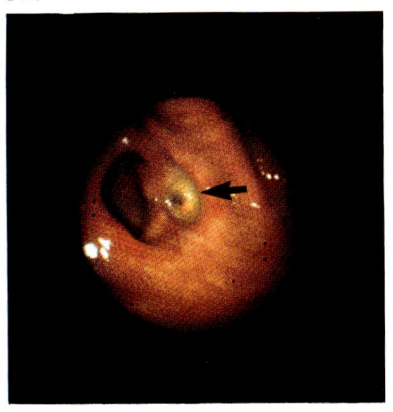

310 Peptic ulceration. Endoscopic photograph of a chronic duodenal ulcer complicated by haematemesis and melena. The exposed vessel in the base of the ulcer is clearly visible.

28 The small intestine

Atresia

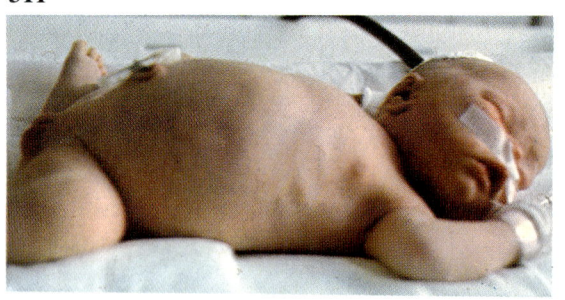

311 Intestinal obstruction. Typical presentation of low small intestinal obstruction in a newborn infant with abdominal distension, bile-stained vomiting and failure to pass meconium. Small amounts of mucus may be passed per rectum and occasionally the mucus is frankly meconium stained even in the presence of a complete atresia.

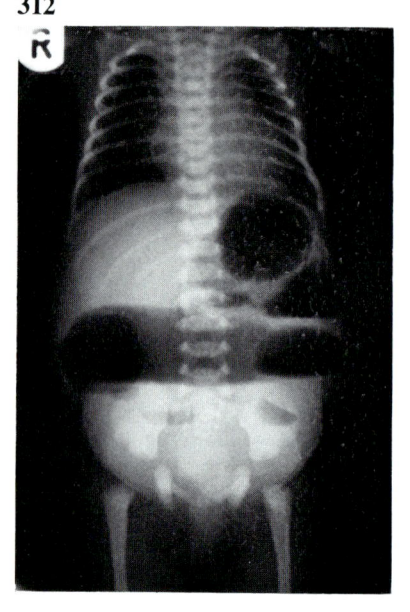

312 Jejunal atresia. Straight erect abdominal xray showing dilated upper intestinal loops with air-fluid levels. The rest of the abdomen is opaque. The appearance is characteristic of a high small bowel obstruction.

313 Intestinal atresia. The various types of atresia are diagrammatically demonstrated:

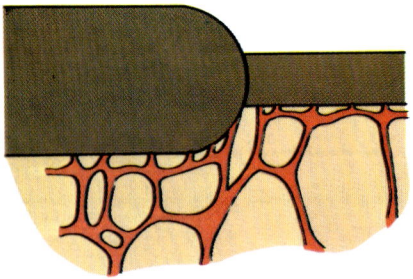

Type I: the proximal and distal ends are contiguous

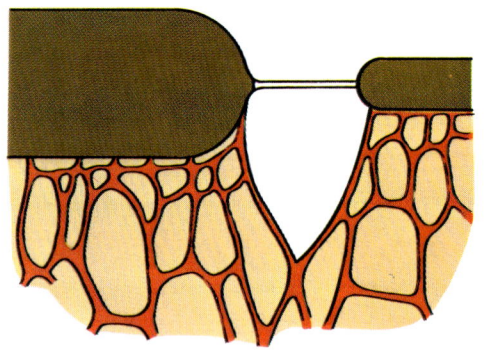

Type II: the proximal bowel is connected to the distal bowel by a fibrous strand

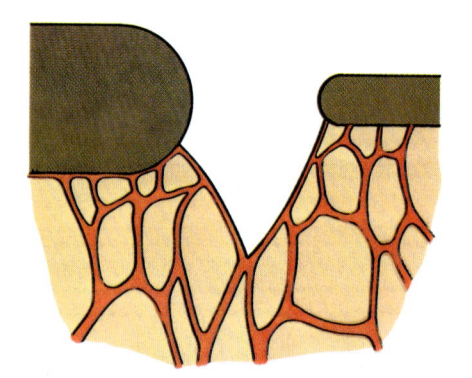

Type III: there is discontinuity between the two ends with an associated gap in the mesentery

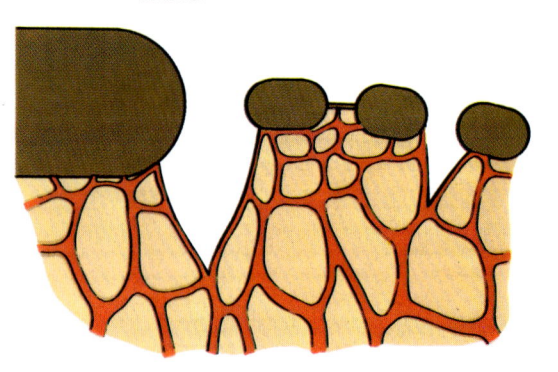

Type IV: multiple intestinal atresias

314 Type I – atresia. Surgically resected specimen showing the dilated hypertrophied proximal small bowel in continuity with the collapsed 'unused' distal intestine.

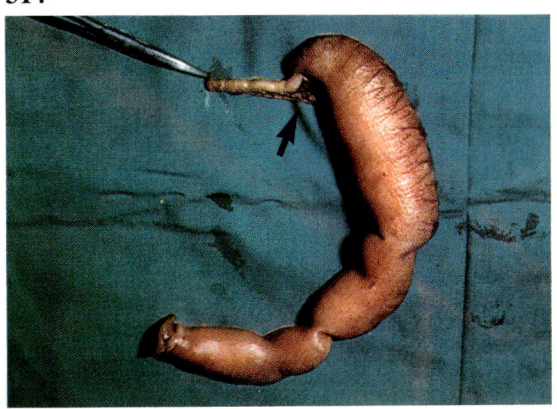

315 Type II – atresia. Operative view showing the dilated proximal jejunum connected to the distal collapsed small bowel by a thin fibrous strand. There is no gap in the mesentery.

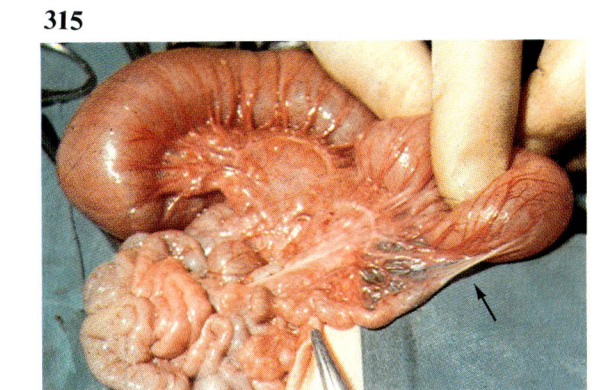

316 Type III – atresia. The proximally dilated intestine is completely separated from the distal bowel and there is a gap in the mesentery at the site of the atresia.

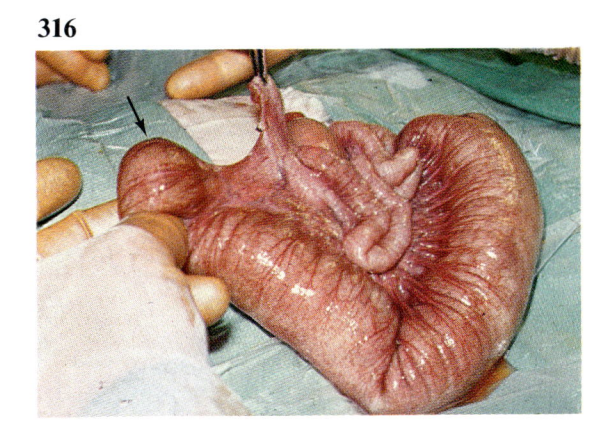

317 Multiple atresia. There are a number of short segments of surviving bowel connected by fibrous bands. If only a short length of intestine is affected the segments should be resected en-bloc and an end-to-end anastomosis performed.

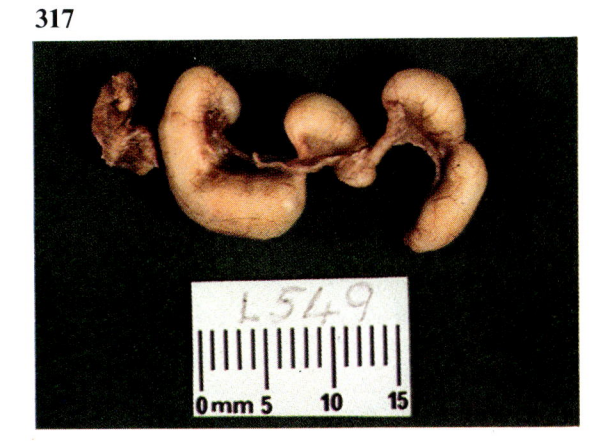

318 'Christmas-tree' deformity ('apple-peel syndrome'). The combination of anomalies includes a high jejunal atresia with enormous distension of the proximal loop and a distal intestine which is arranged in a spiral around the nutrient blood vessels. The blood supply to the distal intestine is derived from the middle colic artery in a retrograde manner. The main trunks of the superior mesenteric vessels are obliterated and the mesentery is totally deficient.

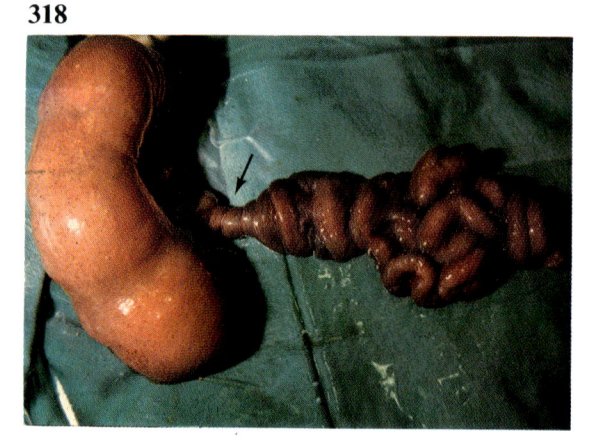

319 Intestinal atresia. Sagittal section through the atresia showing the fibrous connection between the two ends. Within the lumen of the distal bowel is a remnant of bowel representing an intrauterine intussusception.

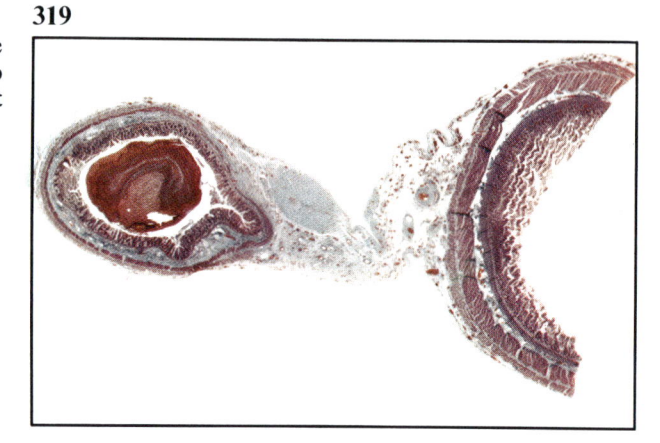

Malrotation

Between the fourth and tenth weeks of intrauterine life growth of the developing intestine proceeds at a rate more rapid than that of the enveloping coelomic cavity. The intestine (particularly the midgut) is forced into a physiological hernia within the umbilical cord. From the tenth week the intestine begins to return to the peritoneal cavity. The small intestine returns first and lies mainly on the left side of the abdomen. The caecocolic loop returns last and initially re-enters the abdomen in the left lower quadrant, but rapidly rotates through 270° to assume its final position in the right iliac fossa by the twelfth week.

320 Malrotation. Rotation of the caecocolic loop has arrested at 180° and the caecum has come to lie in the right hypochondrium in front of and adjacent to the duodenum. Note the narrow base of the mesentery of the entire midgut. Bands (Ladds) from the caecocolic loop cross and compress the second part of the duodenum causing intermittent obstruction.

321 Midgut volvulus. This is the most dreaded complication of a malrotation. The narrow-based mesentery and malfixation predisposes towards the volvulus which interferes with the blood supply to the midgut. Only urgent surgery at an early stage will prevent gangrene of a large section of the involved intestine.

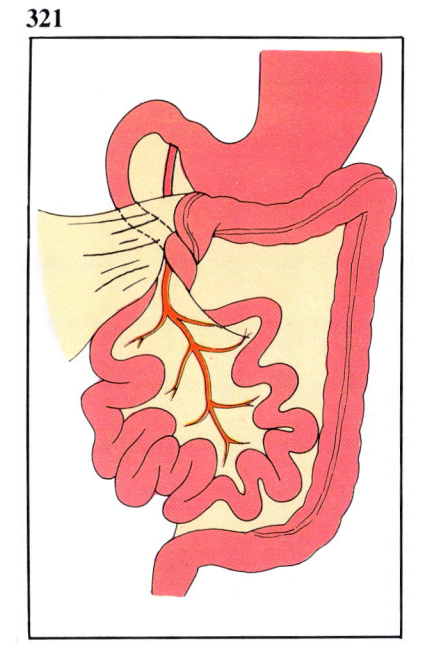

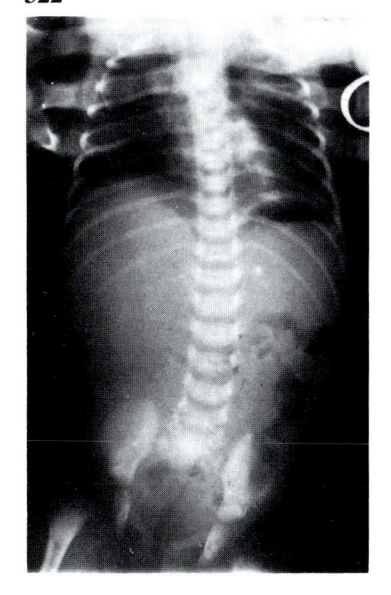

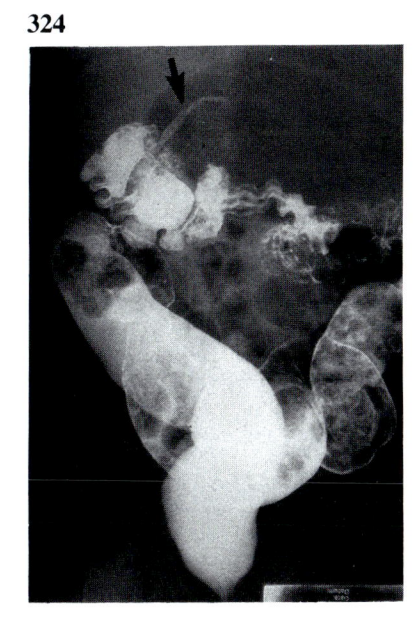

322 Malrotation. The infant with an uncomplicated malrotation presents with intermittent bile-stained vomiting as the only significant symptom. As volvulus occurs, the infant becomes shocked and hypothermic and passes blood per rectum or has a haematemesis. Straight xray of the abdomen reveals a paucity of gas shadows in the intestine beyond the duodenum. This relatively 'gasless' abdomen is an important sign and warrants further investigation.

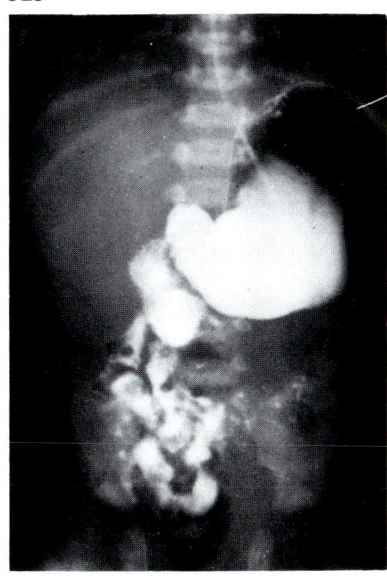

323 Malrotation. Barium meal and follow through examination showing a dilated stomach and proximal duodenum. The duodenum empties caudally into the small intestine which is predominantly located on the right side of the abdomen. There is incomplete rotation of the duodenum which has failed to develop the normal C-configuration.

324 Malrotation. Barium enema examination showing the caecum and appendix lying in the right upper quadrant under the right lobe of the liver.

325 Malrotation with volvulus. Volvulus of the midgut loop but without intestinal gangrene has taken place. The loop has twisted four times around the axis of the narrow-based mesentery.

326 Malrotation and volvulus. Necropsy appearance of midgut volvulus and total midgut gangrene. Note the twist of the intestine at the base of the mesentery.

Duplications

Duplications of the alimentary tract may be cystic or tubular and can be found at any site from the tongue to the anus. There are three cardinal characteristics of a duplication:
  i) they are firmly attached to a particular part of the gastrointestinal tract;
  ii) they possess a well-developed smooth muscle layer;
  iii) the epithelial lining is representative of some part of the alimentary tract.

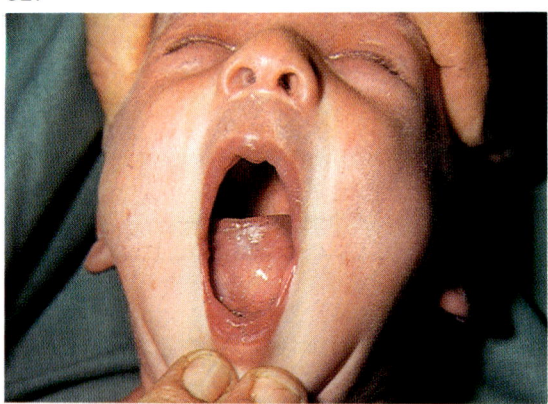

327 Duplication cyst of the tongue. There is a large cyst in the floor of the mouth displacing the tongue posteriorly. Obstruction to the airway is a potential risk in such cases.

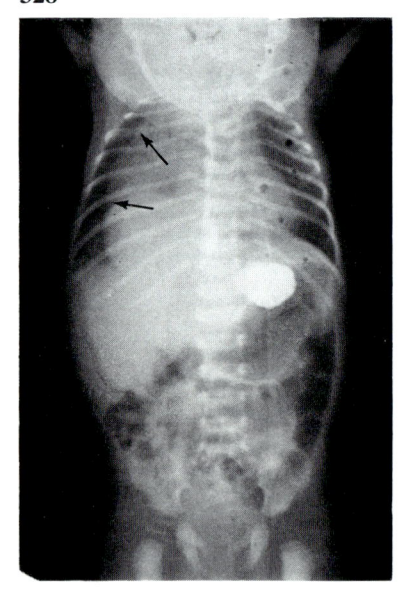

328 Oesophageal duplication cyst. Xray of the chest of a newborn infant presenting with respiratory distress. A radio-opaque mass is visible in the right hemithorax. The presence of vertebral anomalies is very suggestive of a duplication. Lateral view will show the mass in the posterior mediastinum.

329 Oesophageal duplication cyst. Necropsy appearance of a large right-sided posterior mediastinal cyst loosely attached to the oesophagus. Commonly associated with an intra-abdominal duplication by means of a stalk traversing through the diaphragm.

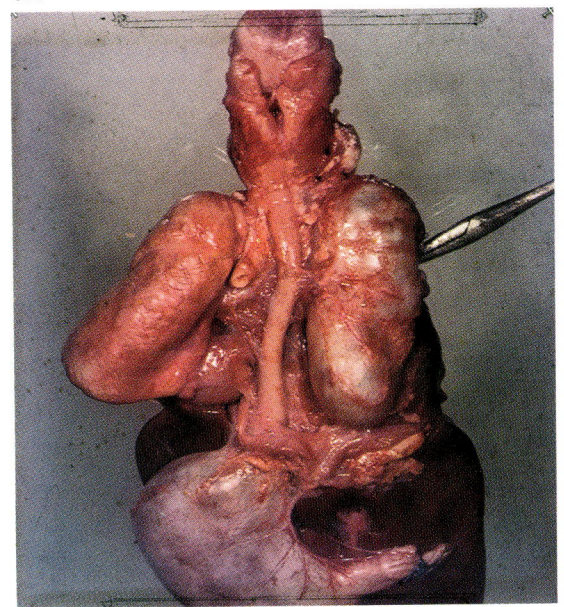

330 Gastric duplication. The operative specimen consists of four cysts connected by a tubular structure. It was situated along the greater curvature of the stomach. The most distally located cyst protruded into the antrum of the stomach causing intermittent gastric outlet obstruction.

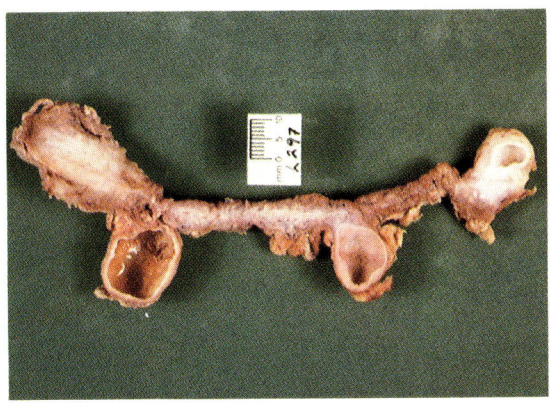

331 Intestinal duplication cyst. Clinical presentation includes the features of an intestinal obstruction in association with a palpable freely mobile cystic mass.

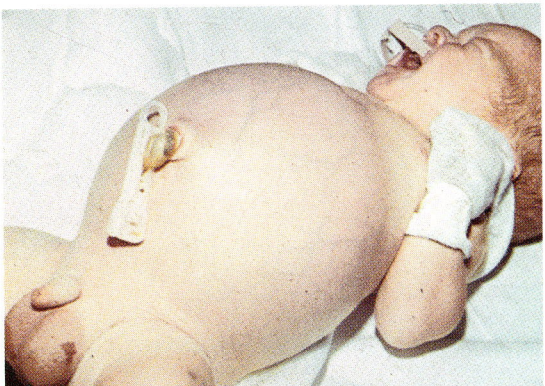

332 Intestinal duplication cyst. Plain xray of the abdomen reveals a centrally located abdominal mass displacing bowel laterally into the flanks.

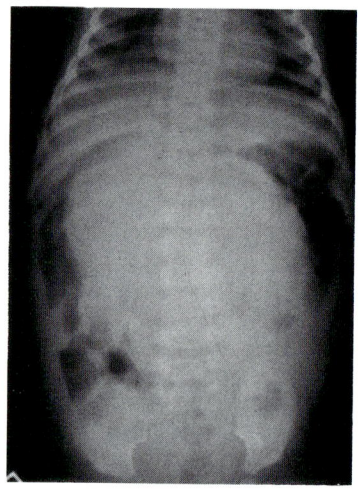

333 Duplication cyst of the jejunum. The large tense cyst is intimately attached to the adjacent jejunum, which is stretched out and compressed by the progressively enlarging cyst. No communication exists between the cyst and the adjacent jejunum.

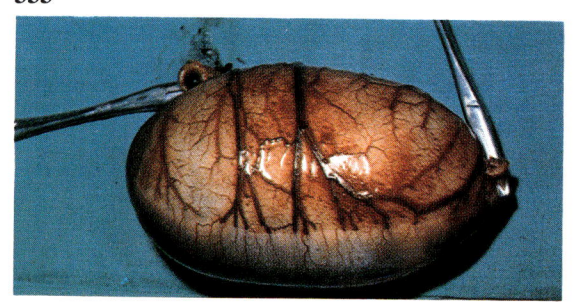

334 Ileal duplication cyst. The cross-section shows the glistening interior surface of the cyst, which is projecting into and impinging upon the lumen of the adjacent ileum. The cyst may appear at the apex of an intussusception.

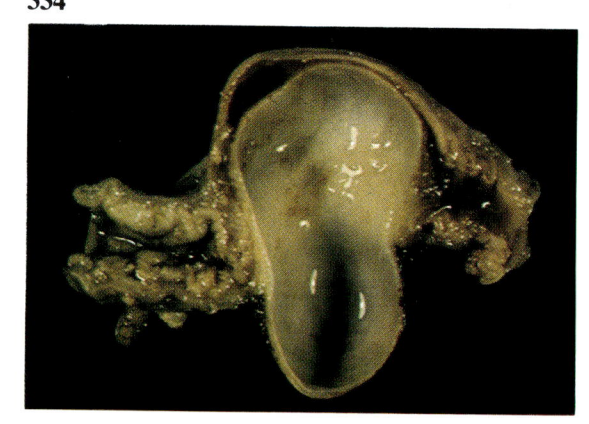

335 Tubular duplication of the ileum. There is a long section involved with the tubular duplication. Note the close proximity of the walls of the duplication and the adjacent ileum. These duplications almost invariably communicate with the adjacent intestine and commonly contain ectopic gastric mucosa.

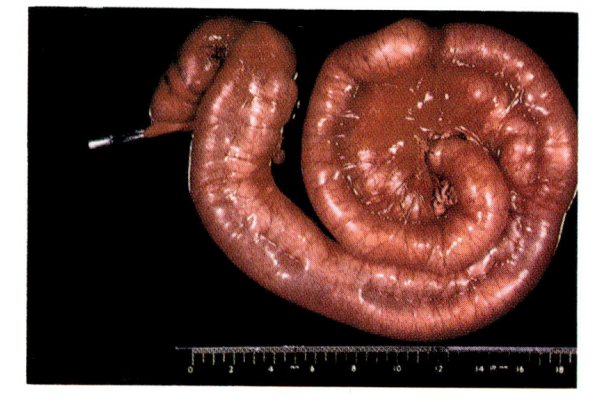

336 Tubular duplication of the colon. The long tubular duplication communicated with the descending colon proximally and was closely attached over a 12 cm length of the left colon. The duplication continued for approximately 20 cm, unattached to the adjacent bowel, to end in a bulbous partially necrotic tip.

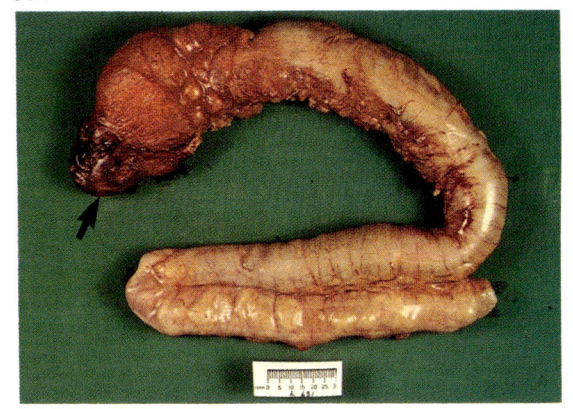

337 Tubular duplication of the colon. The resected specimen has been opened to show the intimate attachment to the adjacent colon and the bulbous end with evidence of a sealed perforation.

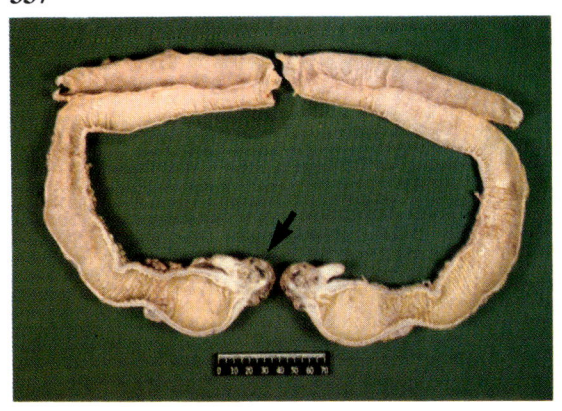

338 Duplication cyst of the transverse colon. The cyst has been opened to show the gastric mucosal lining. There is an active peptic ulcer, which caused profuse rectal haemorrhage, in the colonic mucosa adjacent to the communication with the cyst.

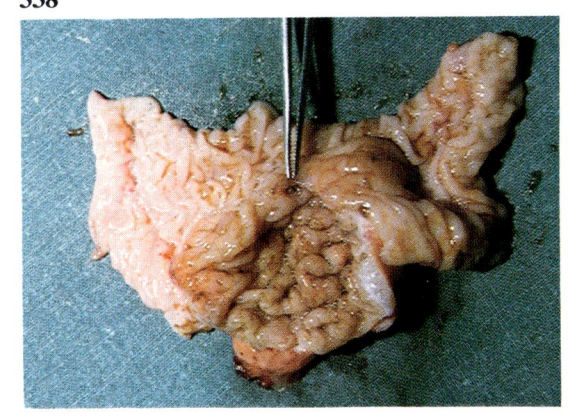

Meconium ileus

Mucoviscidosis is the commonest form of intraluminal intestinal obstruction in the neonatal period. The mucous glands all over the body are affected and they produce secretions which are abnormally viscid. This applies particularly to the bronchi and gastrointestinal tract and results in fibrocystic disease of the lung and intestinal obstruction respectively. The pancreatic involvement and the consequent lack of exocrine secretion leads the meconium in the small intestine to change from a semi-fluid consistency to a thick, tenacious and sticky mass which impacts and obstructs the lumen of the ileum. Volvulus, gangrene, perforation and atresias are possible complications.

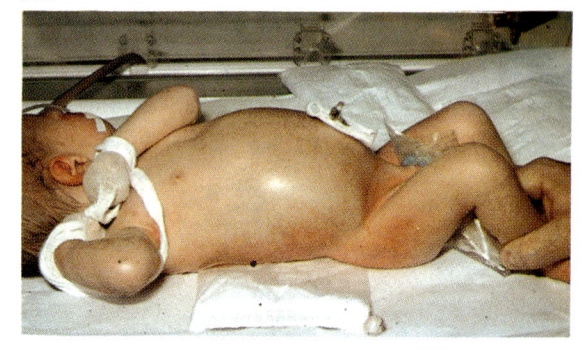

339 Meconium ileus. The clinical presentation is that of a low small intestinal obstruction with pronounced abdominal distension. Palpation reveals distended loops of intestine filled with a 'putty-like' material which indents on pressure.

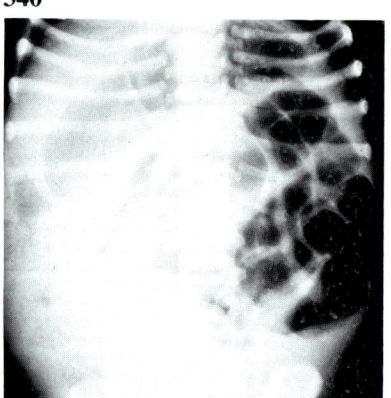

340 Meconium ileus. Abdominal xray shows dilated loops of bowel of varying calibre and usually without air-fluid levels (unless complicated by atresia or volvulus). There may be a coarse granular appearance in the right iliac fossa caused by the admixture of air and meconium within the lumen of the distended bowel.

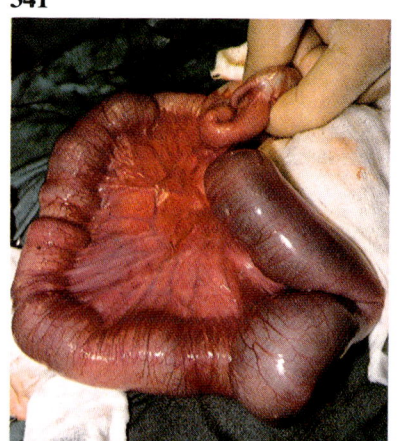

341 Meconium ileus. Operative view showing the tensely distended meconium-filled ileum terminating in a collapsed distal ileum and caecum.

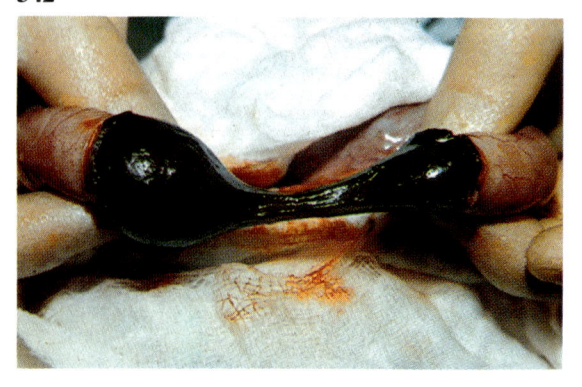

342 Meconium ileus. The intestine has been opened to reveal the thick, tenacious meconium adherent to the bowel wall. Infusion of gastrografin rapidly liquifies the meconium mass by a combination of the emulsifying properties of the material and the attraction of water into the intestinal lumen by the hyperosmolarity of the solution.

343 Meconium ileus. Rabbit-like greyish pellets of meconium evacuated from the distal ileum and colon in an infant with meconium ileus.

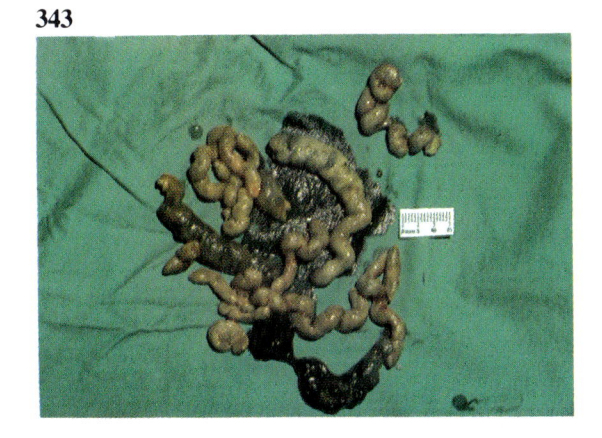

344 Mucoviscidosis. Photomicrograph ($H\&E \times 10$) of the bowel wall showing the distended submucous glands filled with mucoid material.

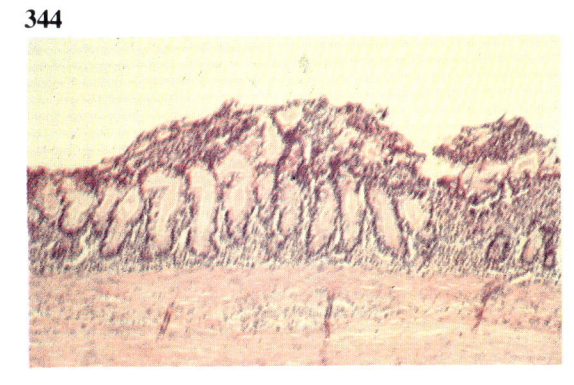

345 Meconium peritonitis. The perforation occurs in-utero and seals before birth. The escaped meconium tends to calcify. Should the perforation remain open, large amounts of swallowed air may enter the peritoneal cavity producing a tension pneumoperitoneum.

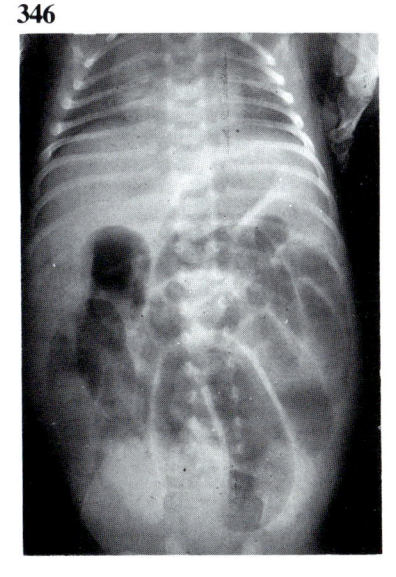

346 Milk inspissation. Confined to artificially fed infants. The baby who is previously perfectly well develops intestinal obstruction between the fourth and sixteenth days of life. Xray of the abdomen shows features similar to meconium ileus with dilated loops of bowel and an absence of air-fluid levels. Gastrografin enema may be therapeutic as well as diagnostic.

347 and 348 Milk inspissation. Operative view of the intraluminal obstruction in the distal ileum with distended proximal small bowel. On opening the bowel (**348**) the coarse granular impacted milk curds are visible.

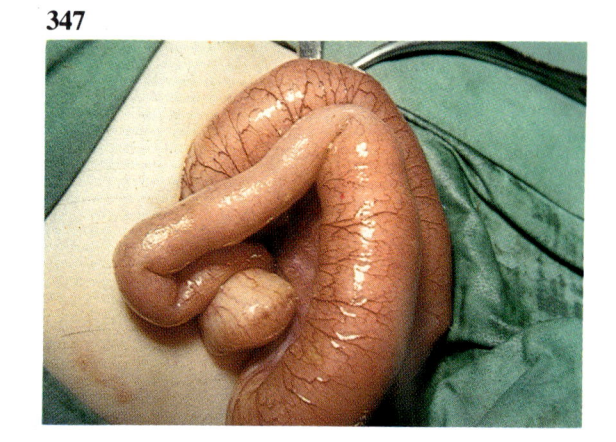

347

348

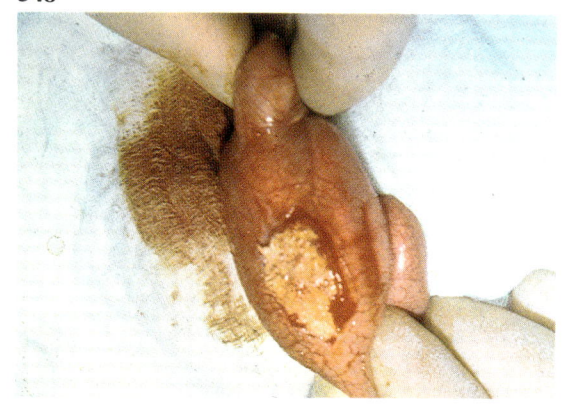

Omphalomesenteric duct
(See also **244**)

349 Omphaloileal fistula. May be simple or associated with prolapse through the umbilicus of adjacent ileum. Symptoms may be merely a leak of faecal material from umbilicus without any other intestinal problems.

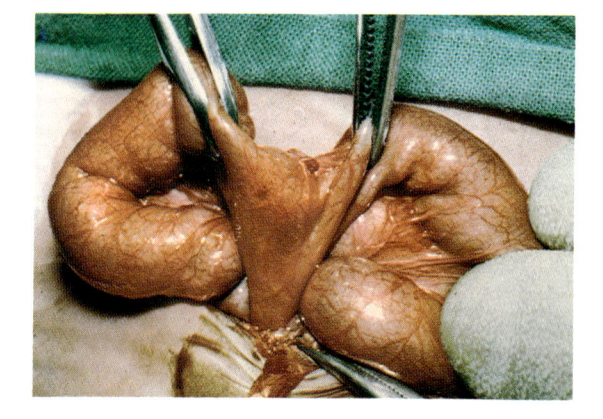

349

350 Omphaloileal fistula. Frequently a degree of intestinal obstruction is evident at the site of the fistulous connection to the ileum. The proximal bowel is dilated while the distal ileum is narrow and collapsed.

351 Meckel's diverticulum. May be an incidental finding at laparotomy, or associated with an anomaly at the umbilicus, or present with a complication, e.g. perforation, haemorrhage, infection, intussusception. Uncomplicated Meckel's lined with normal ileal mucosa and possessing a wide neck. This type of diverticulum is incidentally discovered at laparotomy and usually remains completely asymptomatic.

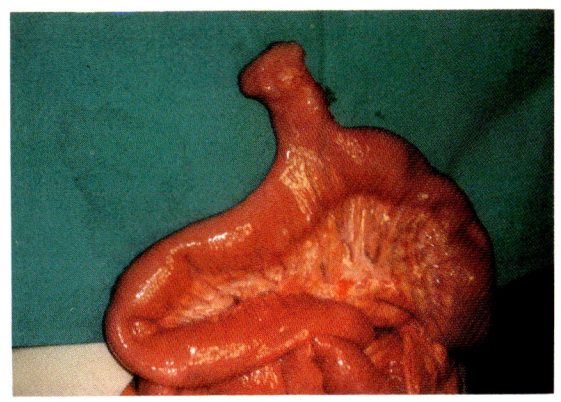

352 Meckel's diverticulum with peptic ulceration. The mucosal lining consists of gastric mucosa and the resultant peptic ulcer develops in the adjacent ileal mucosa at the neck of the diverticulum. Presents with rectal haemorrhage which may be profuse and life-threatening.

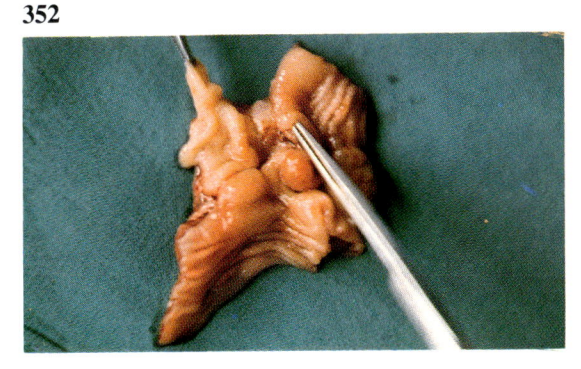

353 Technetium scan (Tc^{99}). The isotope is selectively taken up by gastric mucosa. The scan shows technetium activity in the stomach and bladder (caused by renal excretion), with further uptake in the right lower quadrant. The ectopic gastric mucosa could either be located in a Meckel's diverticulum or in an intestinal duplication.

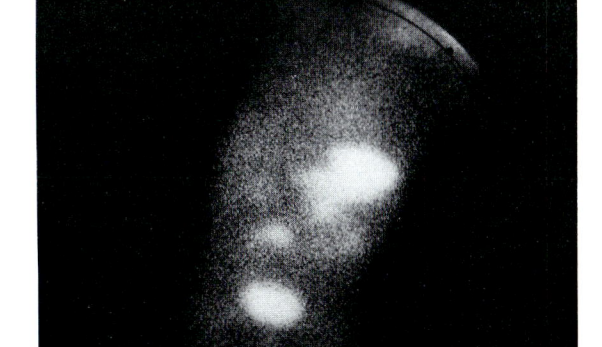

354 Meckel's diverticulitis. Symptomatology and physical findings closely resemble that of acute appendicitis. Laparotomy reveals a non-inflamed appendix but on further exploration an inflamed Meckel's diverticulum with adjacent ileitis may be discovered.

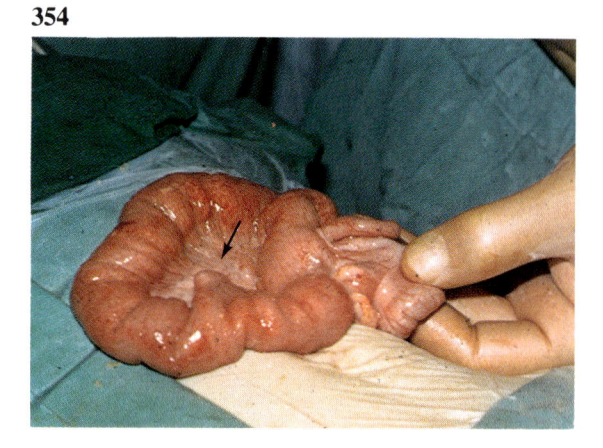

355 Intestinal obstruction. May arise secondary to intussusception, band obstruction or to volvulus. The commonest obstructing band extends from the apex of the diverticulum to the base of the mesentery on the posterior abdominal wall. Volvulus, with or without strangulation, can occur around the connection to the umbilicus. The plain erect abdominal xray shows numerous air-fluid levels in the small intestine.

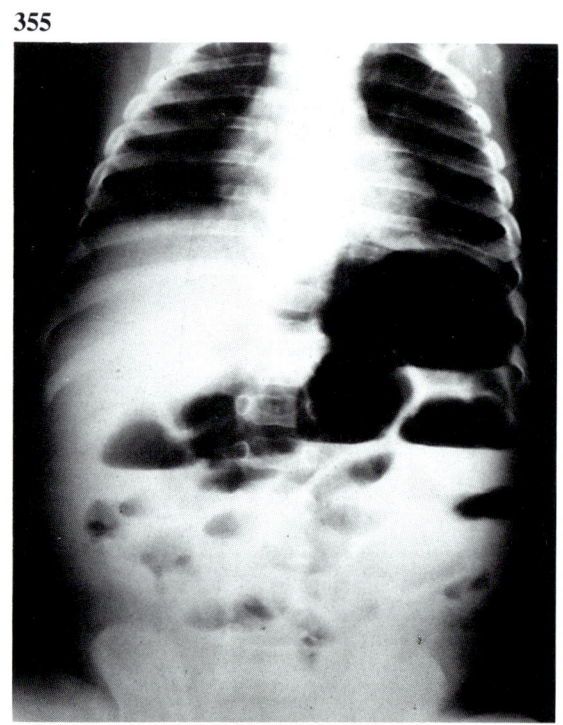

356 Gangrenous Meckel's diverticulum. The gangrene followed volvulus and resection of a large amount of adjacent intestine was necessary.

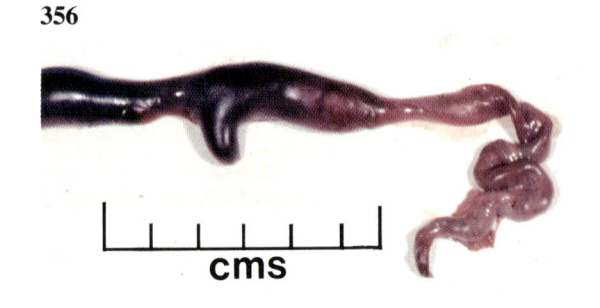

Intussusception

357 Intussusception. This results from the invagination of one part of the intestine (usually the ileocoecal region) into the adjacent distal bowel (caecum and colon). The invaginated bowel is termed the intussusceptum and the bowel into which the intussusception occurs is the intussuscipiens.

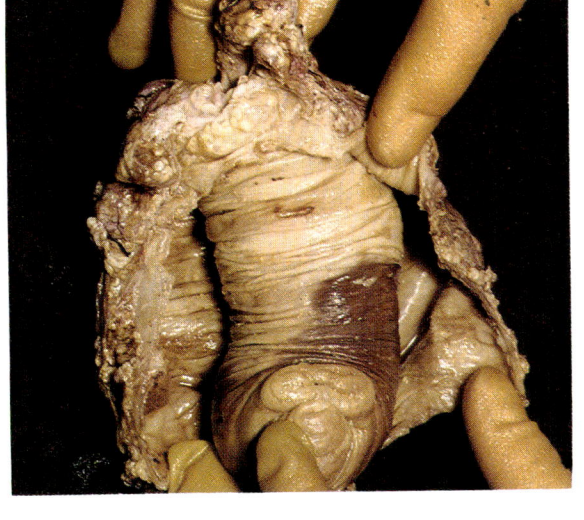

358 Intussusception – barium enema. The classical 'coiled-spring' appearance of contrast tracking around the invaginated bowel in the right transverse colon. The infant (3 to 12 months of age) presents with severe colicky abdominal pain, vomiting and/or the passage of blood per rectum. A 'sausage-shaped' abdominal mass may be palpable.

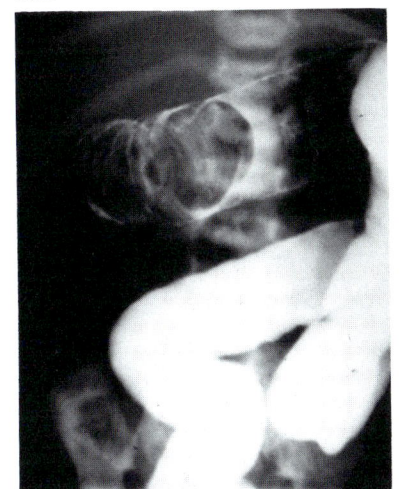

359 Intussusception. The xray of the abdomen on admission shows the typical features of a small bowel obstruction. This is an absolute contraindication for hydrostatic reduction. Other contraindications are a shocked critically ill patient or clinical evidence of peritonitis.

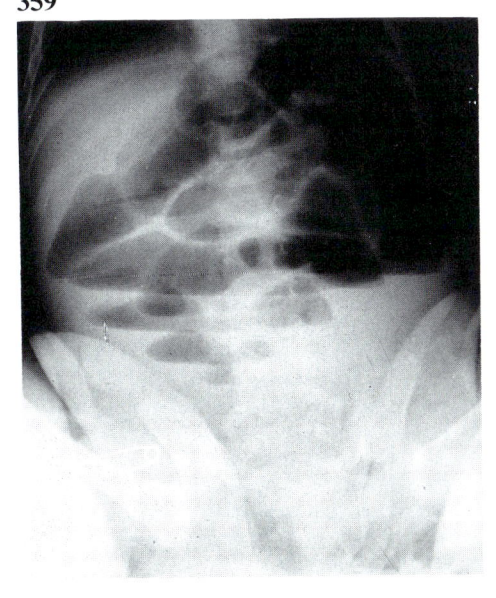

360 Intussusception. Treatment is either by hydrostatic reduction (barium enema) in the uncomplicated case or by manual reduction as shown. In the latter, the apex of the intussusception is gently squeezed or 'milked' out of the distal intestine.

361 Ileo ileal intussusception. Occurs most frequently after a recent major abdominal procedure e.g. resection of a tumour, anorectal 'pull-through' procedure etc. The patient experiences an abnormally prolonged post-operative ileus.

362 Gangrenous intussusception. Delayed treatment with prolonged compression of the vascular supply results in necrosis of the intussuscepted bowel. Treatment is by resection and immediate end-to-end anastomosis.

363 Intussusception. In five to ten per cent of childhood cases there is a primary cause for the intussusception (most of the remainder are idiopathic). The primary lesion may be a polyp, Meckel's diverticulum, duplication or tumour. The specimen shows a duplication cyst at the ileocaecal junction.

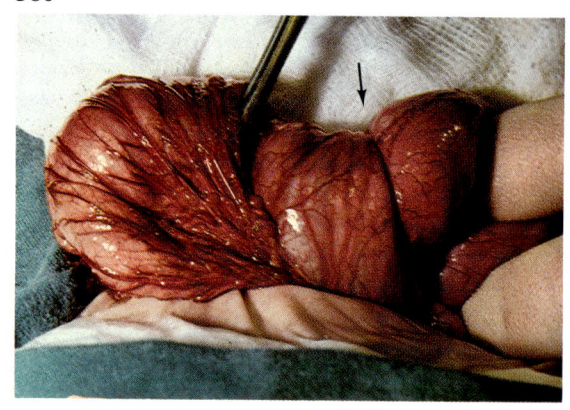

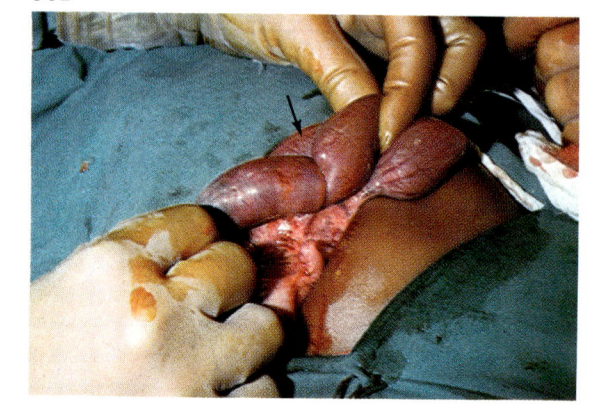

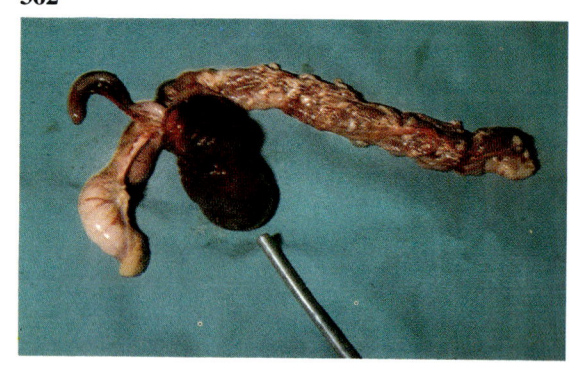

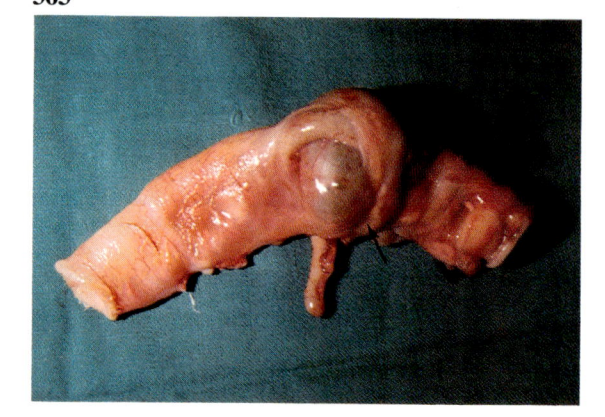

364 Intussusception. Severely congested and partially gangrenous intestine is seen prolapsing through the anus of a three-year-old girl. A Meckel's diverticulum was found at the apex of the intussusception.

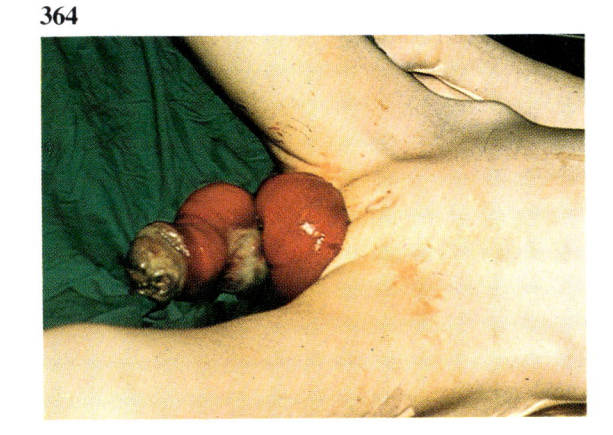

365 Henoch-Schonlein purpura. Acute vasculitis, manifesting with a diffuse purpuric rash and swelling of the ankles and knees. Commonly occurs after an upper respiratory tract infection. Clinical presentation may resemble acute appendicitis. Haemorrhage into the bowel wall may precipitate an intussusception.

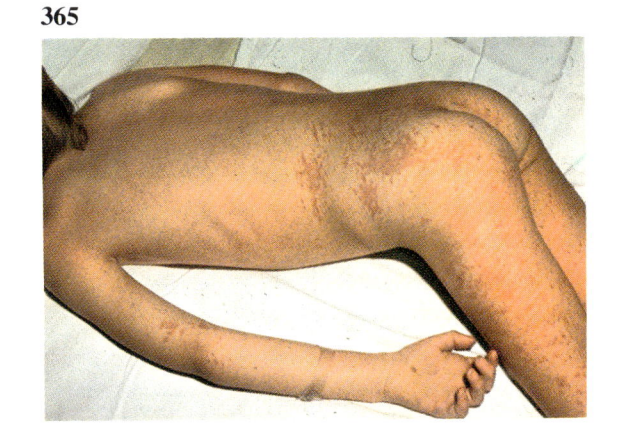

Small intestinal conditions

366 Acute ileitis. A long segment of terminal ileum is acutely inflamed. Usually accompanied by mesenteric lymphadenopathy. Yersinia infection has been implicated. Clinical presentation is indistinguishable from acute appendicitis.

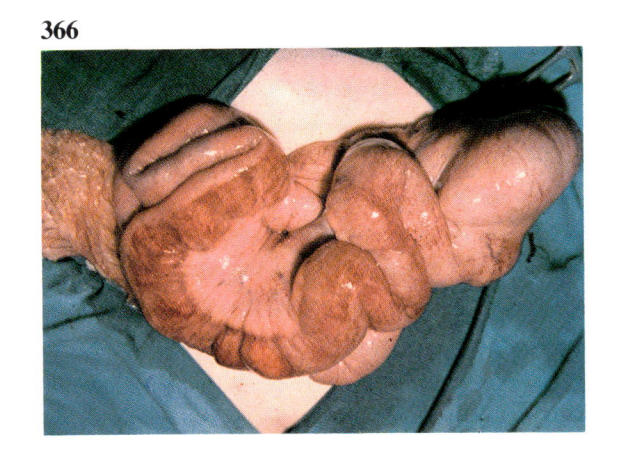

367 Tuberculous peritonitis. Ileocaecal tuberculosis presents with pain in the right iliac fossa, weight loss and pyrexia. Tender mobile mass may be palpable. The ulcerative form may progress to intestinal perforation with resulting fibrinous peritonitis. Diagnosis depends on the demonstration of acid-fast bacilli in the bowel lesions.

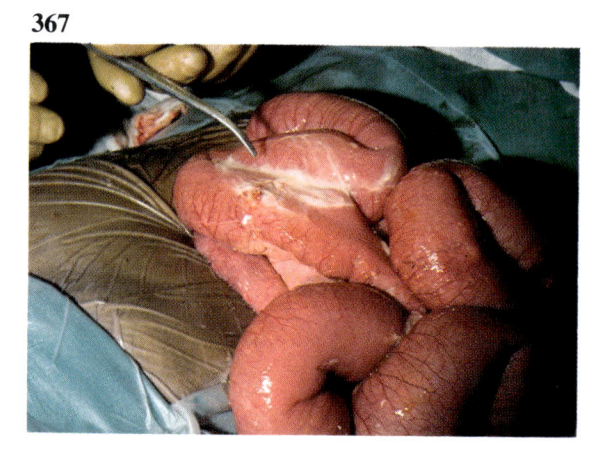

368 Tuberculous mesenteric adenitis. The lymph nodes in the ileocaecal region are enlarged and are liable to undergo caseous necrosis. Rupture may occur. Acute pulmonary infection may be evident. A tender mobile nodular mass is felt in the right iliac fossa. Acid-fast bacilli may be present in the stools.

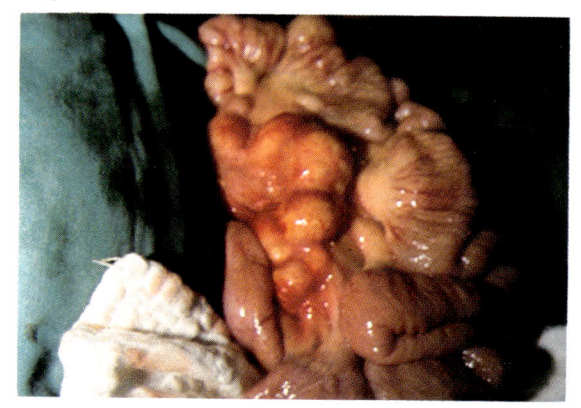

369 Perianal lesion of Crohn's disease. The lesions consist of deep fissures, superficial ulcers with undermined edges, fistulae and skin tags. May precede abdominal manifestations by months or years. Biopsy and histological examination may be helpful in establishing the diagnosis.

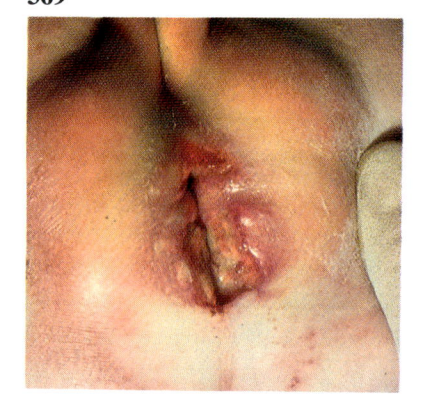

370 Crohn's stomatitis. There is dryness and scaling of the lips. Aphthous ulceration is rare in childhood. May progress to severe ulcerative stomatitis.

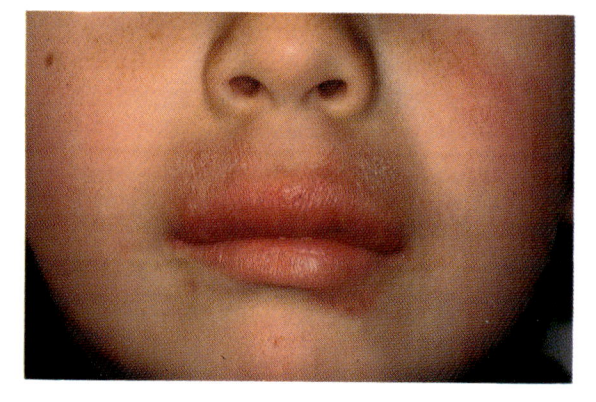

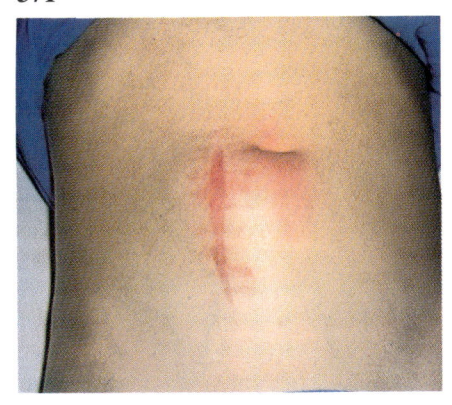

371 Incisional abscess (Crohn's). The wound abscess developed shortly after appendicectomy for mistaken diagnosis. Contrast radiography reveals local ileocaecal disease. Growth retardation and delayed puberty were also present. There was a dramatic response to surgical resection of the diseased intestine.

372 Multiple fistulae (Crohn's). Complete necrosis of the abdominal wall and multiple small intestinal fistulae in a 10-year-old girl who had undergone total procto-colectomy for advanced ileocolic Crohn's disease. There was a dramatic response to prolonged total parenteral nutrition.

373 Ileocolic Crohn's disease. The contrast study of distal small intestine shows extensive involvement with long segments of luminal stenosis. The involved loops are rigid and widely separated by oedema of the bowel wall. Note the intervening area of dilated bowel indicating 'skip lesions'.

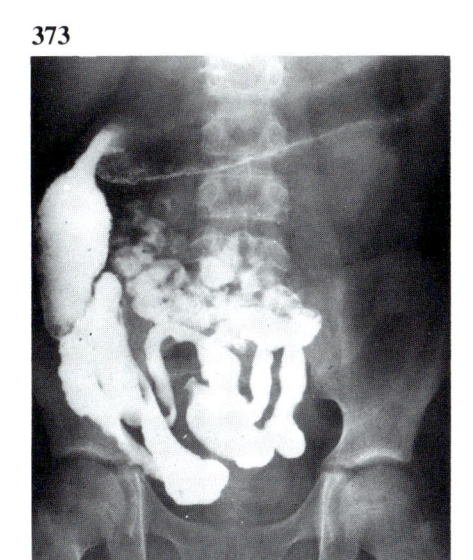

374 Crohn's colitis. Extensive involvement of the large bowel from the caecum to the sigmoid colon. There is loss of haustral pattern, shortening and thickening of the bowel wall. The rectum appears to be uninvolved.

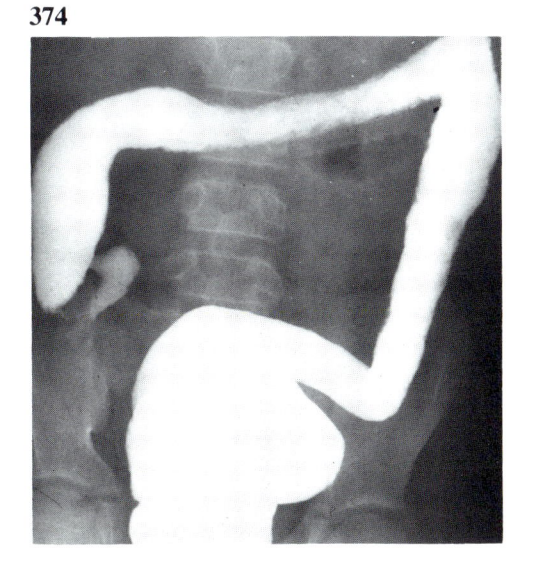

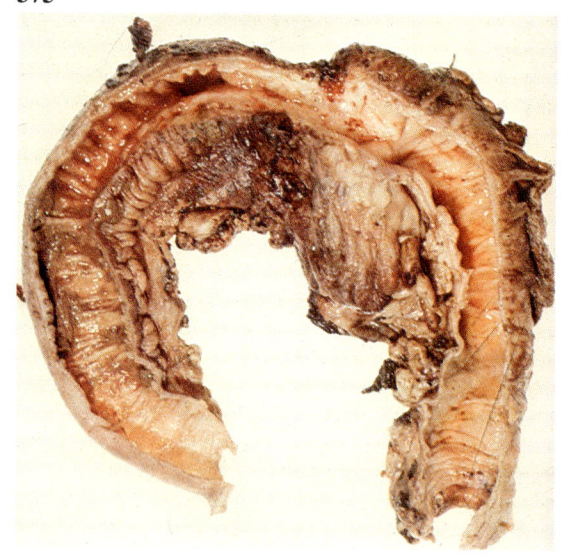

375 Crohn's disease. The resected specimen consists of a strictured area in the distal ileum. The bowel wall is enormously thickened by transmural involvement. The mesentery is thickened and oedematous.

376 Ascariasis (round worm). Prevalent in the tropics. The parasite normally lives in the lumen of the host's small intestine where it causes bouts of colicky abdominal pain. Bowel lumen may be occluded by a mass of writhing worms. Abdominal xray shows an incomplete small bowel obstruction. The large bolus of worms is visible in the right upper quadrant. Conservative management was successfully carried out.

377 Ascariasis with volvulus. The loop of intestine impacted with the conglomerate of worms is liable to undergo a volvulus with resultant necrosis from vascular insufficiency. Perforation may occur as in the case of the child shown in the operation photograph. Note the area of full-thickness necrosis and the exposed worms.

378 Ascariasis. Barium examination showing the intraluminal filling defect indicating the round worm. The worm itself has swallowed the barium which clearly outlines the length of the parasite.

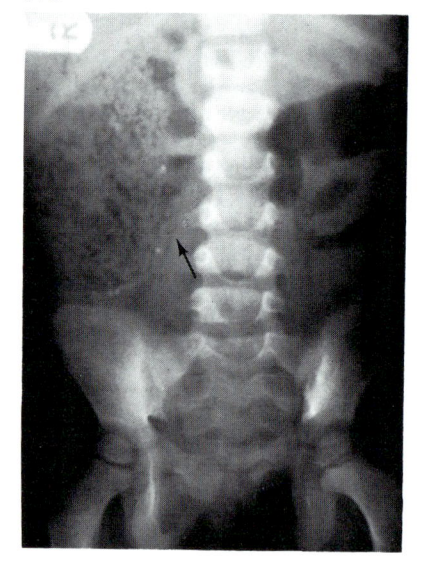

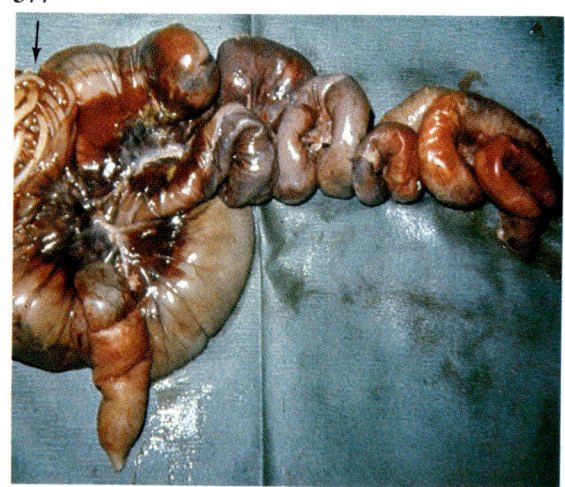

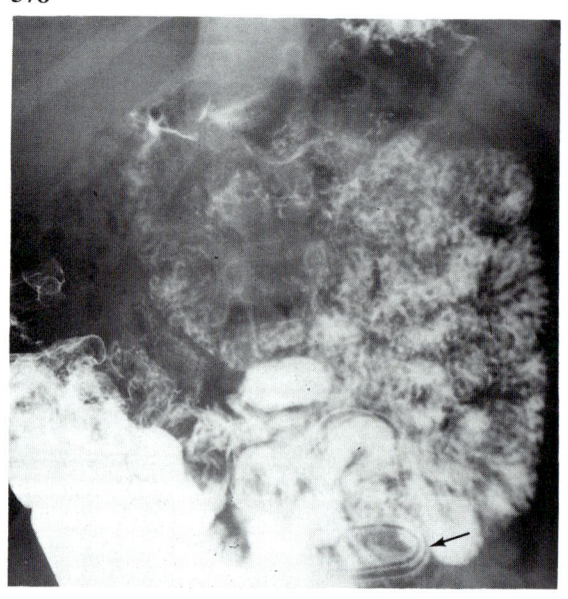

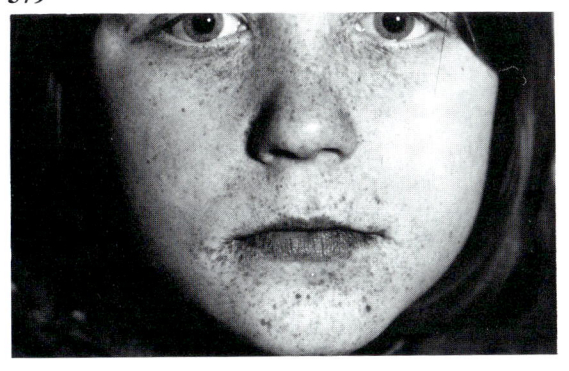

379 Peutz-Jeghers syndrome. Refers to the association of intestinal polyps with mucocutaneous pigmentation. Autosomal dominant inheritance. Areas of pigmentation affect the lips and buccal mucosa. Prominent freckles are seen over the nose and infraorbital areas.

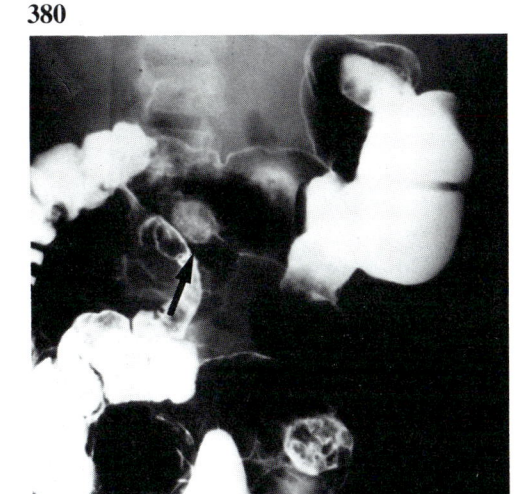

380 Peutz-Jeghers syndrome. The polyps are usually confined to the small intestine. Microscopically the polyps are hamartomata. Malignant degeneration is rare. The polyps may present with recurrent episodes of intussusception or gastrointestinal haemorrhage with hypochromic anaemia.

381 Ileocaecal lymphoma. Most common malignant tumour of the small intestine in childhood is the non-Hodgkins lymphoma. The patient presents with abdominal pain, vomiting and diarrhoea. A large abdominal mass is commonly present. May present with an intussusception or acute gastrointestinal bleeding. Is almost always only part of more generalised disease. Specimen shows ileocaecal tumour which was found at the apex of an intussusception.

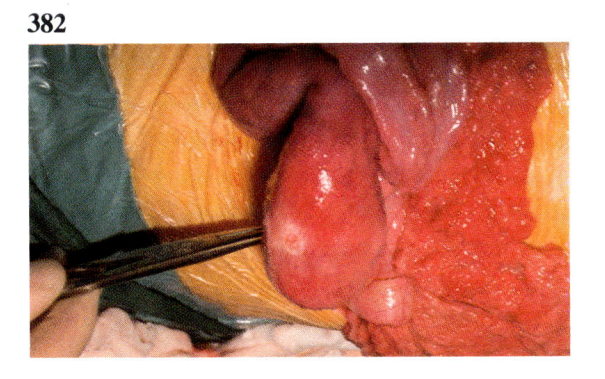

382 Ileocaecal lymphoma. May present with intestinal colic which progresses to subacute incomplete intestinal obstruction. An irregular nodular abdominal mass is palpable. The resected specimen shows the terminal ileum expanded and thickened with tumour infiltration. There were numerous nodular infiltrates in the omentum.

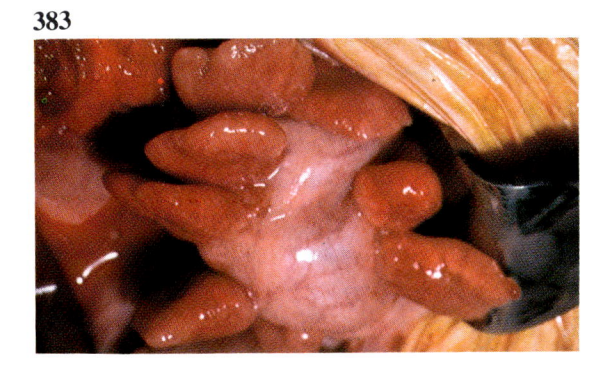

383 B-cell lymphoma (non-Hodgkins). Characteristic appearance of the taenia of the sigmoid colon in disseminated abdominal disease. The individual taenia are swollen, tumescent and erythematous. Histological examination reveals diffuse infiltration of the taenia with tumour cells.

29 The appendix

384 Acute suppurative appendicitis. Acute appendicitis is the most common condition requiring abdominal surgery in childhood. Classical history consists of vague central abdominal pain radiating to and localising in the right iliac fossa. Nausea and vomiting are invariably present. There is tenderness in the right iliac fossa with muscle 'guarding' or rigidity. The appendix lumen is filled with suppurative material but perforation of the wall has not occurred.

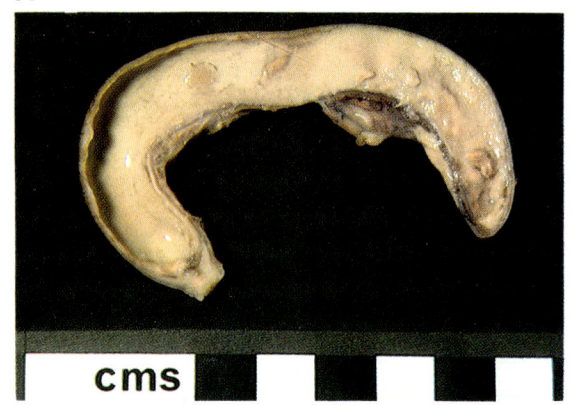

385 Gangrenous appendicitis. May occur with localised or generalised peritonitis. Local signs of peritonitis, i.e. muscular rigidity, indicate the advanced stage of the condition. Resuscitative measures are required before surgery.

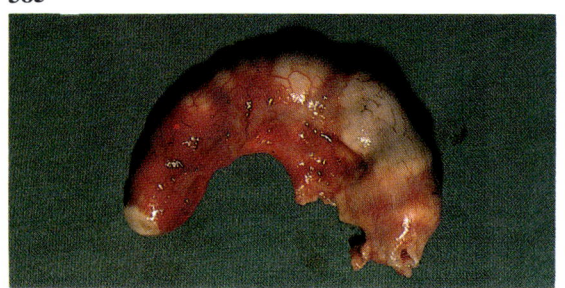

386 Appendicolith. The resected appendix shows evidence of gangrenous appendicitis with a localised perforation at the site of impaction of a faecolith.

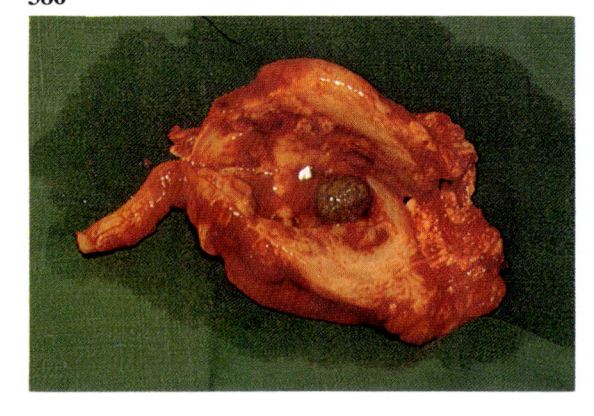

387 Appendicitis. Abdominal xray in a child with acute abdominal pain showing the calcified appendicolith in the right iliac fossa. In addition the psoas shadow is absent on the right and localised ileus in the right lower quadrant is evident.

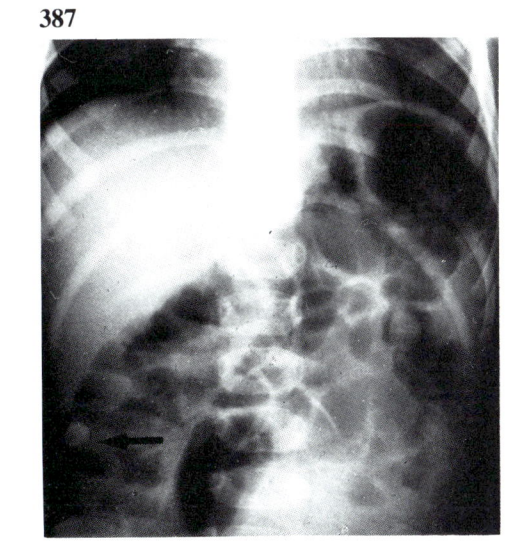

388 Perforated appendicitis. The erect abdominal xray shows numerous air-fluid levels in the small intestine with evidence of free intraperitoneal fluid. This presentation is not uncommon in the young infant under two years of age who invariably presents with one of the complications of acute appendicitis.

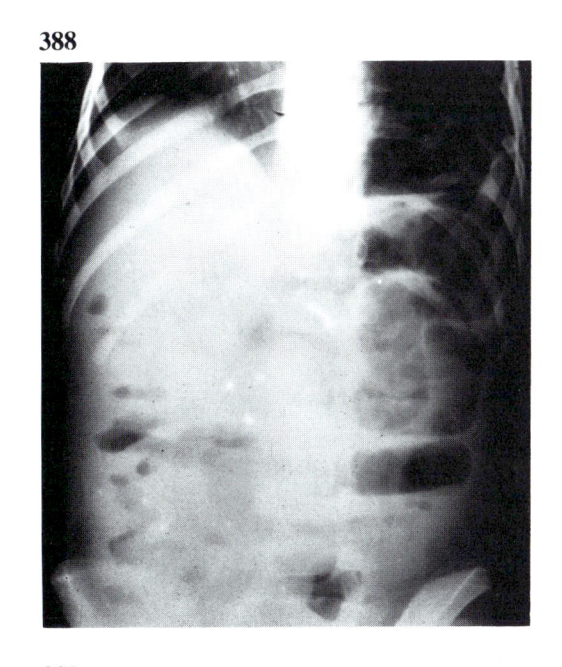

389 Carcinoid of the appendix. Rare in childhood. In most cases the tumour is confined to the tip of the appendix and is an incidental finding at laparotomy for acute appendicitis. Distant metastases are rare. Symptoms related to circulation of excessive amount of 5-hydroxytryptamine (5-HT) only occur in the presence of hepatic metastases.

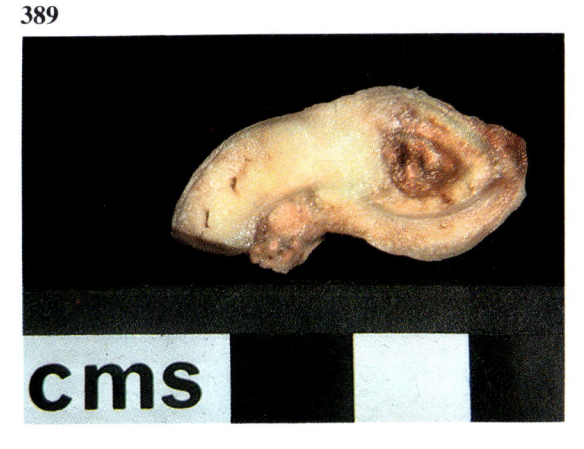

30 The colon

Necrotising enterocolitis

Neonatal necrotising enterocolitis is commonly encountered in neonatalogy practice. It particularly affects severely premature infants or infants who have experienced significant perinatal stress such as asphyxia, shock, hypothermia or septicaemia. Exchange transfusions have also been implicated in the aetiology of the condition. Interference with the blood supply to the intestinal with mucosal ulceration and secondary bacterial invasion would appear to be the most acceptable pathogenetic explanation for the condition. All parts of the gastrointestinal tract may be involved, but the ileocaecal region and colon are most commonly involved.

390 Necrotising enterocolitis. The infant presents with reluctance to feed, vomiting with or without bile-staining, passage of blood and mucus per rectum and abdominal distension. Intensive conservative treatment with broad-spectrum antibiotics, nasogastric decompression and parenteral nutrition is successful in most cases.

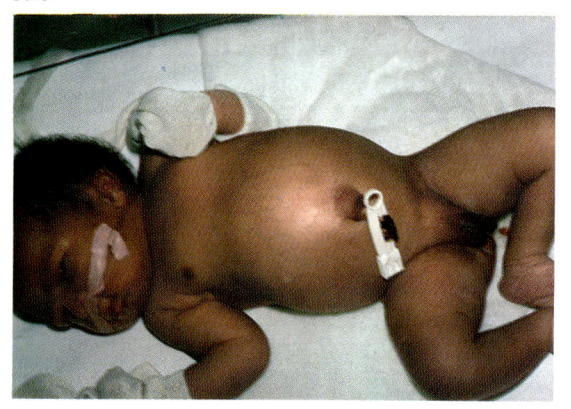

391 Necrotising enterocolitis – periumbilical erythema with or without oedema of the anterior abdominal wall is a sign of intestinal necrosis and impending perforation. In itself it is not an indication for surgical intervention and intensive conservative management at this stage may be successful.

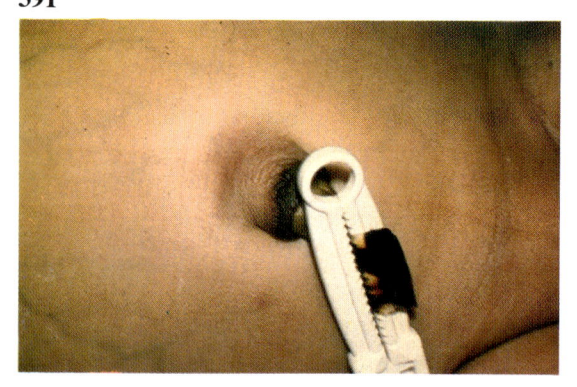

392 Erythema of anterior abdominal wall. There is gross abdominal distension and widespread redness of the abdominal wall. The infant was shocked on admission. Laparotomy revealed extensive mid small-bowel necrosis and gangrene with generalised peritonitis.

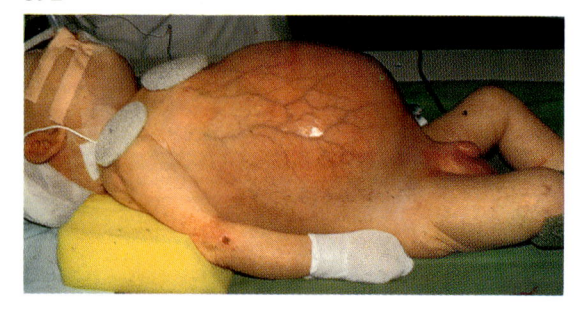

393 Pneumatosis intestinalis. The presence of intramural gas on plain abdominal xray is diagnostic for necrotising enterocolitis. The intramural gas may produce crescentic shadows around the involved loop of intestine, linear shadows along and parallel to the bowel wall producing a 'tramline' effect or give a diffuse granular appearance.

394 Gas in the portal venous system. In addition to the coarse granular appearance in the mid-abdomen, there is evidence of gas in the portal venous system in the right lobe of the liver. This is not necessarily a fatal prognostic sign.

395 Pneumoperitoneum. The presence of free gas in the peritoneal cavity is indicative of an intestinal perforation. Intestinal perforation, intestinal obstruction and failure to respond to conservative measures should be regarded as indications for operative intervention.

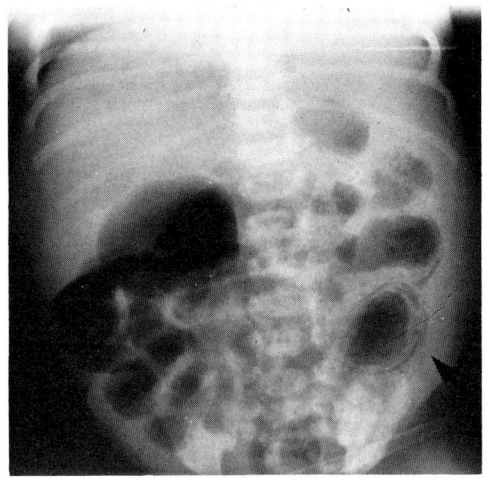

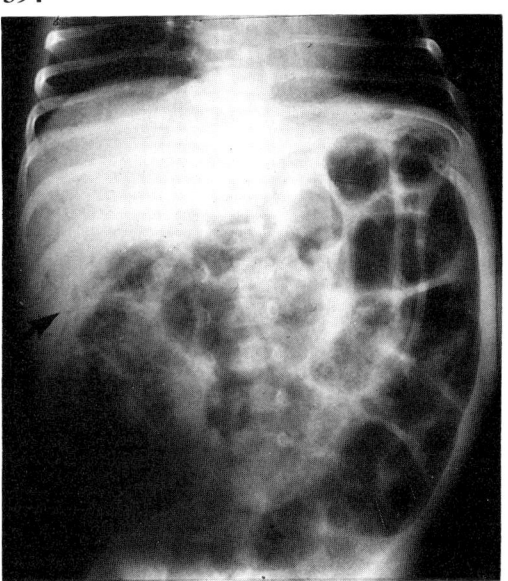

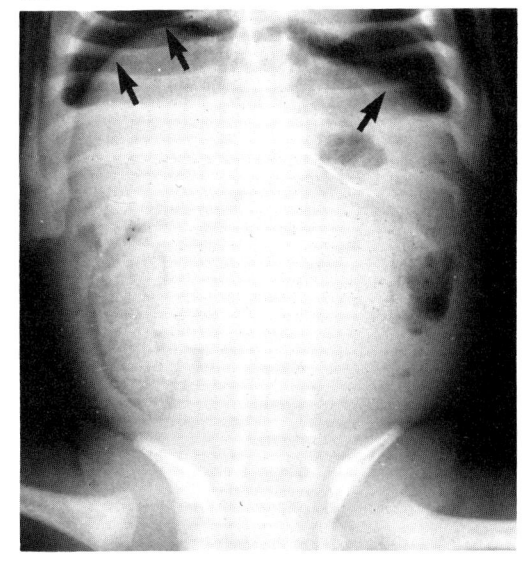

396 Enterocolitis. Necropsy appearance of the exposed intestine showing extensive subserosal gas bubbles.

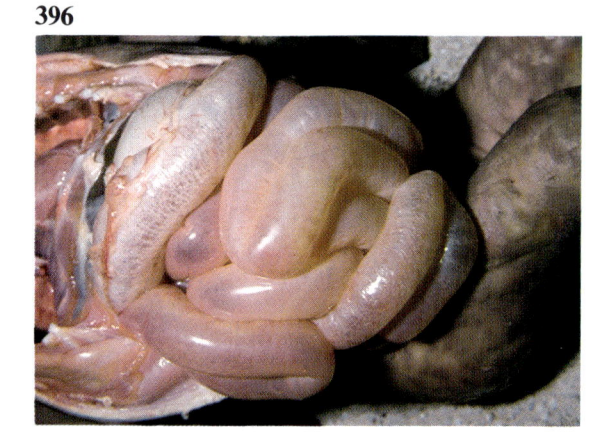

397 Enterocolitis. Specimen of a subtotal colectomy showing extensive involvement of the bowel wall and areas of partial and full-thickness necrosis. Frank perforation has occurred in the mid-transverse colon.

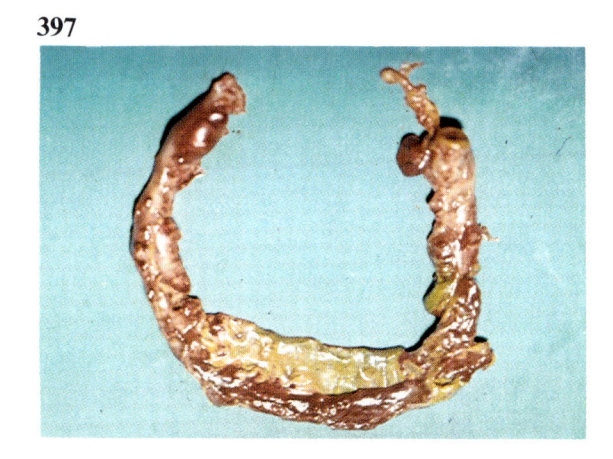

398 Enterocolitis. Operative specimen of the caecum and ascending colon in an infant presenting with massive rectal bleeding. Extensive haemorrhagic and ulcerative changes in the mucosa can be seen.

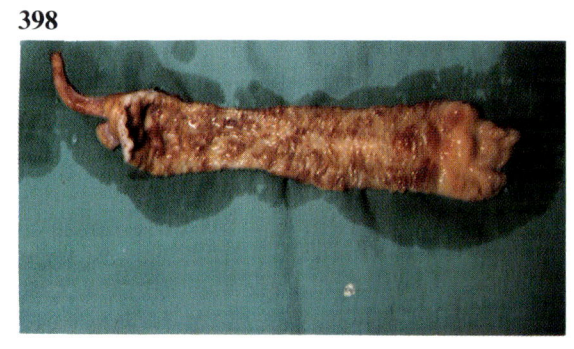

399 Enterocolitis. Microscopic examination reveals multiple loculi of gas within the bowel wall and an intense acute inflammatory reaction.

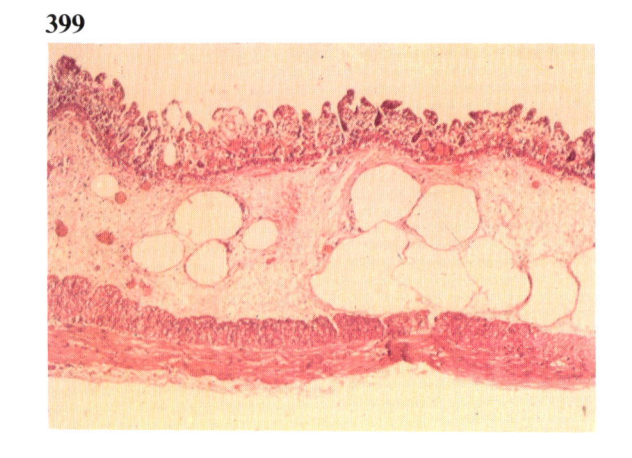

Hirschsprung's disease

Hirschsprung's disease is associated with the absence of ganglion cells within the wall of the distal intestine. This leads to a functional intestinal obstruction at the transition between normal and aganglionic bowel. The rectum is always involved, to a greater or lesser extent, and the abnormality extends proximally for a varying distance. In about five per cent of cases there is total colonic involvement. The condition presents in the neonatal period either with: i) complete intestinal obstruction or ii) delayed passage of meconium ('meconium plug syndrome'). Enterocolitis, a dreaded complication which is responsible for most deaths in Hirschsprung's disease, usually occurs in infants over two or three weeks of age.

400 Hirschsprung's disease. There is abdominal distension and visible colonic peristaltic waves in the epigastric region. The infant manifested delayed passage of meconium in the immediate newborn period.

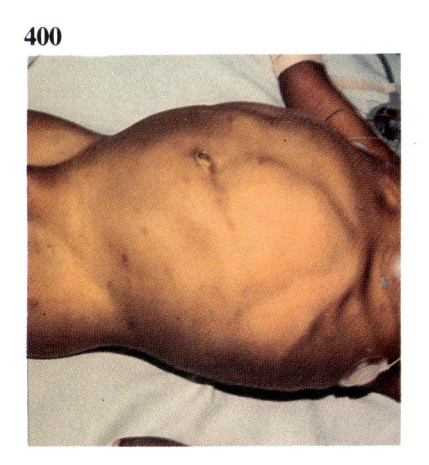

401 Hirschsprung's disease. In the older child there is marked abdominal distension, severe intractable constipation and mild malnutrition. A search through neonatal records will often reveal a history of delayed passage of meconium which resolved spontaneously. These cases should be regarded as missed neonatal diagnoses.

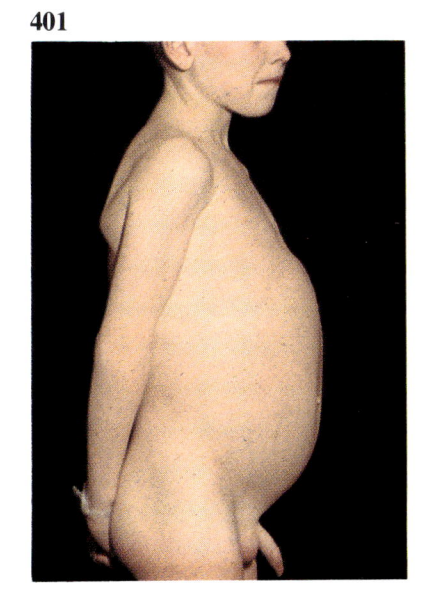

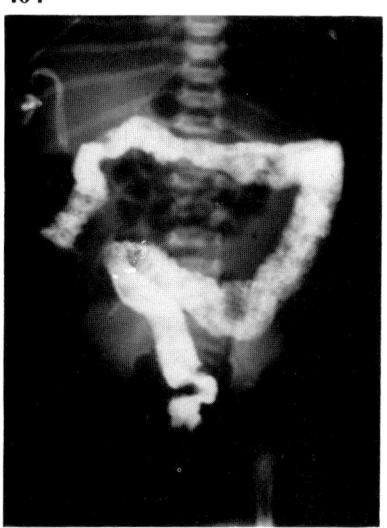

402 Hirschsprung's disease. Erect abdominal xray showing massive colonic distension with long air-fluid levels. Note the elevation of the diaphragm and the absence of gas in the pelvis. *NB* It is difficult to distinguish small from large intestine on plain abdominal xray in the infant.

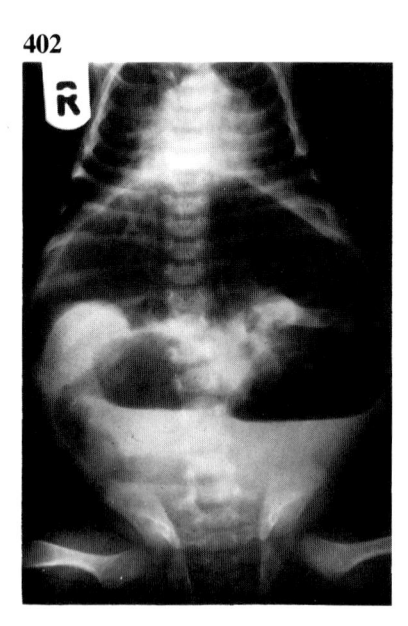

403 Barium enema. The barium outlines the narrow distal (aganglionic) segment and widens in a cone-like fashion into the proximal dilated sigmoid colon (ganglionic). Note the irregular outline of the lower rectum indicative of abnormal contractility.

404 Barium enema. There is considerable retention of barium within the large bowel 24 hours after the examination. This is highly suspicious of Hirschsprung's disease in infancy. Normally most of the contrast will have been evacuated within 24 hours of the investigation.

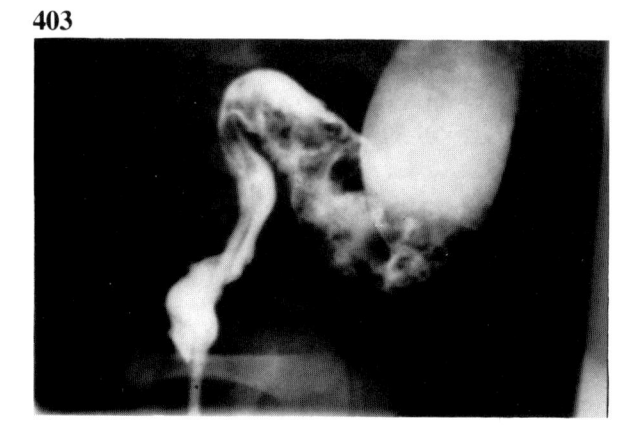

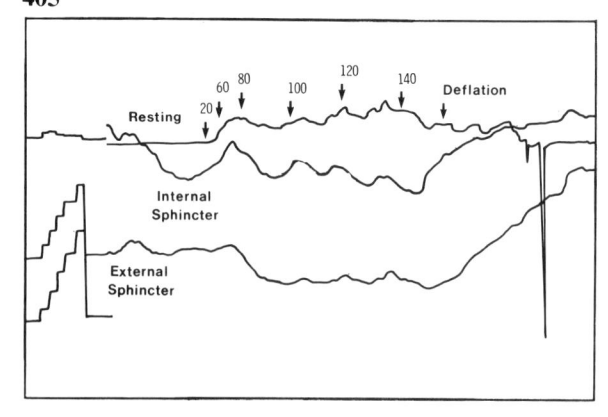

405 Anorectal manometry. Normal physiological response of the internal sphincter to rectal distension. There is a relaxation wave in the internal sphincter zone.

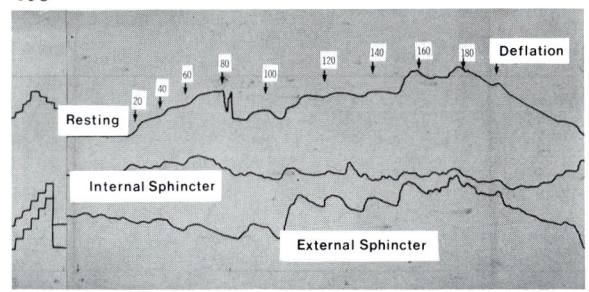

406 Anorectal manometry. In patients with Hirschsprung's disease the internal sphincter zone fails to exhibit a relaxation wave in response to rectal distension. There is also an abnormal motor response in the rectum. The diagnostic value of anorectal manometry is suspect in the immediate neonatal period.

407 Suction rectal biopsy. Normal microscopic appearance of an adequate rectal suction biopsy (taken at least 3 cm above the anal verge to avoid the normal hypoganglionic zone) showing a group of four ganglion cells in Meissner's plexus in the submucosal layer. Cryostat section of suction rectal biopsy (*H&E × 100*).

408 Rectal biopsy (normal). Photomicrograph of an acetylcholinesterase preparation (× 100). The ganglion cells in Meissner's plexus stain dark brown. Note the paucity of nerve fibres in the muscularis mucosae.

409 Rectal biopsy (normal). Acetylcholinesterase stain (× 40) showing only a few nerve fibres in the lamina propria and muscularis mucosae.

410 Rectal biopsy (Hirschsprung's). Acetylcholinesterase preparation (× 40) showing numerous darkly stained nerve fibres in the lamina propria and muscularis mucosae. There are no ganglion cells in the submucosa.

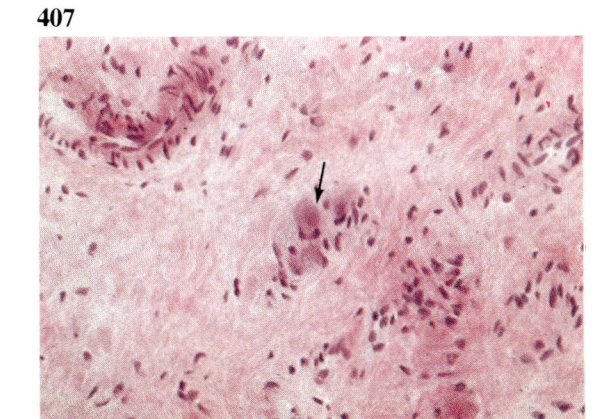

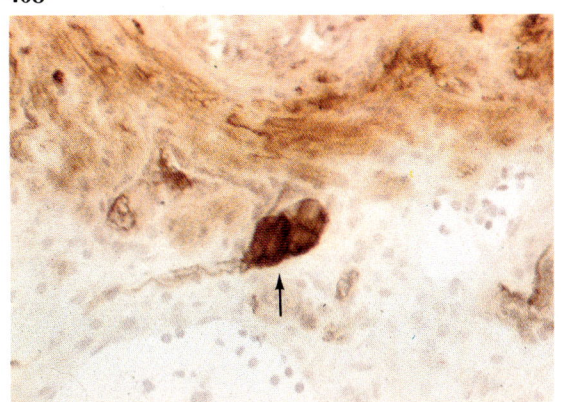

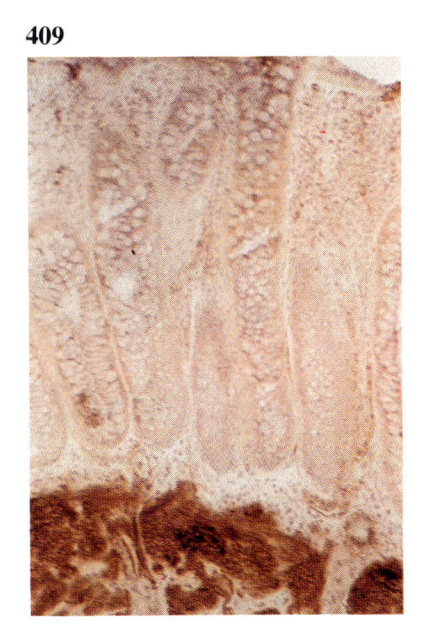

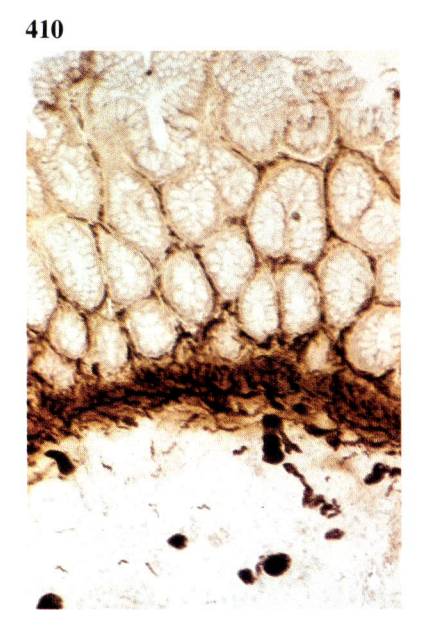

411 Hirschsprung's disease. Operative view of the proximally distended and hypertrophied large intestine. The distension ends abruptly at the junction with the aganglionic distal bowel which is narrow and collapsed. The junctional zone is not always obvious and frozen section histological examination of extramucosal intestinal biopsies may be necessary to establish the level of the transitional zone.

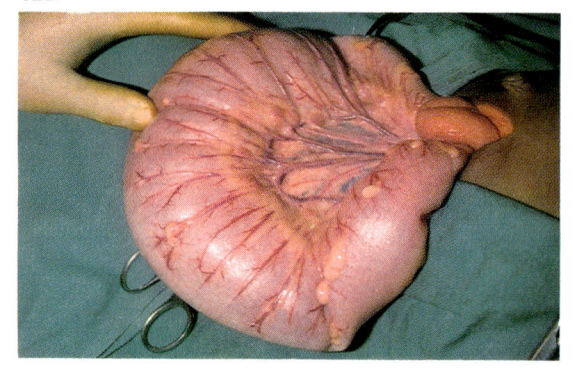

412 Meconium plug syndrome. The lateral abdominal xray shows a plug in the presacral portion of rectum. The infant presents with abdominal distension, vomiting (may contain bile) and delayed passage of meconium. Hirschsprung's disease must be excluded in these patients.

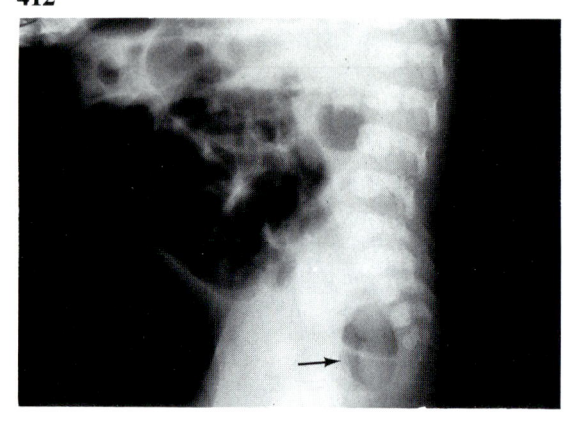

413 Meconium plug syndrome. The gastrografin enema outlines the mass of meconium within the distal colon and rectum. This contrast material serves as a liquifying and emulsifying agent which is often therapeutic in effecting expulsion of the meconium plug.

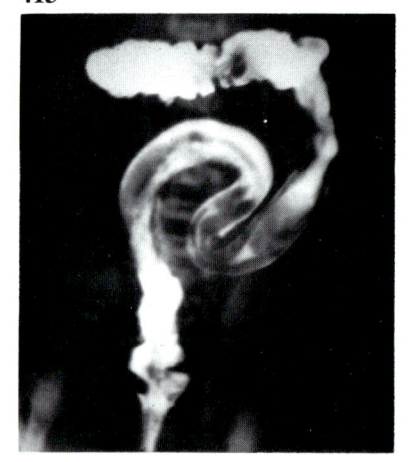

414 Meconium plug. There is a whitish mucoid plug at the head of the mass followed by a large volume of thick tenacious black meconium. Relief of the obstructive symptoms after evacuation of the meconium plug is often dramatic. Hirschsprung's disease must be excluded in these patients.

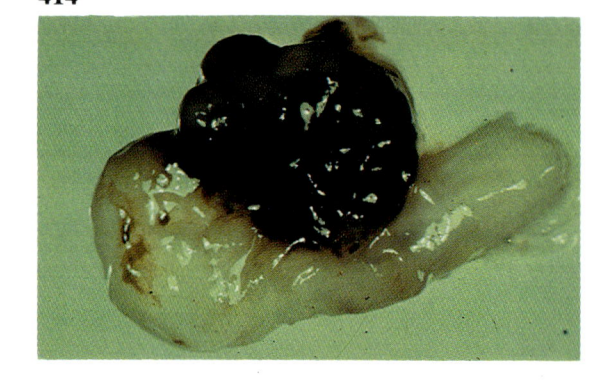

Miscellaneous conditions

415

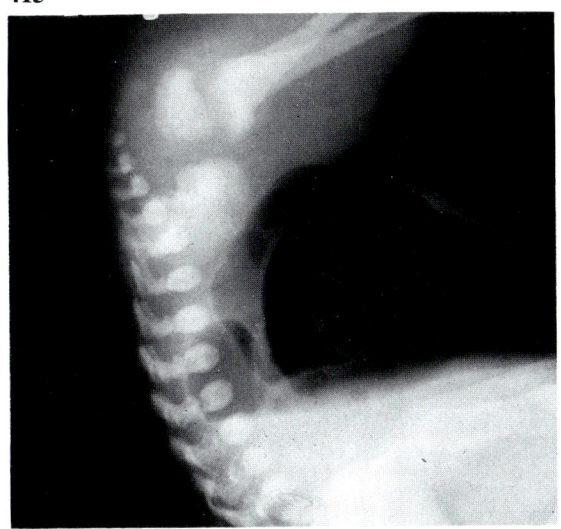

415 Colonic atresia. Accounts for less than five per cent of gastrointestinal atresias. Pathogenesis is similar to that of small bowel atresia. Presents with massive abdominal distension and failure to pass meconium. Bile-stained vomiting occurs late. The inverted lateral xray shows the enormously distended colonic loop with a long air-fluid level. Contrast enema will distinguish colonic atresia from Hirschsprung's disease.

416

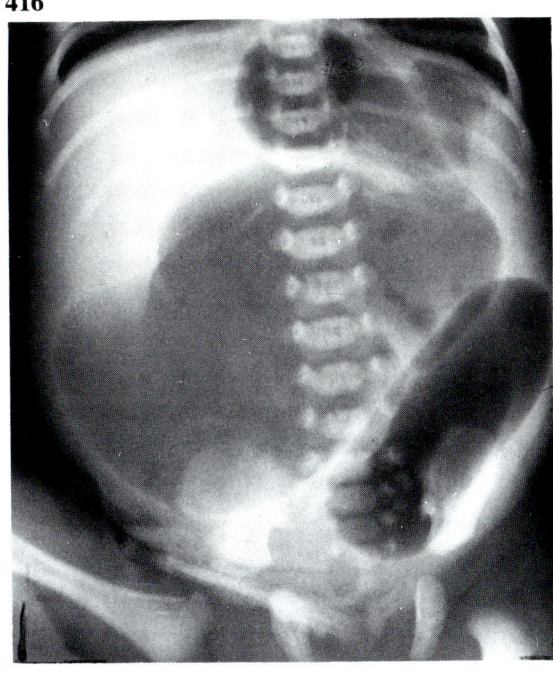

416 Colonic atresia. Abdominal xray shows distension virtually confined to the colon. This is caused by the competent ileocaecal valve.

417 Meconium peritonitis. A clearly demarcated perforation is visible in the transverse colon with soiling of the peritoneal cavity. Evidence of necrotising enterocolitis is absent. In these cases it is mandatory to exclude a distal obstruction, e.g. atresia, Hirschsprung's disease, mucoviscidosis etc, as the aetiological factor.

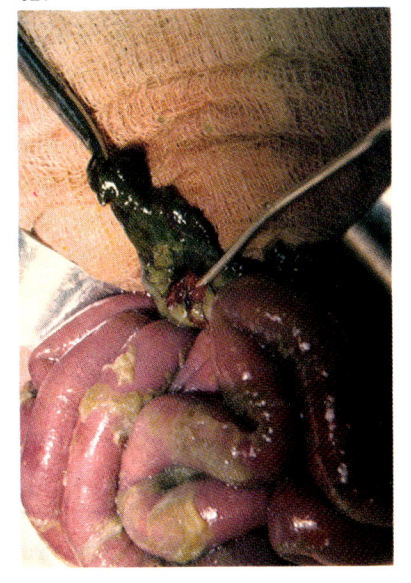

417

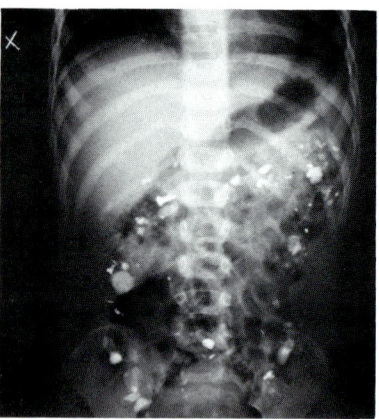

418 Ingested foreign body. The plain xray shows multiple radio-opaque foreign bodies studded throughout the large intestine (nails, screws, washers, etc). Surgery is rarely required and spontaneous evacuation without intestinal injury is the expected outcome.

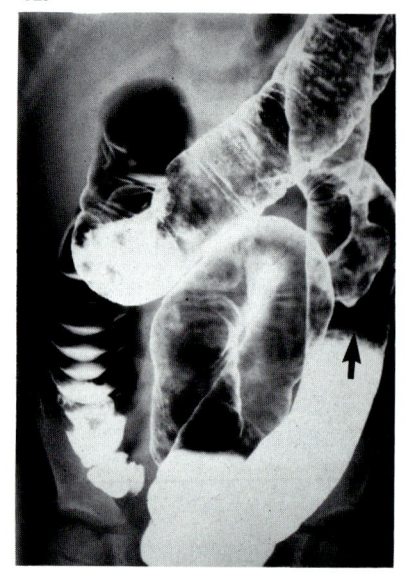

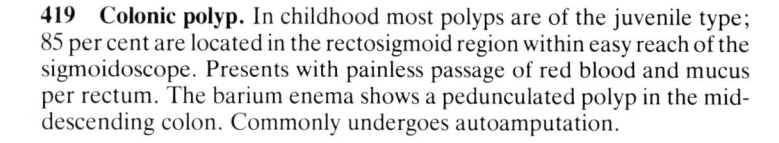

419 Colonic polyp. In childhood most polyps are of the juvenile type; 85 per cent are located in the rectosigmoid region within easy reach of the sigmoidoscope. Presents with painless passage of red blood and mucus per rectum. The barium enema shows a pedunculated polyp in the mid-descending colon. Commonly undergoes autoamputation.

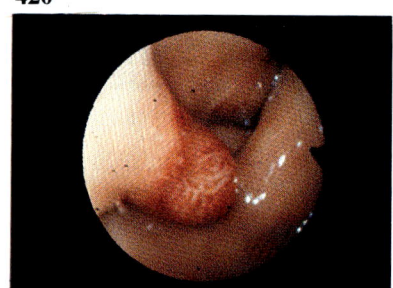

420 Colonic polyp. Seen at colonoscopy. The surface of the lesion is erythematous and friable. The attachment to the colonic wall is broad based (sessile) as opposed to the more usual pedunculated polyp.

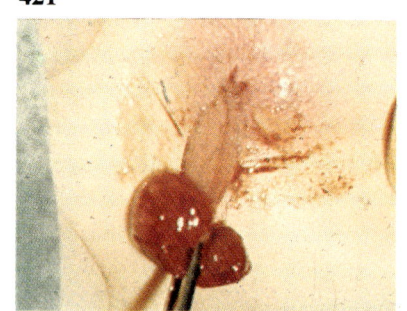

421 Rectal polyp. The polyp may prolapse out of the anus. Note the oval-shaped glistening cherry red appearance of the polyp and the long smooth pedicle. Polypectomy by transfixion ligation at the base of the pedicle is easily performed.

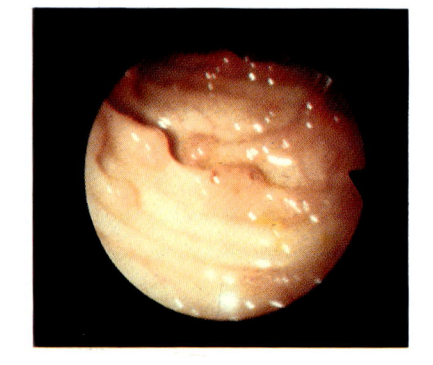

422 Polyposis coli. Multiple mucosa-lined polyps covering the colon from the anus to the caecum. Pathologically the lesions are adenomatous polyps. Familial adenomatous polyposis (Mendelian dominant) presents in mid-teens with diarrhoea, rectal bleeding and abdominal pain. High (50 per cent) risk of malignant degeneration. Should be distinguished from lymphoid polyposis, Gardner's syndrome and pseudopolyps of ulcerative colitis.

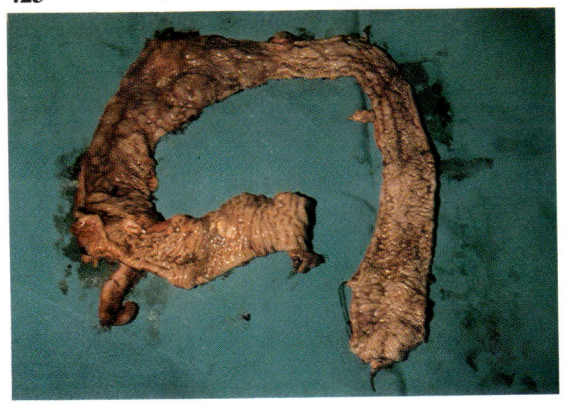

423 Amoebic colitis. Caused by the parasite *Entamoeba histolytica* and common in the tropics. Symptoms vary from mild colitis with blood and mucus in the stools to overwhelming involvement of the entire colon with extensive mucosal destruction. Total colectomy in a child with fulminating amoebic colitis showing extensive full-thickness necrosis of the right colon and haemorrhagic ulcerative changes in the rest of the colon.

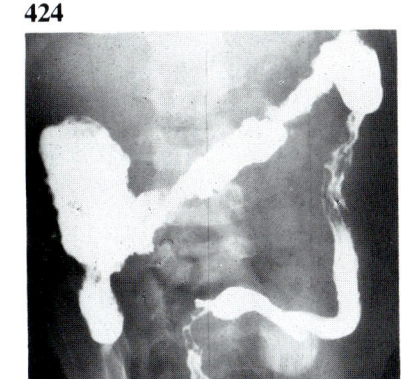

424 Amoebic colitis. Barium enema showing extensive strictures and areas of mucosal damage in the recovery phase of fulminating amoebic colitis.

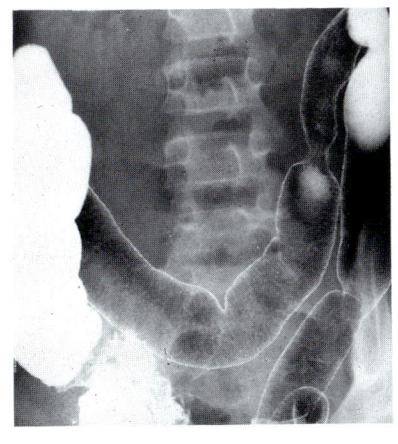

425 Ulcerative colitis. 10 to 15 per cent of ulcerative colitis begins in childhood. Presenting symptoms include diarrhoea containing blood and mucus accompanied by colicky abdominal pain. Extraintestinal manifestations, i.e. growth retardation, joint and skin involvement, are common. Barium enema shows fine serrations ('sawtooth' appearance) with loss of haustral pattern. Late sequelae include colonic shortening, narrowing and stricture formation.

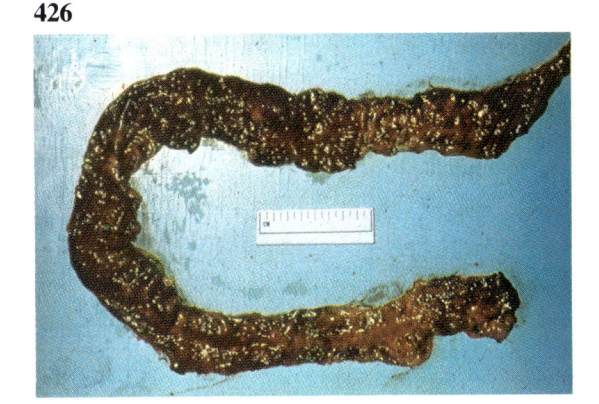

426 Ulcerative colitis. Resected specimen in a three-year-old child manifesting toxic dilatation of the colon. Extensive mucosal haemorrhage and ulceration is evident. No recognisable mucosa remains. The disease process is confined to the mucosa and transmural inflammation does not occur.

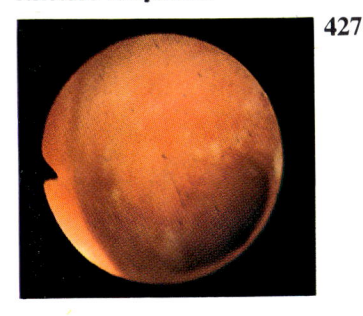

427 Ulcerative colitis. Endoscopic appearance showing a diffusely hyperaemic mucosa, oedema and friability. The whitish areas represent superficial ulcerations but discrete ulcers are not seen.

31 Rectum and anus
Anorectal malformations

Diagnostic approach to the male anorectal anomaly

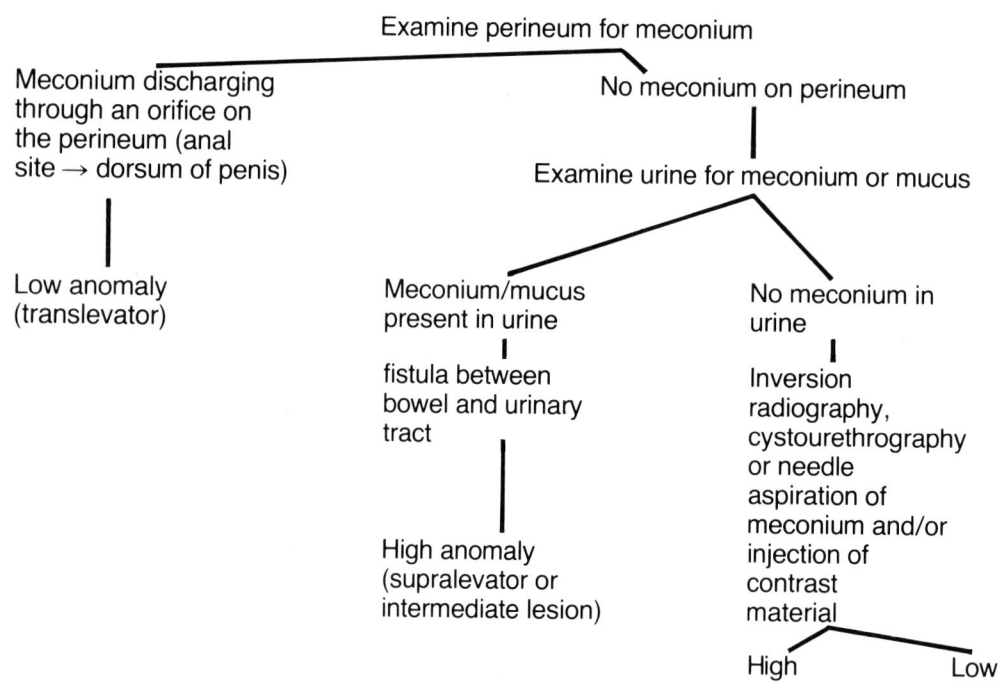

Examine perineum for meconium

- **Meconium discharging through an orifice on the perineum (anal site → dorsum of penis)**
  - Low anomaly (translevator)

- **No meconium on perineum**
  - Examine urine for meconium or mucus
    - **Meconium/mucus present in urine**
      - fistula between bowel and urinary tract
      - High anomaly (supralevator or intermediate lesion)
    - **No meconium in urine**
      - Inversion radiography, cystourethrography or needle aspiration of meconium and/or injection of contrast material
        - High
        - Low

Diagnostic approach to female anorectal anomalies

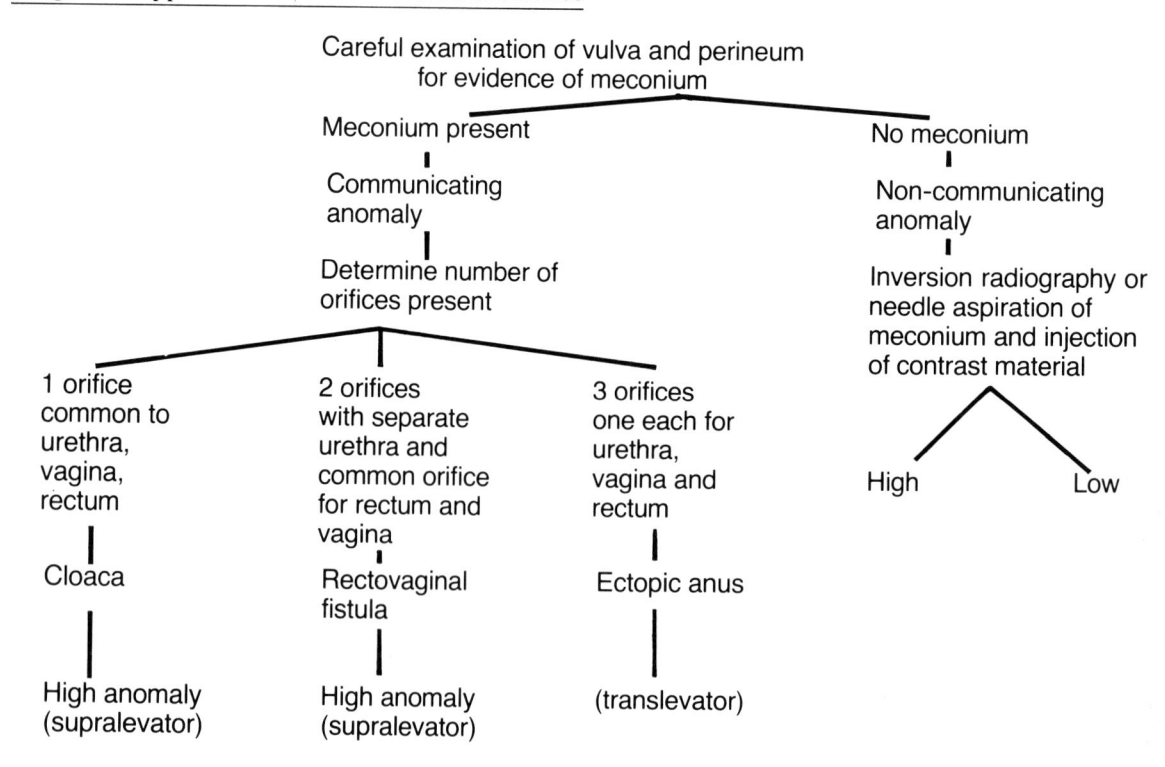

Careful examination of vulva and perineum for evidence of meconium

- **Meconium present**
  - Communicating anomaly
  - Determine number of orifices present
    - **1 orifice common to urethra, vagina, rectum**
      - Cloaca
      - High anomaly (supralevator)
    - **2 orifices with separate urethra and common orifice for rectum and vagina**
      - Rectovaginal fistula
      - High anomaly (supralevator)
    - **3 orifices one each for urethra, vagina and rectum**
      - Ectopic anus
      - (translevator)

- **No meconium**
  - Non-communicating anomaly
  - Inversion radiography or needle aspiration of meconium and injection of contrast material
    - High
    - Low

428 High (supralevator) anomaly in the male. The commonest type is an anorectal agenesis with a rectourethral fistula. Note the fistulous end of the rectum ending in the prostatic portion of the posterior urethra above the puborectalis part of the levator ani muscle. Meconium can be seen entering the urethra and being passed during micturition.

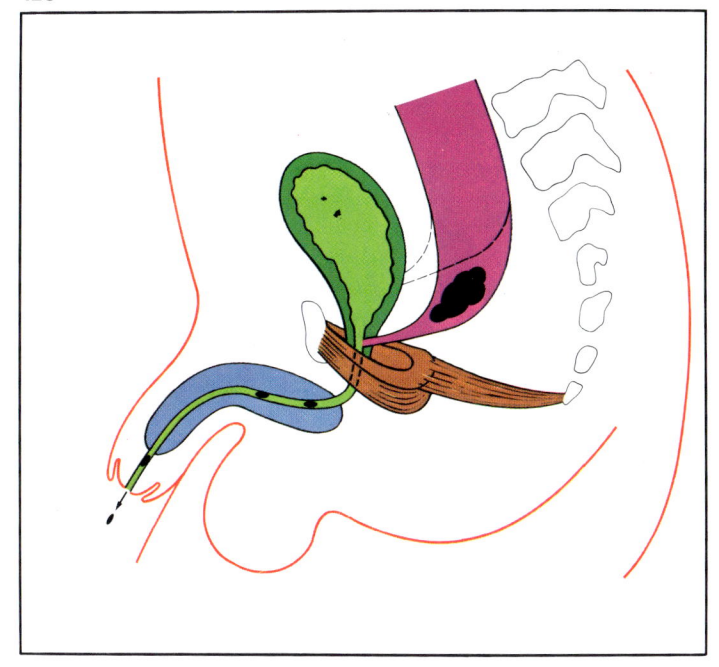

429 Low (translevator) anomaly in the male. The commonest type is a covered anus with an anocutaneous fistula discharging meconium on the perineum at any one of a variety of sites from the anal region to the base of the penis. Note the rectum traversing through the puborectalis sling.

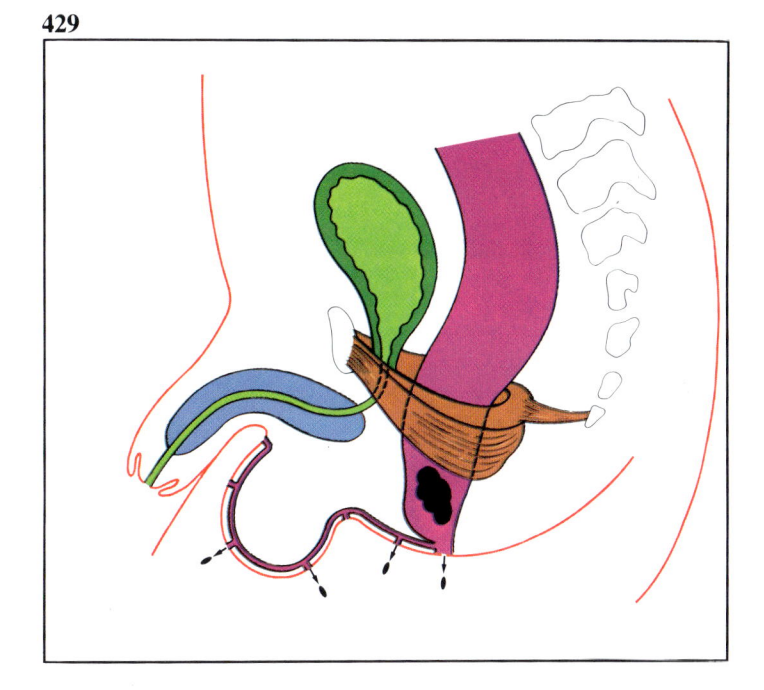

129

430 High (supralevator) anomaly in the female. Cloacal anomaly in which there is a common opening on the perineum for the urethra, vagina and rectum.

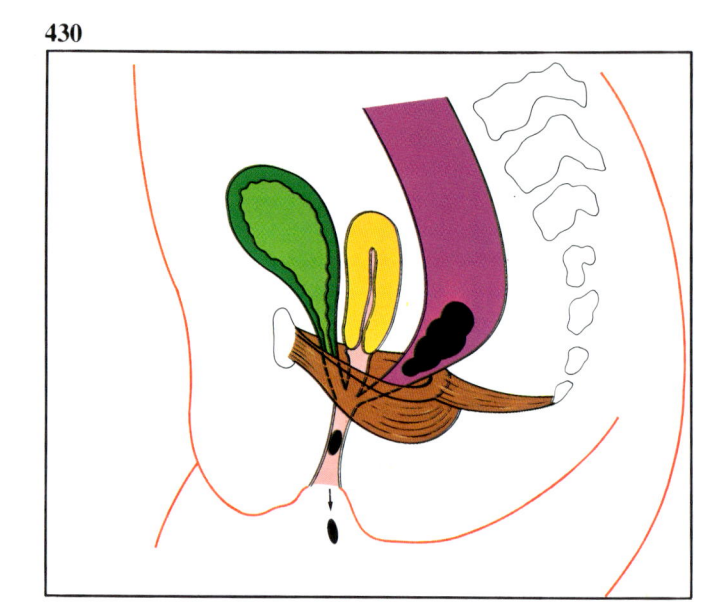

431 High (supralevator) anomaly in the female. High (and low) rectovaginal fistula with an anorectal agenesis. The fistula either enters the posterior vagina well above the puborectalis muscle or enters lower down in the vagina where the bowel itself ends above the pelvic diaphragm and the fistulous tract only penetrates the puborectalis sling. There are two openings in the vulva – urethra and a common orifice for the vagina and rectum.

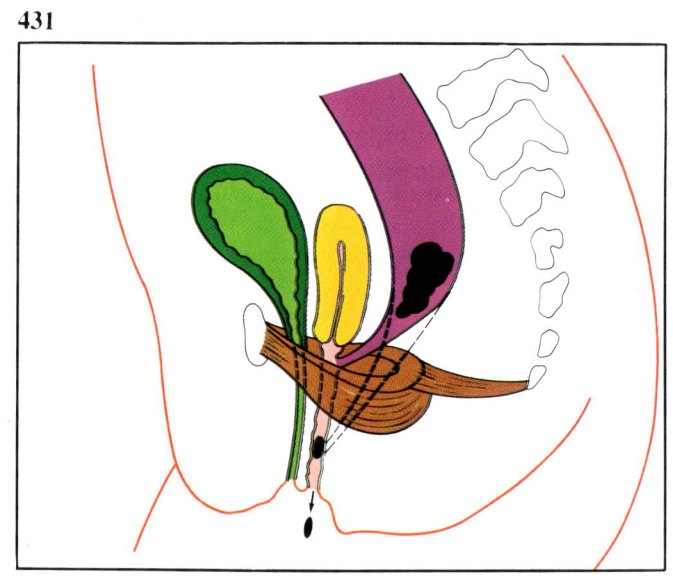

432 Low (translevator) anomaly in the female. The commonest type is an ectopic anus where the orifice is either in the posterior fourchette or in the perineum anterior to the normal anus site. Note the presence of three separate perineal orifices – urethra, vagina and ectopic anus.

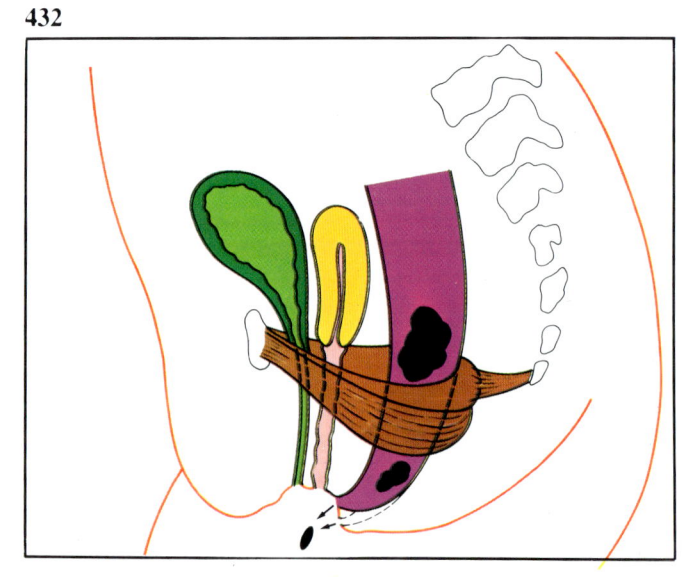

433 Anorectal agenesis with rectourethral fistula in a newborn male infant. Frank meconium is being passed per urethra.

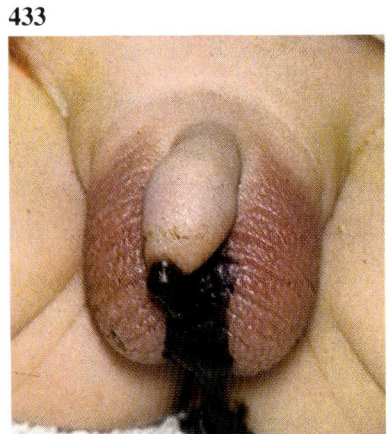

434 Covered anus with an anocutaneous fistula extruding a spot of meconium in the midline of the perineum.

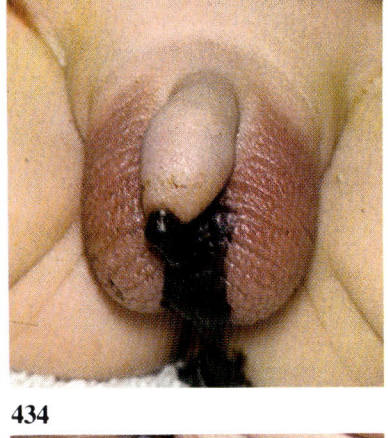

435 Covered anus and anocutaneous fistula containing meconium and extending to the base of the scrotum.

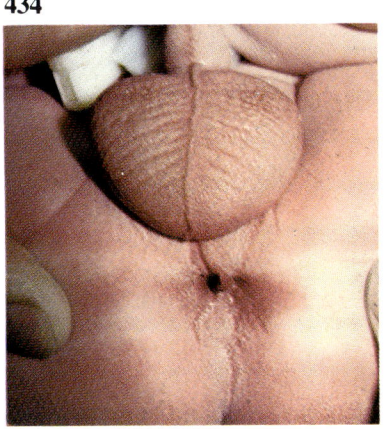

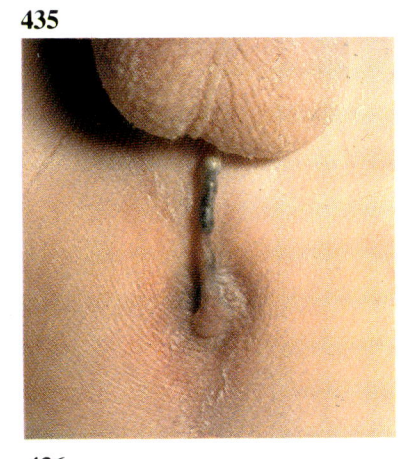

436 Cloaca. There is a single vulval orifice through which urine and meconium are passed. An example of an anorectal agenesis and rectocloacal fistula.

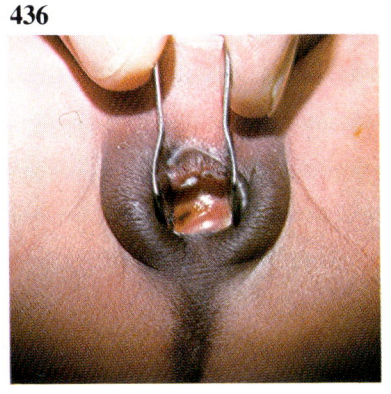

437 Anorectal agenesis and rectovaginal fistula. There are two openings in the vulva – one being the urethra (anteriorly) and the second a common orifice for the vagina and rectum.

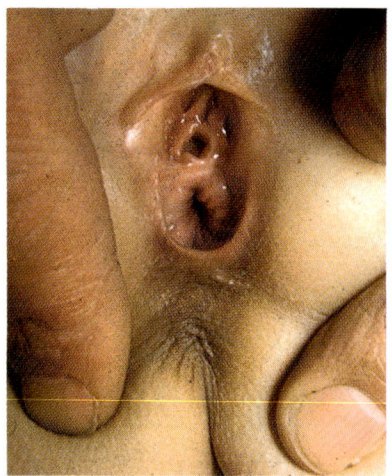

438 Ectopic anus with anovulvar fistula. Note the presence of three orifices – urethra, vagina and ectopic anal orifice in the posterior fourchette (containing meconium).

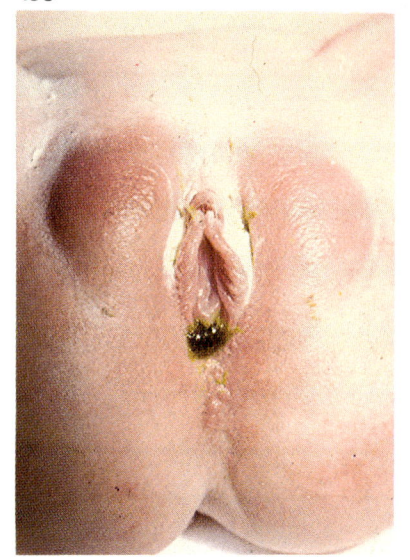

439 Anterior perineal anus. There is a fully formed, patent and functioning anus in the anterior perineal region just posterior to the vulva.

440 Covered anal stenosis in the female. On straining the perineum is shown to bulge and a spot of meconium is expelled through the narrow anocutaneous fistula.

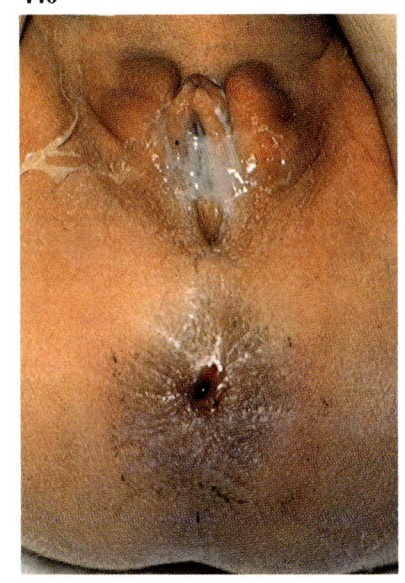

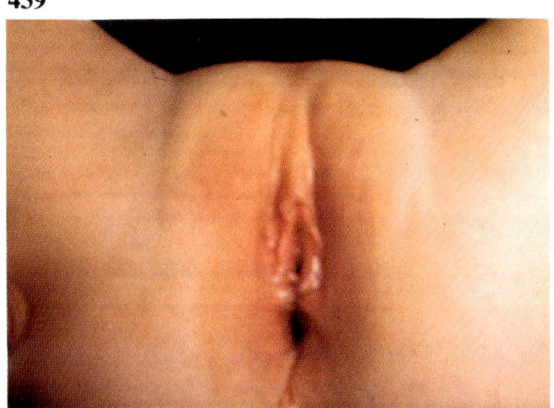

441 Rectal atresia. There is a normally formed anal canal which ends blindly just above the internal sphincter (2.5 cm from the anal verge). There is no fistulous connection between the rectum and urinary tract.

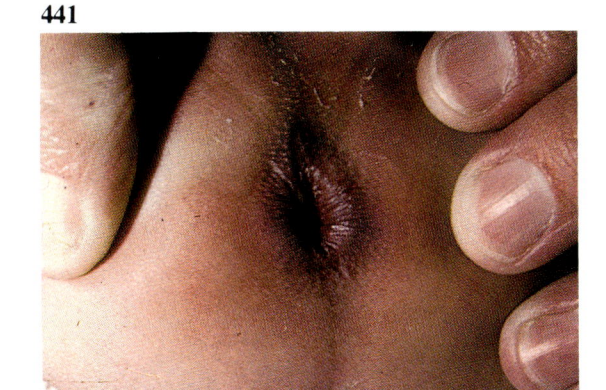

442 Perineal canal. There is an anovestibular fistula in the presence of normal anal and vaginal orifices.

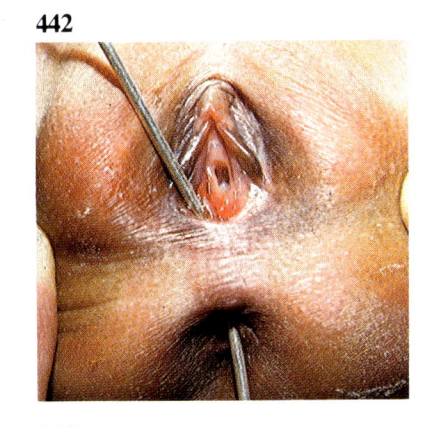

443 Anorectal agenesis with a hamartomatous malformation at the anal site. Note the presence of associated ambiguous genitalia.

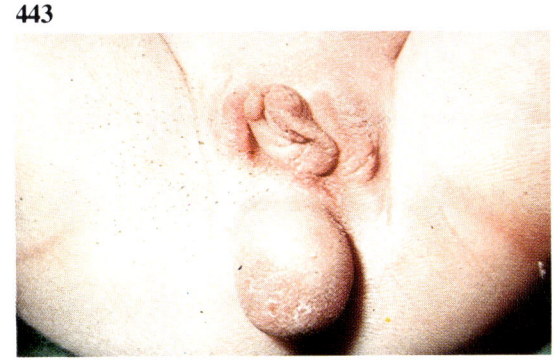

444 Translevator anorectal anomaly. Inversion radiograph showing the bowel gas well below the pelvic floor. Three lines have been drawn on the xray. The upper line (3) is the pubococcygeal line which extends from the pubic bone to the sacrococcygeal junction. The lower line (1) is the I line running parallel to (3) at the level of the lowest point of the ischium. The M line (2) is parallel to (3) and transects the ischium at the junction of the upper two-thirds and lower third (neck of the pear). This latter line is approximately at the level of the puborectalis muscle.

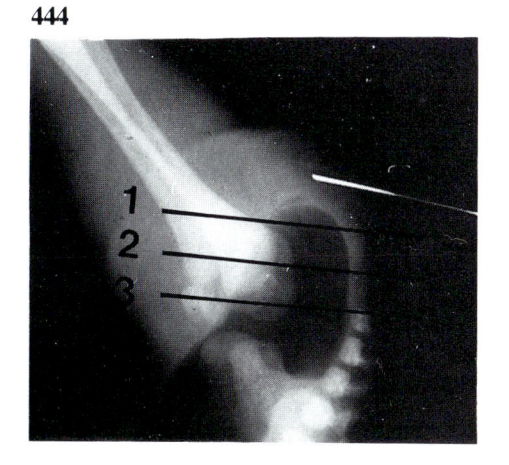

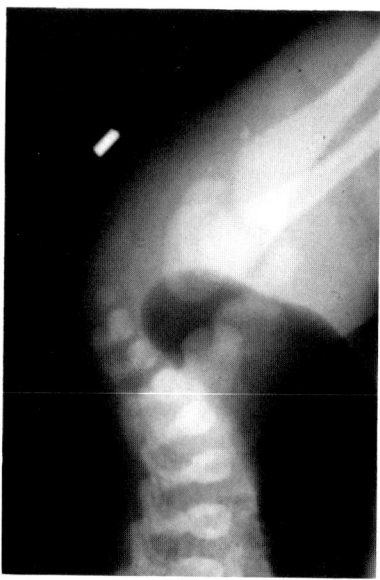

445 Supralevator anorectal anomaly. Inversion radiography showing gas in the terminal rectum ending well above the pelvic floor.

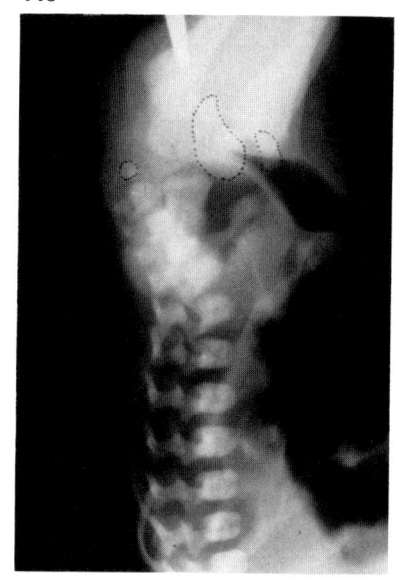

446 Anorectal agenesis and rectourethral fistula. The bony landmarks, i.e. symphysis pubis, ileum and fifth sacral vertebra have been outlined. The gas in the rectum ends above the pelvic floor and the presence of gas in the urinary bladder denotes the existence of a fistulous communication between the rectum and urinary system.

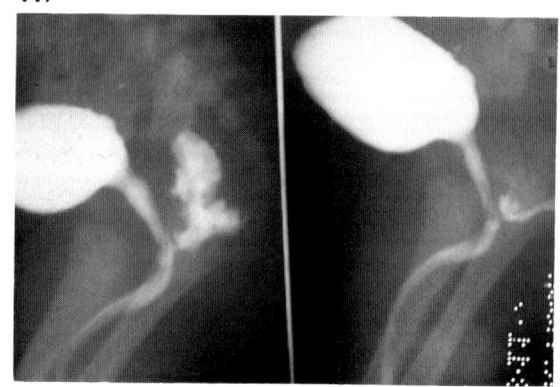

447 Rectourethral fistula. A micturating cystourethrogram shows the entrance of the rectourethral fistula in the posterior aspect of the bulb of the urethra.

Miscellaneous conditions

448 Rectal prolapse. Usually involves only the loosely attached rectal mucosa. The prolapse is seldom more than 2 to 3 cm in length. Appears on straining during defecation and commonly reduces spontaneously.

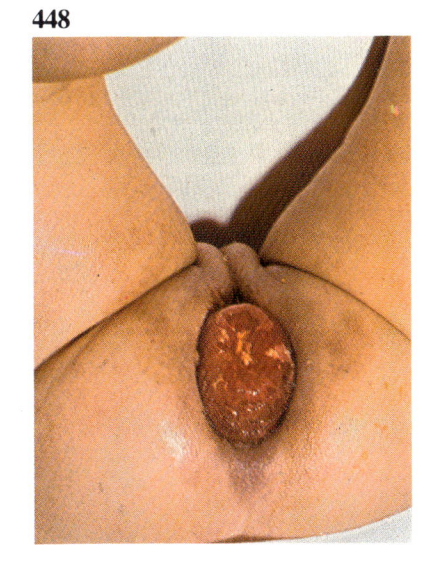

449 Rectal prolapse (procidentia). The full-thickness of the rectal wall prolapses out of the anal orifice for a varying distance. Frequently seen in children with major neuromuscular disorders, e.g. myelomeningocoele, ectopia vesicae, etc.

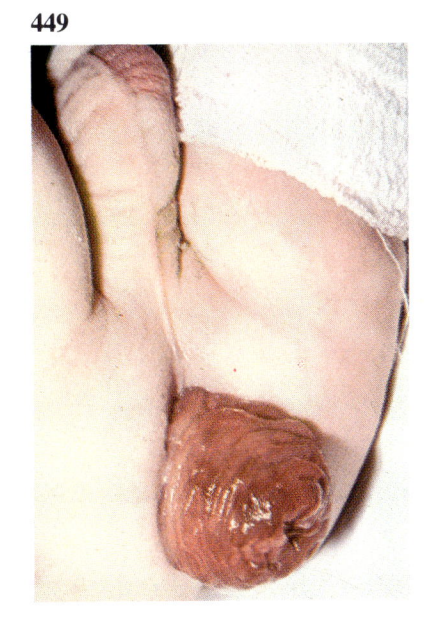

450 Anal fissure. Most common cause of rectal bleeding in first year of life. Usually located in the midline of the anus – anterior or posteriorly. Develops after the passage of a large constipated stool. Acute pain with defecation and a few drops of bright red blood follow the stool. Untreated, may result in secondary megacolon.

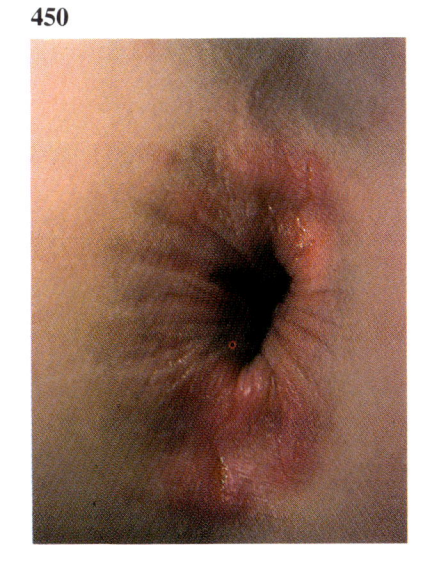

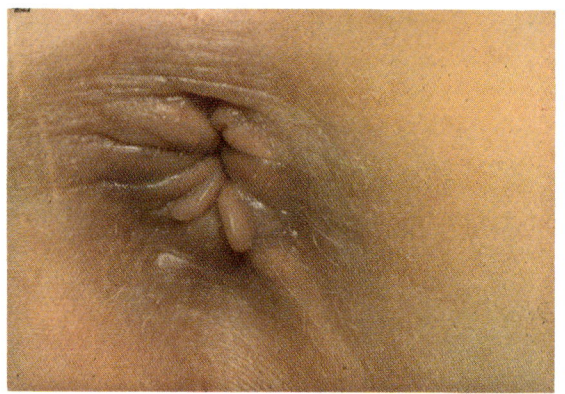

451 'Sentinel' anal tag. Indicates presence of a chronic fissure-in-ano. The edges of the fissure become thickened and oedematous thus forming a tag of skin at the distal end of the fissure. Usually responds to conservative measures but occasionally excision combined with anal dilatation or partial sphincterotomy may be required.

452 Posterior anal 'pit'. Common condition. There is an epithelial lined depression overlying the coccyx posterior to the anal orifice. No risk of meningitis (caused by connection with lumbar theca) if base can be accurately viewed. Has been implicated in the pathogenesis of pilonidal sinus.

453 Fistula-in-ano. Usually occurs after spontaneous rupture or inadequate drainage of an anorectal abscess. The tract is lined by granulation tissue. There may be recurrent abscess formation or intermittent purulent discharge. Where the external opening is related to the anterior half of the anus, the fistulous tract tends to enter into the anal canal radially opposite. Posterior located fistulae have tracts pursuing a more tortuous course with the internal orifice lying on the posterior midline of the anal canal (Goodsall's rule). Treatment is by laying open of the fistulous tract. Crohn's disease, ulcerative colitis and tuberculosis should be excluded.

454 Ischial hernia. There is a bulge in the left ischiorectal space caused by protrusion of peritoneum and abdominal content through a defect in the line of origin of the levator ani muscle from the fascia covering the obturator internus (hiatus of Schwalbe).

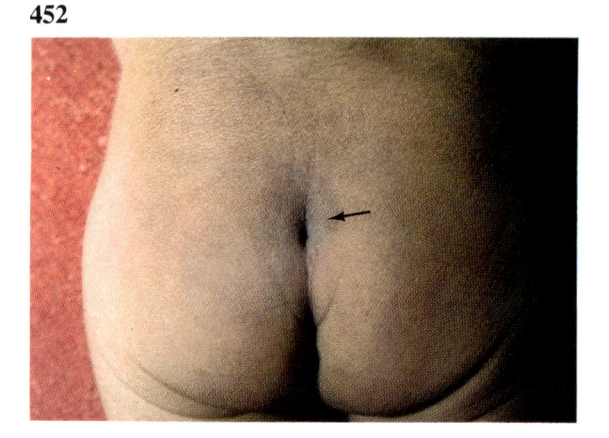

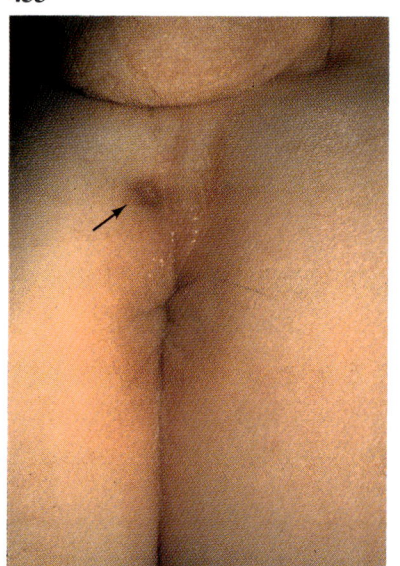

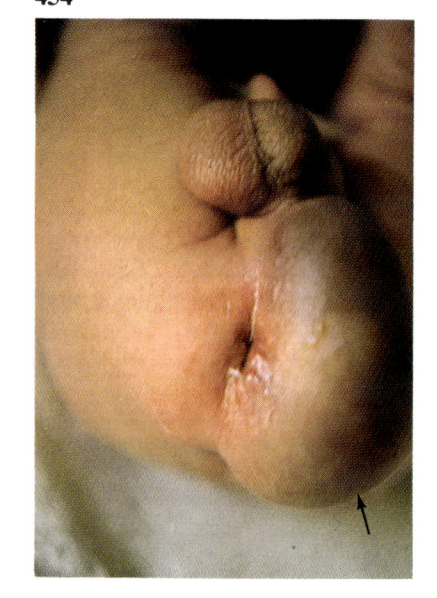

32 Liver and biliary tract

455 Jaundice. Yellow discoloration of the sclera (skin and other tissues) as a result of excessive accumulation of bilirubin. Caused by disorder of the hepatic, biliary or haematological systems. Conjugated hyperbilirubinaemia is always pathological. The most common causes are neonatal hepatitis syndromes (alpha-1-antitrypsin deficiency, metabolic disorders, cytomegalovirus, rubella virus, hepatitis B virus, etc) and lesions of extra-hepatic biliary tree (biliary atresia, choledochal cyst).

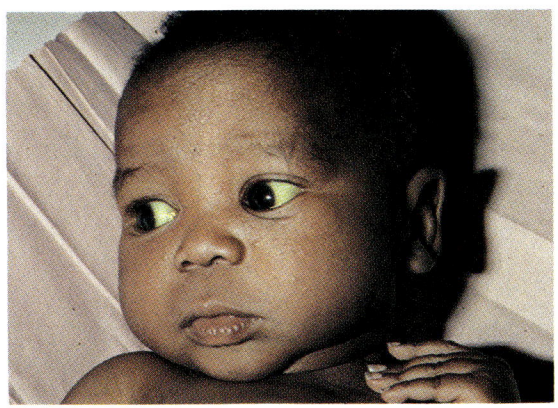

456 Normal cholangiogram. Laparotomy and operative cholangiography before the age of 60 days is indicated in any infant with persistent conjugated hyperbilirubinaemia and acholic stools in whom: a) infections, metabolic and genetic causes have been excluded; b) the percutaneous liver biopsy shows features compatible with extrahepatic biliary atresia, and c) I^{131} Rose Bengal faecal excretion is <10 per cent in 72 hours.

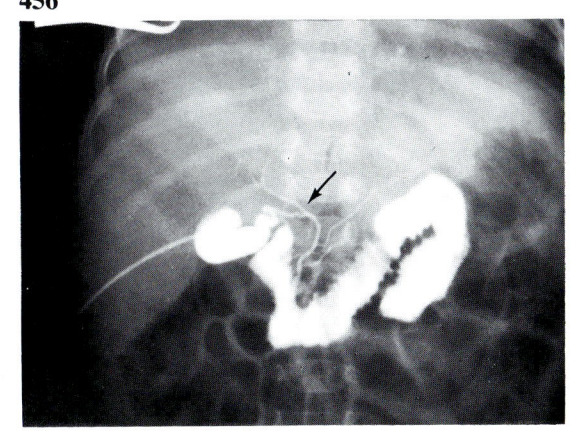

457 Atresia of the common hepatic duct. The operative cholangiogram shows good flow of contrast from the gall bladder into the duodenum. No contrast can be seen in the proximal bile ducts above the junction of the cystic and common bile ducts.

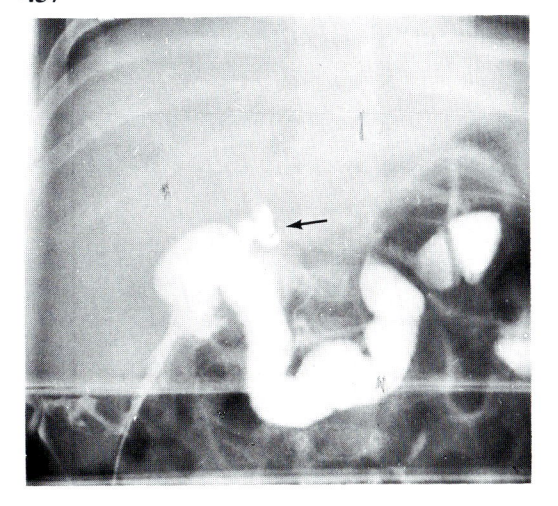

458 Choledochal cyst. The operative cholangiogram via the gall bladder shows massive cystic dilatation of the common bile duct. The duodenum is displaced downwards by the partially outlined choledochal cyst. No contrast has entered the duodenum. The proximal ducts are outlined and are moderately dilated.

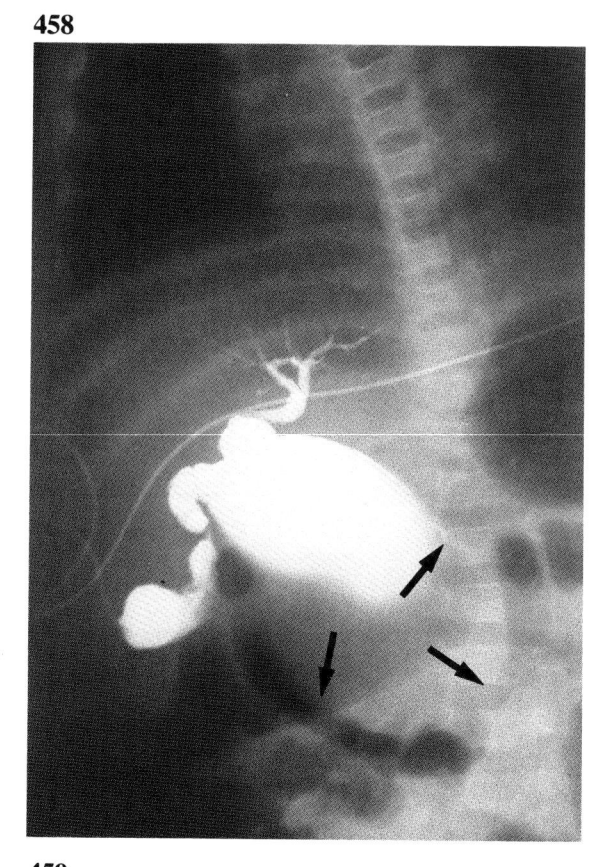

459 Inspissated bile syndrome. The cholangiogram via the gall bladder shows a uniformly dilated extrahepatic biliary system with filling defects in the lower end of the common bile duct. No contrast has entered the duodenum. Exploration of the common duct revealed the presence of 'biliary mud' and three calculi. There was a tight stenosis of the lower end of the common duct.

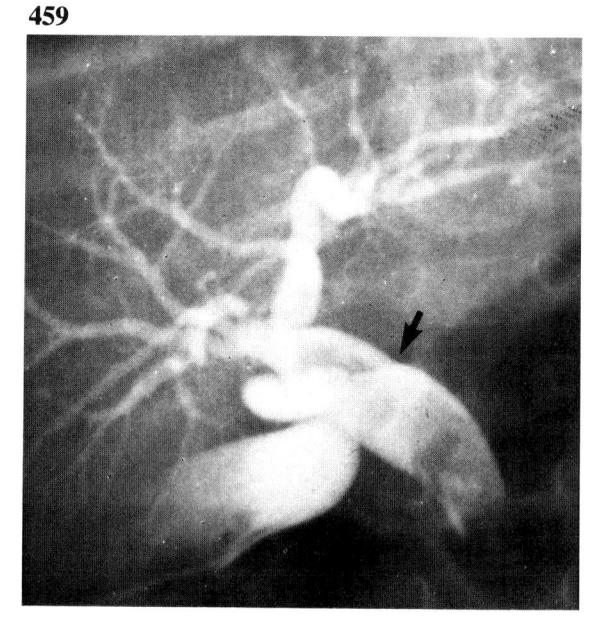

460 Biliary atresia. There is no evidence of the extrahepatic biliary ducts. Note the advanced degree of cirrhosis of the liver. For surgical correction of biliary atresia to be successful it is essential that the procedure is carried out before three months of age. In the 'uncorrectable' type a portoenterostomy should be performed.

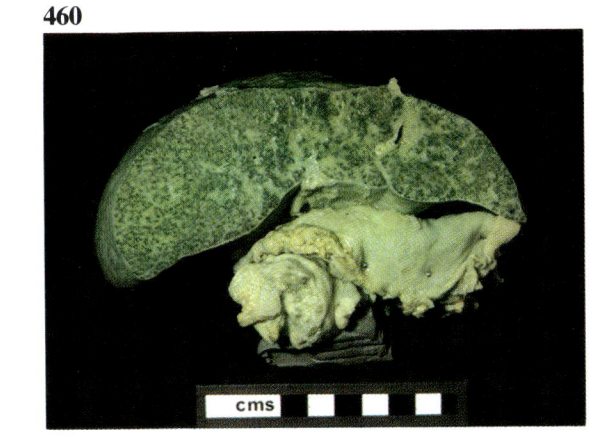

461 Biliary atresia. Photomicrograph of a liver biopsy showing widening of the portal tracts by proliferating small bile ductules and fibrous tissue. Although there is fibrous linking of adjacent portal tracts, cirrhosis has not yet developed. Bile stasis is seen in the large portal tract (*PAS × 40*).

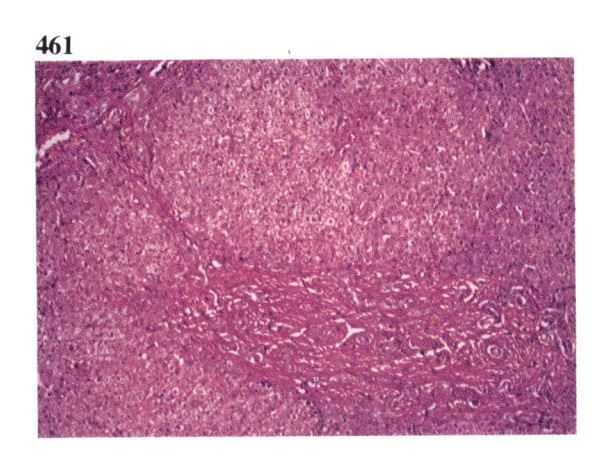

462 Choledochal cyst. Necropsy specimen showing the cystic dilatation of the common bile duct, the collapsed and fibrotic gall bladder and the greenish cirrhotic liver. Treatment of choice is excision of the choledochal cyst and Roux-en-Y choledochojejunostomy.

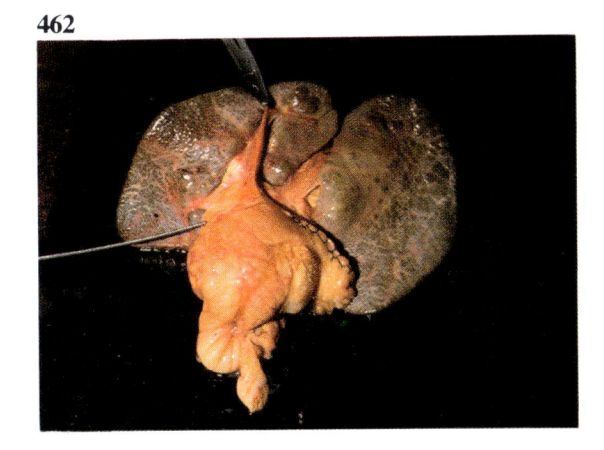

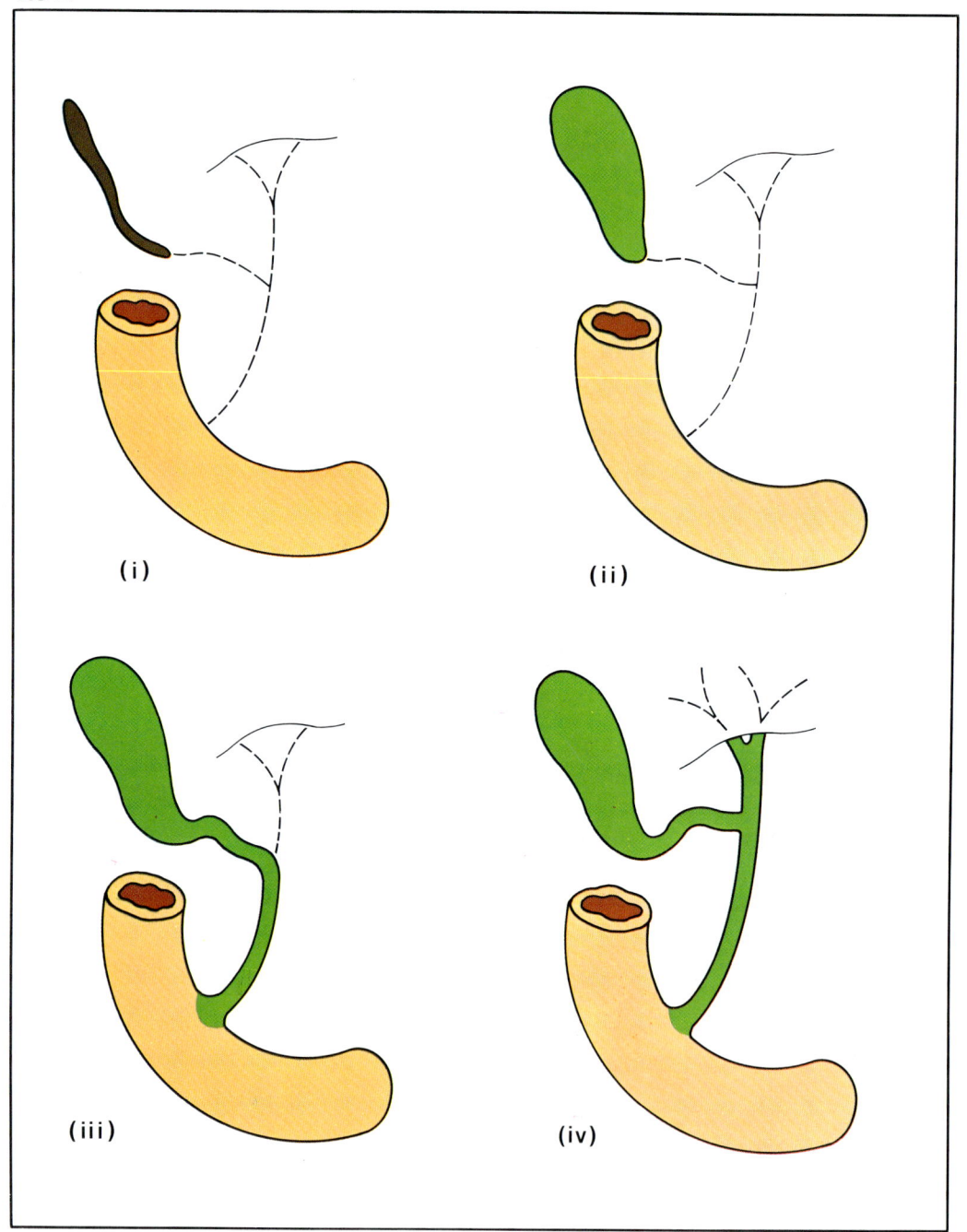

463 Biliary atresia and choledochal cyst.
a) 'Uncorrectable' form.
  i) atresia of the entire extrahepatic bile ducts with a fibrotic remnant of the gall bladder.
  ii) atresia of the extrahepatic bile ducts with a patent gall bladder containing mucus only.
  iii) patent gall bladder and common bile duct with atresia of the hepatic ducts.
  iv) normal extrahepatic biliary system with intrahepatic biliary atresia.

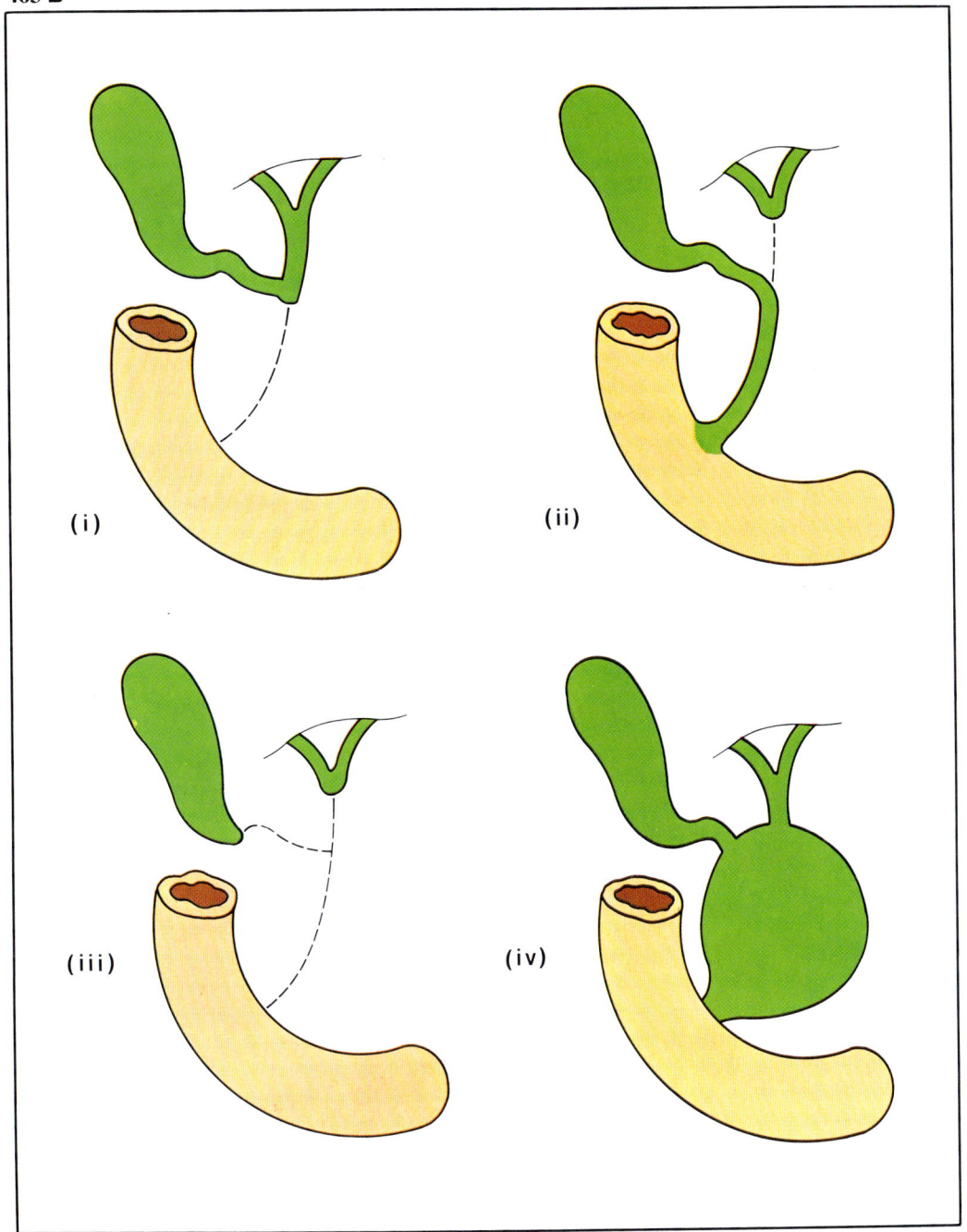

b) correctable form:
  i) patent gall bladder and proximal bile ducts with atresia of the common bile duct.
  ii) patent gall bladder and common duct with atresia of the common hepatic duct. The right and left hepatic ducts in the porta hepatis are patent.
  iii) patent gall bladder with atresia of the common hepatic and common bile ducts but with patent hepatic ducts in the porta hepatis.
  iv) cystic dilatation of the common bile duct (choledochal cyst).

464 Neonatal hepatitis. Photomicrograph of a liver biopsy showing extensive nucleated giant-cell transformation, ballooning of the cytoplasm and rosette formation. Foci of extramedullary haematopoesis is seen. Kupffer's cells are prominent (*PAS × 100*).

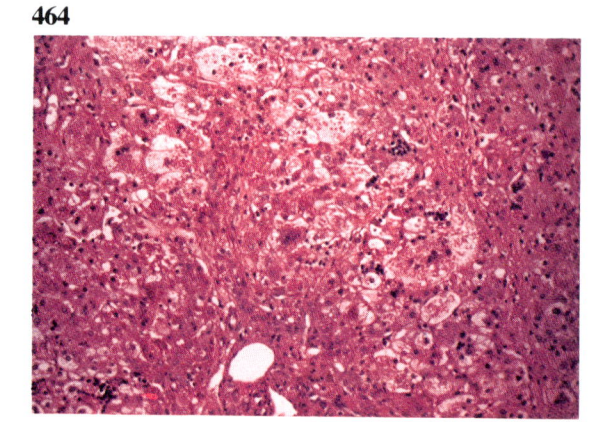

465 Congenital hepatic cyst. Large solitary cyst in the right lobe of the liver. Usually asymptomatic except for presence of a large mass in the right hypochondrium. More frequent in the female. Usually easily resectable especially if superficially situated.

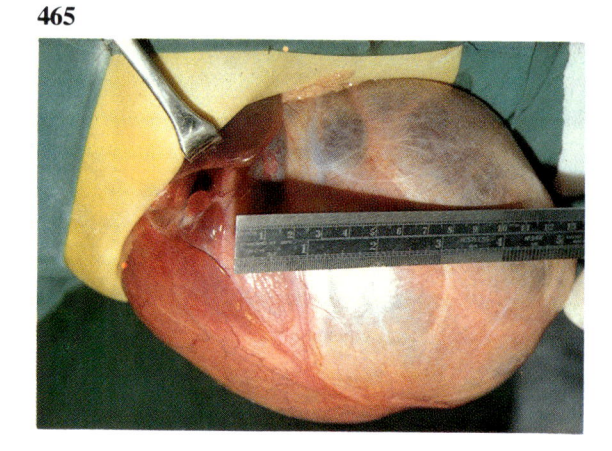

466 Multilocular liver cyst. A large cyst attached to the inferior surface of the right lobe of the liver in a newborn infant. Enucleation of the cyst was easily accomplished.

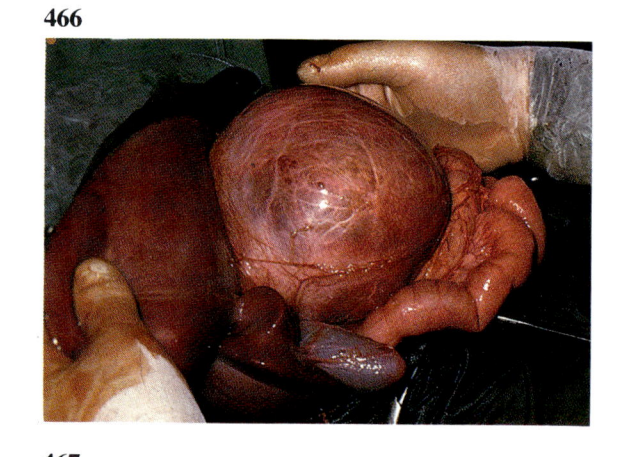

467 Hamartoma of the liver. Presents in the neonatal period with a large mass in the right lobe of the liver. Usually clearly demarcated from surrounding normal liver tissue. Excision should be performed mainly because of problems related to the size of the lesion.

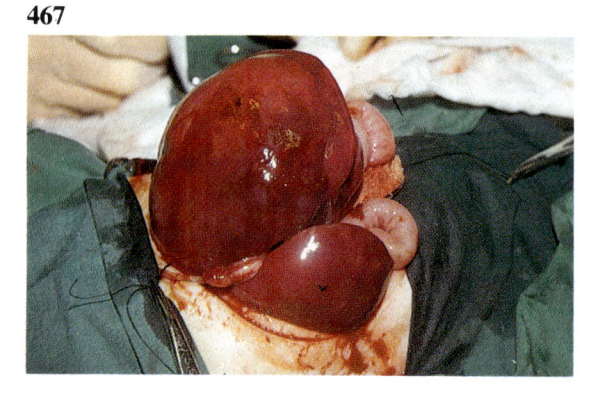

468 Hepatoblastoma. Most cases present before three years of age. More commonly involves the right lobe of the liver. Thrombocytosis is commonly present. Alphafoetoprotein is elevated in two-thirds of the cases. Ultrasonography reveals solid mass. Hepatic angiography shows a 'tumour' circulation in the right lobe of the liver, with extension of the lesion across the midline into the left lobe.

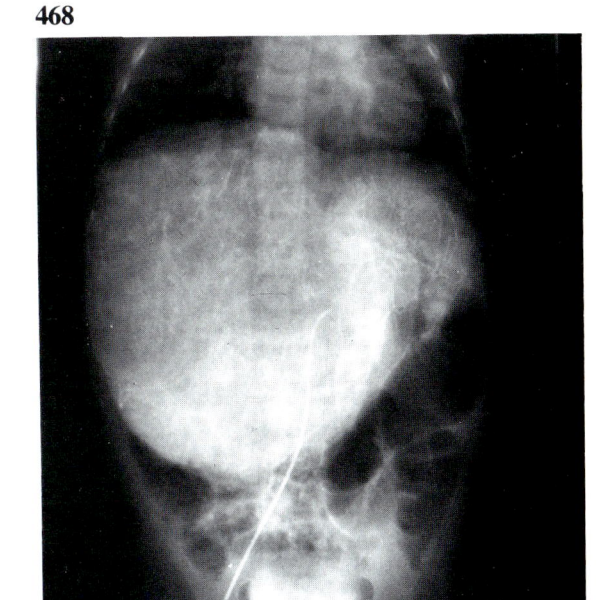

469 and 470 Hepatoblastoma. A large yellowish mass involving most of the right lobe of the liver is evident. Resection, if possible, should be performed. Radiotherapy and chemotherapy will often reduce the size of an 'inoperable' tumour and make subsequent surgery feasible.

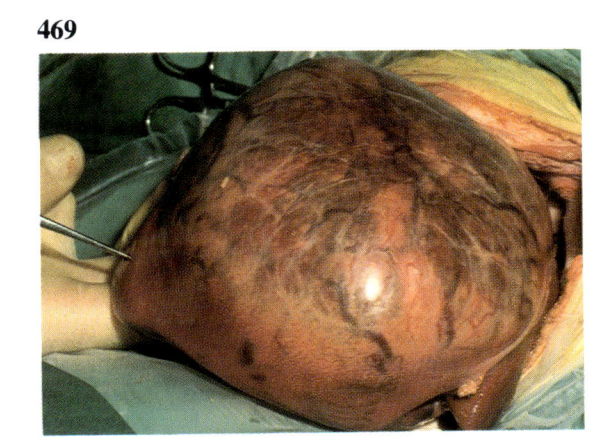

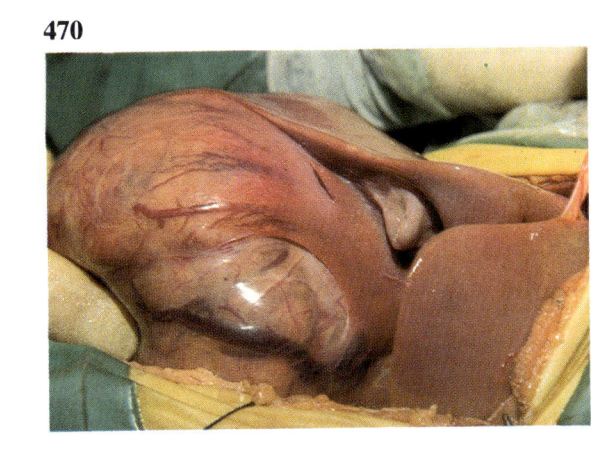

471 Hepatocellular carcinoma. Most cases of this rare condition in paediatrics appear between 10 to 15 years of age. Tumour is often multicentric so that hepatic resection is rarely possible. Frequently involves a liver with underlying cirrhosis. Overall prognosis is poor.

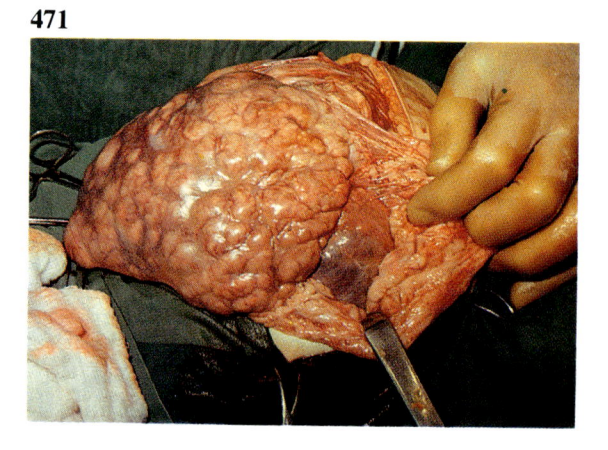

472 Absent gall bladder. May occur as a rare isolated asymptomatic abnormality. Often associated with other anomalies such as absence of common bile duct. Important to exclude intrahepatic gall bladder and secondary atrophy after cholecystitis.

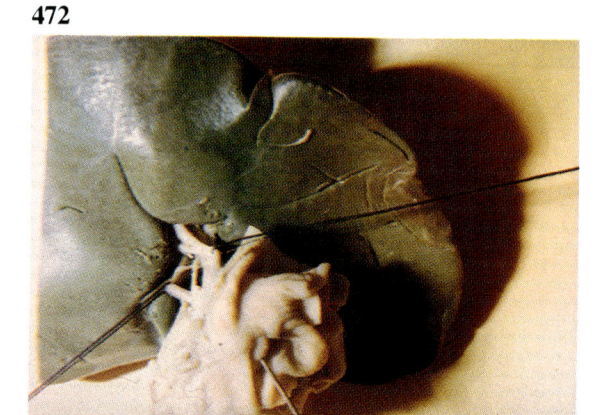

473 Septate gall bladder. May contain one or more chambers. Septum is more commonly longitudinal than transverse. May produce symptoms such as recurrent right hypochondrial pain and fat dyspepsia.

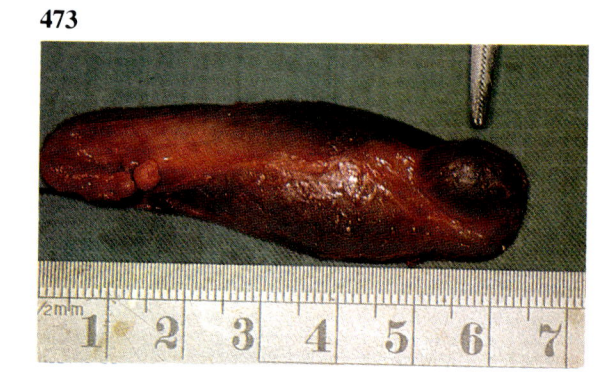

474 Acute acalculous cholecystitis. The tensely distended gall bladder contains clear fluid. Usually a complication of severe illness or injury. Presenting features are jaundice and pyrexia. The gall bladder may be palpable on abdominal examination. Treatment of choice is simple tube cholecystostomy.

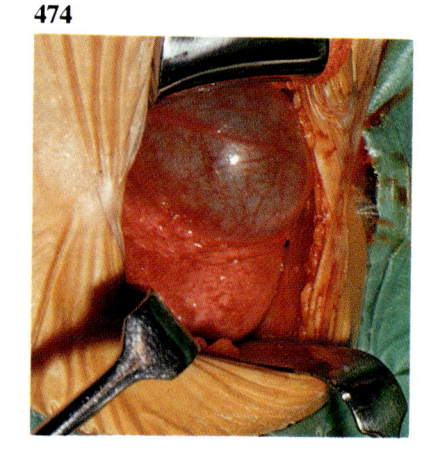

475 Spontaneous perforation of the common bile duct. Idiopathic perforation at the junction between the cystic duct and common hepatic duct occurs in the infant between the ages of one week and two months. There is mild jaundice, pale stools and progressive abdominal distension caused by increasing biliary ascites. Treatment consists of drainage of the area of perforation and tube cholecystostomy (for postoperative contrast studies).

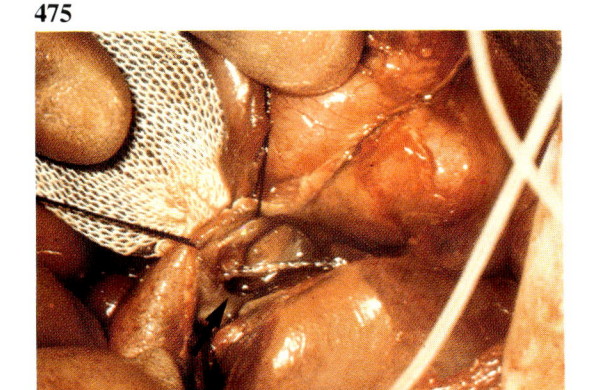

476 Cholelithiasis. Cholecystogram showing presence of filling defects in the gall bladder. May be associated with haemolytic disease (sickle-cell disease, spherocytosis, thalassaemia), congenital malformation of the biliary tract (choledochal cyst), but most appear to be of idiopathic origin. Symptoms consist of right hypochondrial pain, nausea, vomiting and occasional fat dyspepsia. Jaundice is fairly common.

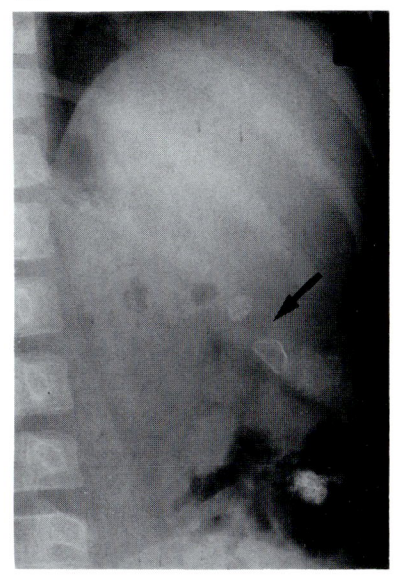

477 Cholelithiasis. Ultrasound scan showing gall stones and 'biliary mud' within the gall bladder.

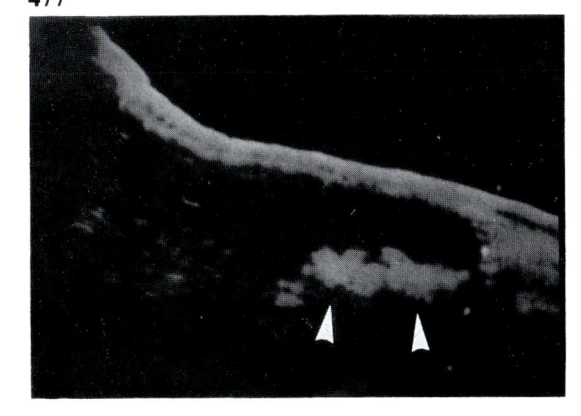

478 Jaundice in sickle-cell anaemia. Genetically determined abnormality of the polypeptide chain of haemoglobin. Usually there is a mild jaundice (mainly unconjugated hyperbilirubinaemia) caused by rapid haemolysis. Extreme hyperbilirubinaemia may occur as a result of viral hepatitis related to transfusions or choledocholithiasis. However, some cases are poorly explained and tend to run a benign course with spontaneous resolution in four to six weeks.

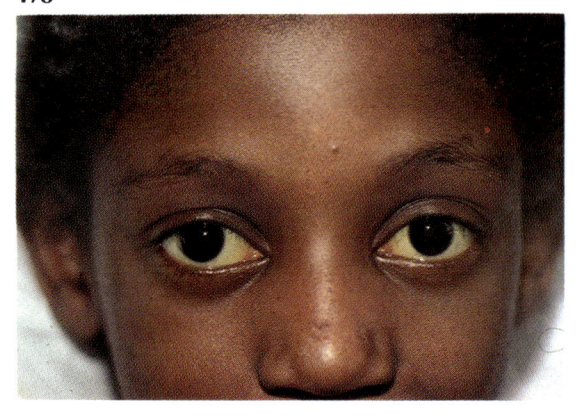

479 Liver abscess. Large solitary abscess in the central portion of the right lobe (may be multiple). Infecting organism may be either aerobic (E. coli, staphylococcus, salmonella, etc) anaerobic (bacteriodes) or mixed. Symptoms include right hypochondrial pain, pyrexia with rigors and hepatomegaly and jaundice. Liver scan (Tc^{99}) or ultrasonography assist with diagnosis. Treatment is by surgical drainage and intensive broad-spectrum antibiotic therapy.

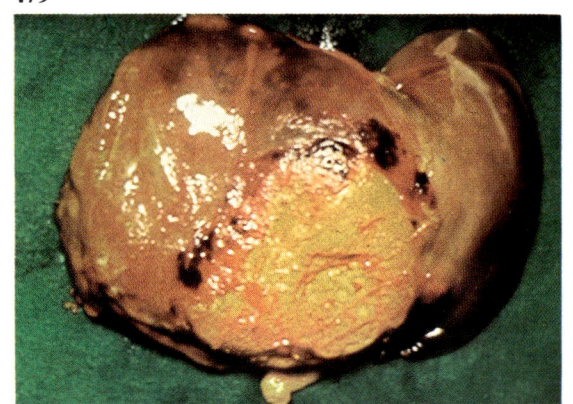

480 Hydatid cyst. Caused by infection with Echinococcus. Definitive host is the dog. Man, sheep and cattle are intermediate hosts. Patient presents with dull right upper quadrant pain and a large tense smoothly rounded swelling continuous with the liver. Rupture can occur. Diagnosis by complement fixation test, xray appearance of calcification in the ectocyst or hepatic scintiscan.

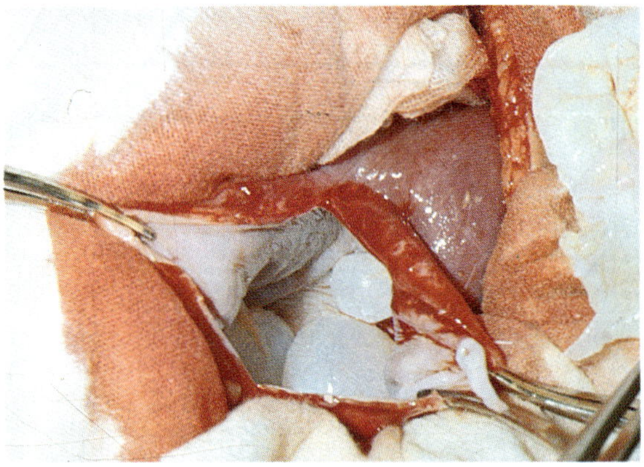

33 The pancreas

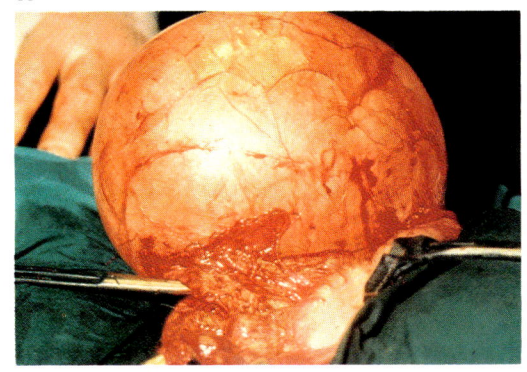

481 Congenital pancreatic cyst. Extremely rare. May be unilocular or multilocular. Lined with epithelium and acinar tissue. Body and tail of pancreas most commonly involved. Symptoms are caused by size or are secondary to compression on neighbouring structures.

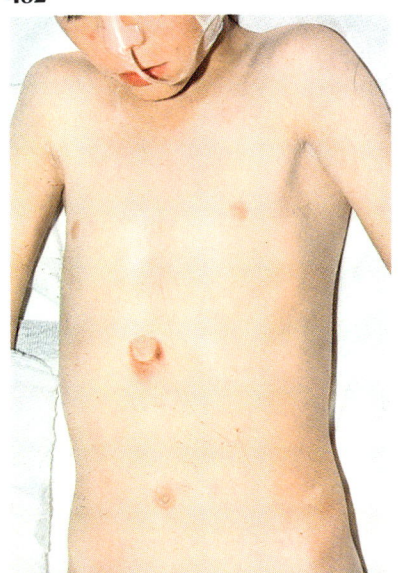

482 Pancreatic trauma. Blunt abdominal trauma is the commonest cause of pancreatitis in childhood. The child frequently gives a history of a fall over the handlebars of a bicycle. Bruising may be evident in the epigastrium at the site of impact. Some time later (days to weeks) symptoms of epigastric pain, nausea and vomiting develop. A mass may be palpable in the epigastrium (pseudocyst).

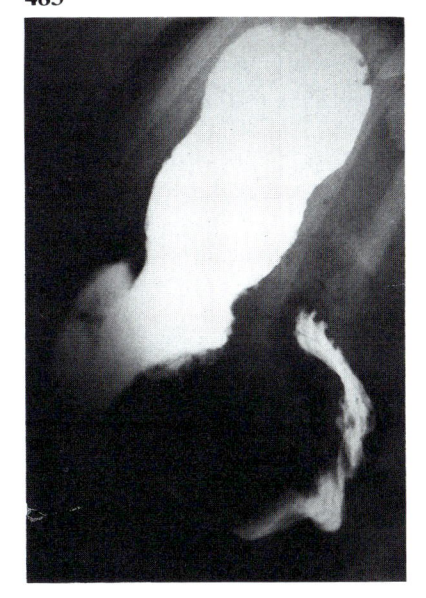

483 Pancreatic pseudocyst. Sixty per cent of cases arise secondary to abdominal trauma. Barium meal shows widening compression and anterior displacement of the duodenal C-loop. The stomach may be displaced superiorly and anteriorly and the colon downwards and forwards.

484 Islet cell adenoma. Rare cause of hypoglycaemia in infancy and childhood. Symptoms may be severe and unremitting or mild and intermittent. The adenoma may be solitary, round, discrete and encapsulated or multiple (14 per cent): 25 per cent are located in the head of the pancreas and 75 per cent in the body and tail. The cells of the adenoma are primarily insulin-secreting B cells. Angiography may be helpful in locating the site of the tumour preoperatively.

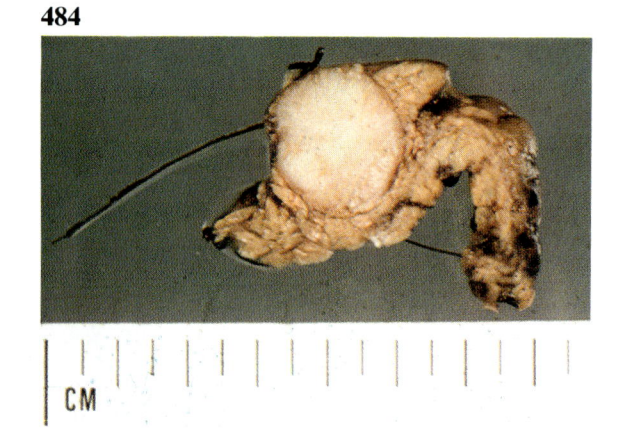

485 'Annular pancreas'. Almost always associated with an underlying abnormality in the second part of the duodenum (stenosis, atresia). The pancreatic tissue extends in a ring around the second part of the duodenum. The proximal duodenum is usually distended and the walls hypertrophied. Treatment is by duodenoduodenostomy (as in duodenal atresia) to bypass the ring of pancreatic tissue.

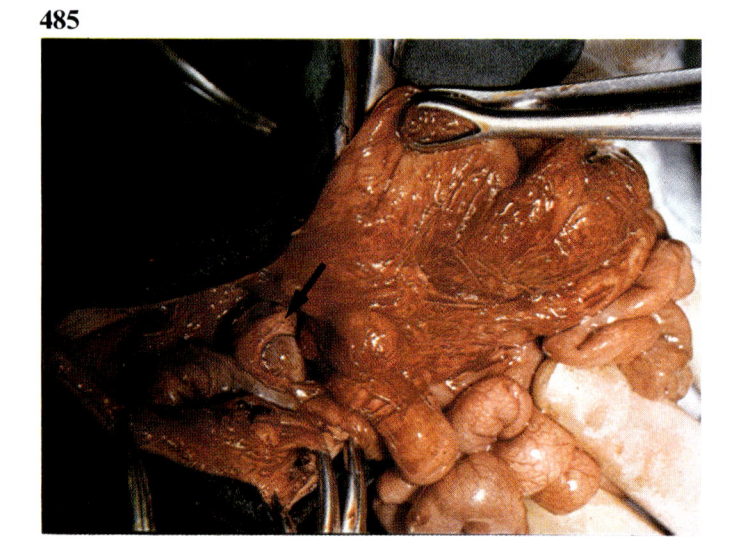

34 The spleen and portal hypertension

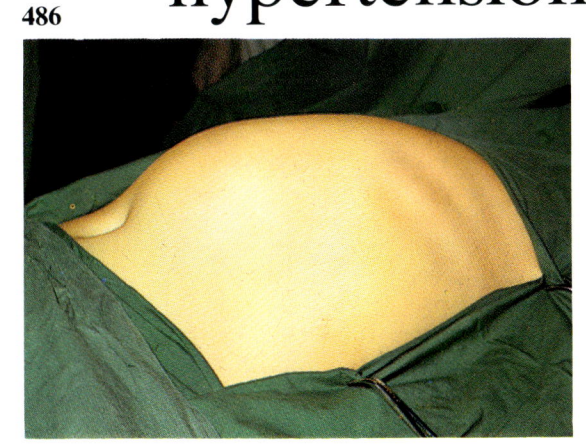

486 Splenic cyst. Rare cause of an asymptomatic dull mass in the left hypochondrium. Usually solitary and unilocular. In one-quarter of the reported cases calcification in the wall permits radiological diagnosis. Splenectomy is required for large cysts.

487 and 488 Splenic cyst. Operative appearance (**487**) of the large serous cyst protruding from the hilar aspect of the spleen. The cyst wall has been opened (**488**) to show the partially lined squamous epithelial inner surface.

489 Ruptured spleen. Traumatic rupture of the spleen after blunt abdominal trauma; one of the commonest accidents in childhood requiring laparotomy. The classical features are abdominal pain, guarding and tenderness in the left hypochondrium, left shoulder tip pain, together with signs of shock and blood loss. Minor lacerations of the spleen may present less dramatically and may be successfully managed conservatively. Lateral decubitus xray with barium in the stomach shows displacement of the greater curvature of the stomach away from the lower rib margin by perisplenic haematoma. The diagnosis can be confirmed by radioisotope scan.

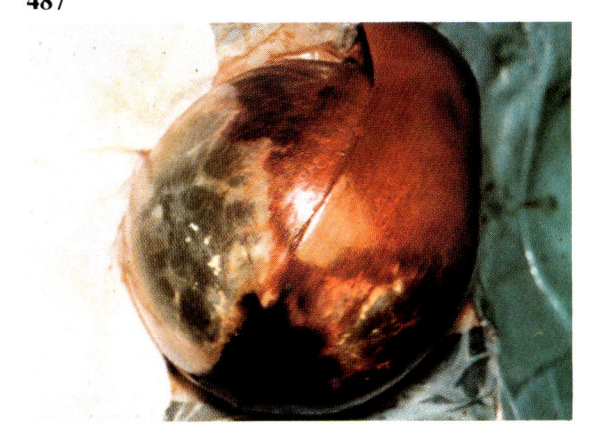

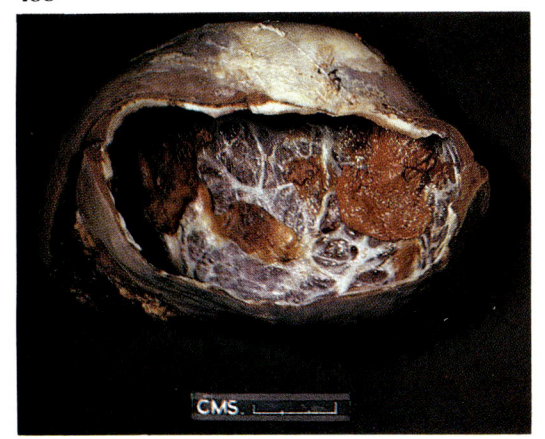

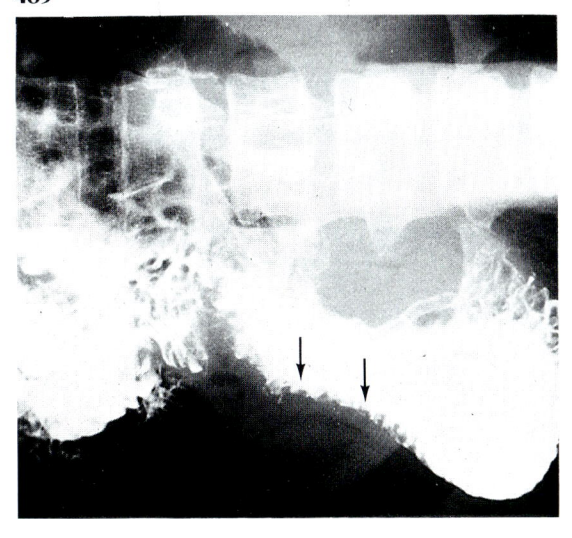

490 Hypersplenism. Haematological indications for splenectomy include:
A Haemolytic disorders.
  i) Hereditary spherocytosis,
  ii) Acquired haemolytic anaemia,
  iii) Selected cases of thallasaemia major and sickle-cell anaemia.
B Hypersplenic syndromes.
  i) Without splenomegaly – chronic idiopathic thrombocytopenic purpura.
  ii) With splenomegaly, e.g. Banti syndrome, splenic neutropenia and pancytopenia, Gaucher's disease, etc.

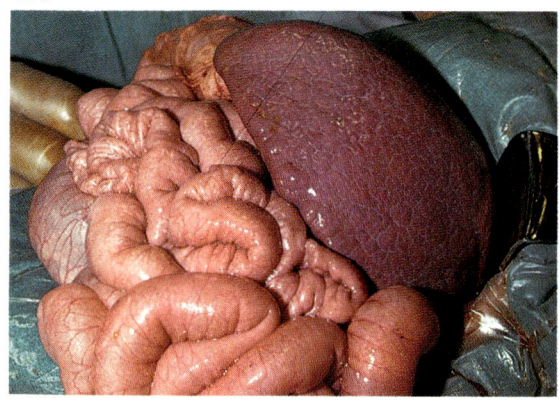

Idiopathic thrombocytopenic purpura. Characterised by petechiae and ecchymoses in the skin and mucous membranes, e.g. lips. There may be internal haemorrhage, e.g. gastrointestinal, renal or central nervous system. Platelet count markedly reduced (below 50,000).

491 a) Submucous haemorrhage in the upper lip and on gingival border.

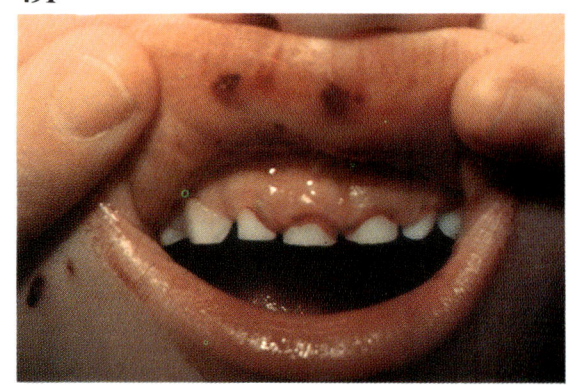

492 b) Purpuric rash on hands. Note subungual haemorrhage on left index finger.

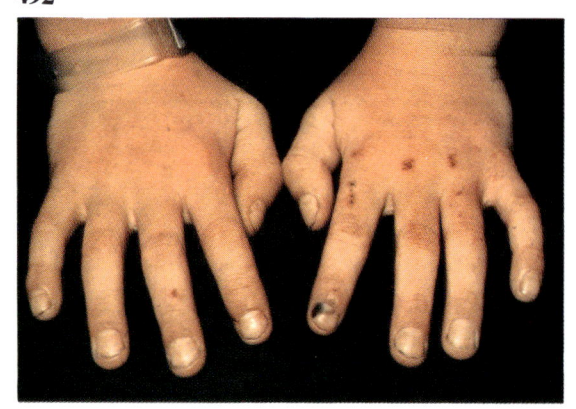

493 Multiple accessory spleens. If splenectomy is performed for a blood dyscrasia a careful search should be made for accessory spleens in the gastrosplenic ligament, greater omentum, splenic pedicle, along the main trunk of the splenic vein, in the mesenteries of the small and large intestine and in the pouch of Douglas. Failure to remove these splenunculi can lead to recurrence of the disease.

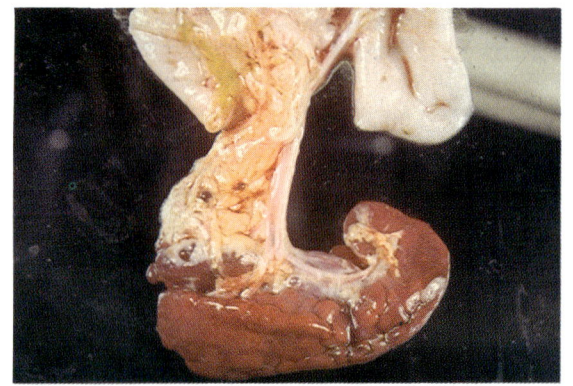

494 Hodgkin's disease. Splenectomy is carried out during staging laparotomy in patients with Hodgkin's disease. Other diagnostic procedures during the laparotomy include excision of any abnormal lymph nodes, random biopsy of para-aortic, portal and splenic hilar nodes, liver biopsy and bone-marrow biopsy.

495 Portal hypertension. Arises secondary to obstruction to the portal venous blood flow caused by:
a) Prehepatic causes, e.g. splenic or portal vein thrombosis.
b) Intrahepatic causes, i.e. cirrhosis (hepatic, biliary, metabolic).
c) Posthepatic causes, e.g. congestive cardiac failure, Budd-Chiari syndrome.
Caput medusae indicates portal hypertension and is signified by the presence of large dilated cutaneous venous collaterals carrying blood away from the umbilicus to the systemic circulation. Ascites is also present.

496 Oesophageal varices. Barium swallow showing linear filling defects in the lower third of the oesophagus. Varices may also be seen in the fundus of the stomach. Haemorrhage from oesophageal varices can be torrential and rapidly exsanguinating. It carries a 10 per cent mortality rate.

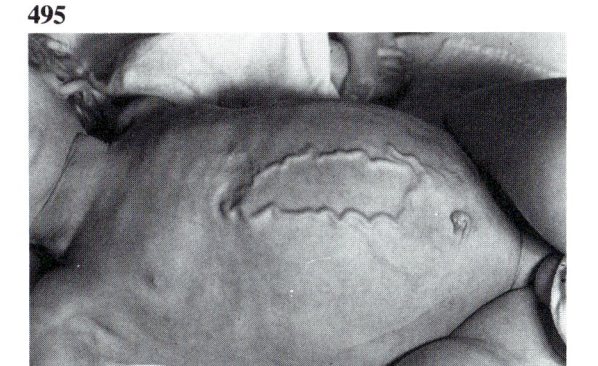

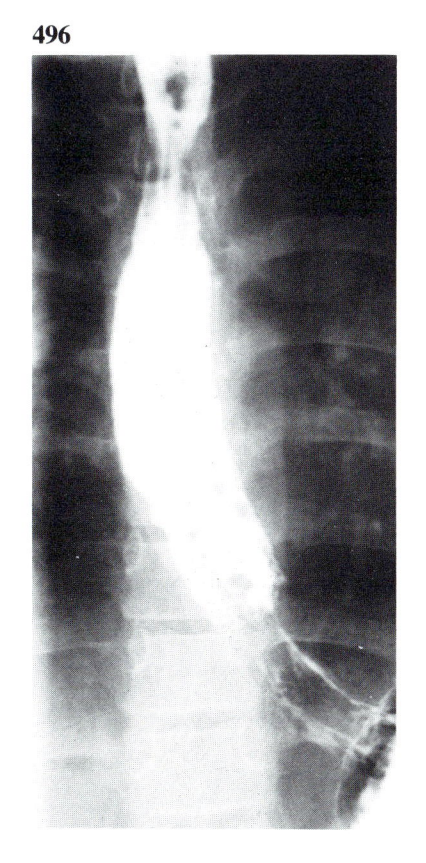

497 Oesophageal varices. Endoscopic appearance of the distal oesophagus showing enormously dilated vascular channels lying immediately deep to the bulging mucosa of the lower third of the oesophagus. Sclerotherapy by perivascular or intravascular injection, via the endoscope, may be carried out as a therapeutic measure in bleeding oesophageal varices.

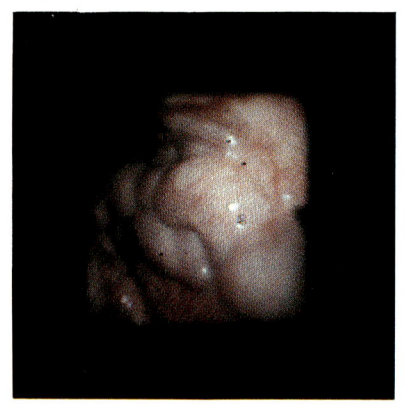

498 Splenoportogram. Contrast is injected into the spleen after the splenic pulp pressure has been measured. Xray shows a dilated splenic vein ending abruptly at the junction with the portal vein (portal vein thrombosis). Note the leash of vessels around the lower end of the oesophagus (oesophageal varices).

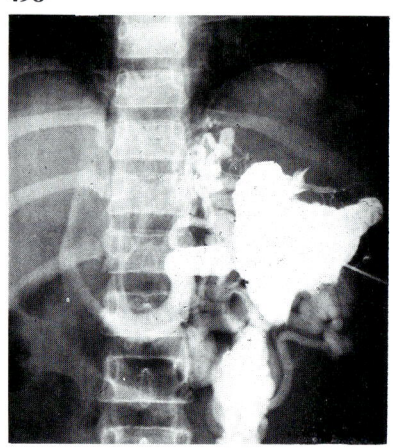

499 Gastric fundal varices. Splenic portovenography showing the dilated tortuous leash of vessels in the fundus of the stomach.

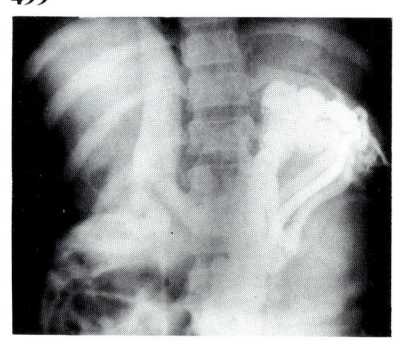

500 Portal vein thrombosis. Necropsy specimen showing the thrombosis and complete obliteration of the portal vein, the dilated splenic vein and the splenomegaly. In infancy the portal vein thrombosis may develop secondary to umbilical sepsis, exchange transfusion or catheterisation, or severe septicaemia.

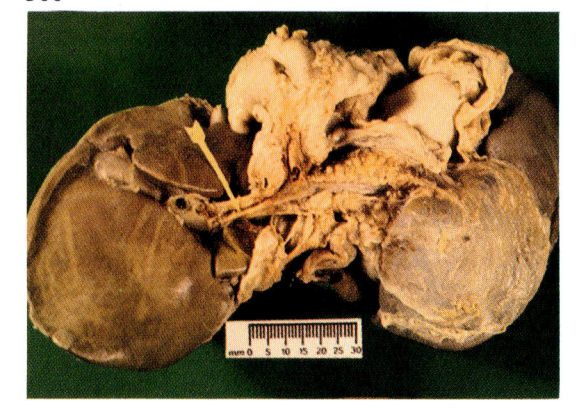

35 Adrenal gland

501 Adrenal haemorrhage. Massive adrenal haemorrhage usually occurs within the first week of life, probably related to birth trauma. A large volume of blood has accumulated within the capsule of the gland. Blood may leak into the retroperitoneal tissues and even into the peritoneal cavity. Seventy per cent of cases occur on the right side: 5 to 10 per cent are bilateral. Treatment is conservative.

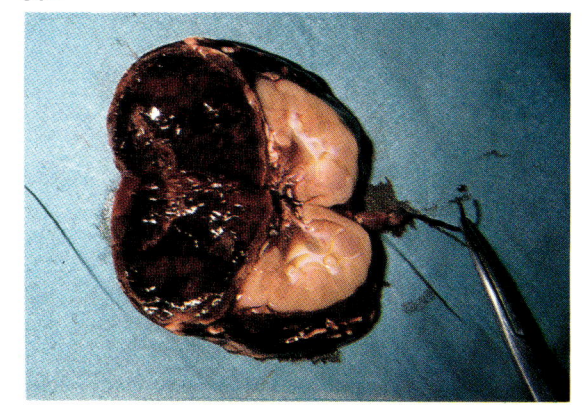

502 Adrenal calcification. Microscopic appearance of extensive calcification of the adrenal gland. Almost always secondary to adrenal haemorrhage. Radiological calcification of an adrenal haemorrhage may be seen as early as 12 days after birth.

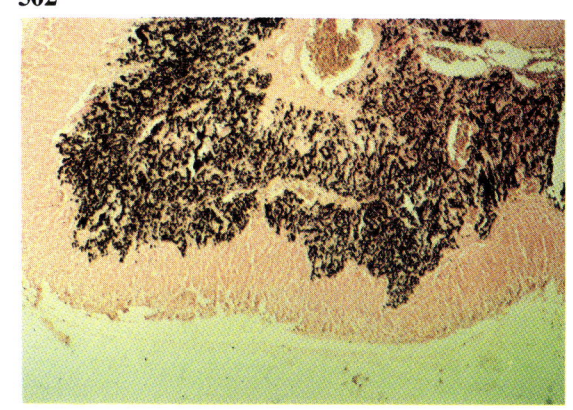

503 Phaeochromocytoma. Rare tumour of childhood. Most are found in the adrenal and abdominal areas. Ninety per cent of childhood cases present with sustained hypertension, but paroxysmal attacks do occur. Attacks of flushing, headaches, blurred vision and sweating occur. Plasma catecholamine levels are raised.

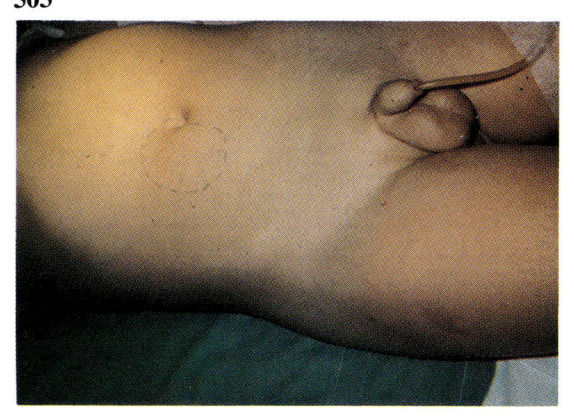

504 Phaeochromocytoma. A discrete tumour is seen in the para-aortic region below the right kidney. There is a high incidence of multiplicity of the tumours and a meticulous search for additional tumours must be made at laparotomy.

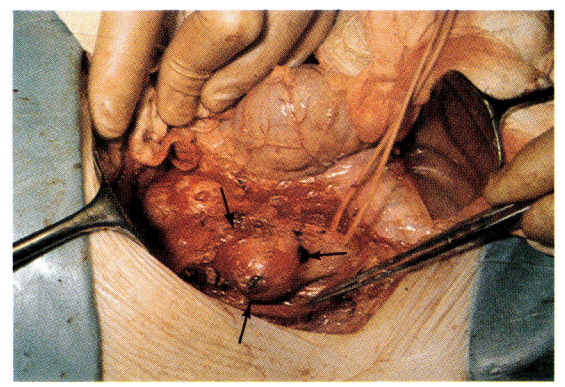

505 Cushing's syndrome. Characteristically an obese, hypotonic, hypertensive infant with an abnormally elevated level of hydrocortisone in the blood. The adrenal lesion may be a functional tumour (carcinoma or adenoma) or bilateral cortical hyperplasia. Pituitary tumour is occasionally present.

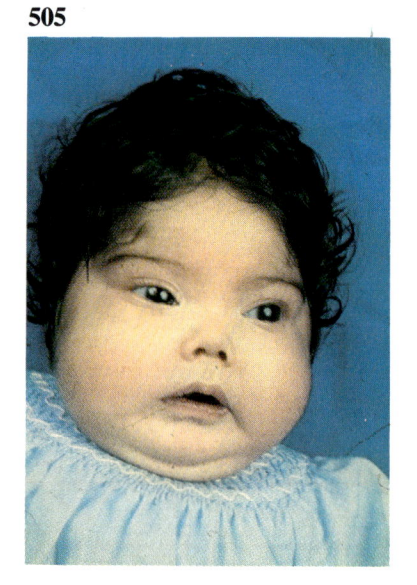

506 Adrenogenital syndrome. Excessive secretion of adrenal androgens during foetal life in the female results in virilisation of the external genitalia. The clitoris is hypertrophied and there is fusion of the labioscrotal folds. Treatment with glucocorticoids early in infancy will prevent progressive virilisation. One-third of patients have 'salt-losing syndrome'.

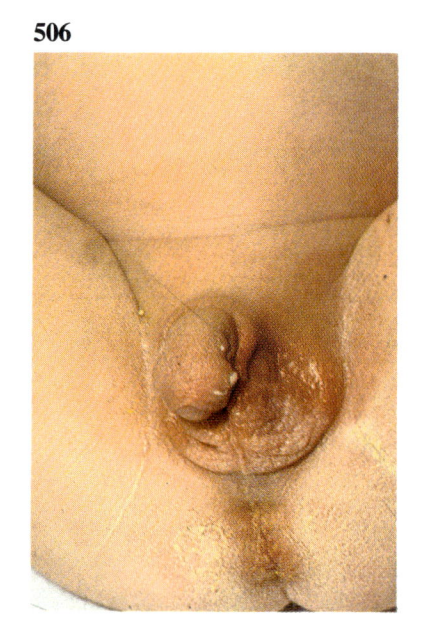

507 Congenital adrenal hyperplasia. A block in the synthesis of cortisol leads to an increased secretion of ACTH by the anterior pituitary because of an impaired negative feedback mechanism. This results in adreno-cortical hyperplasia and an excessive secretion of adrenal androgens. Bilateral enlargement of the adrenal glands in the necropsy specimen is shown.

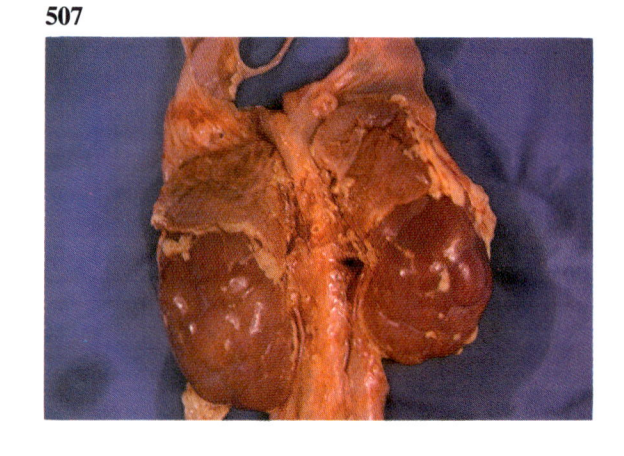

508 Waterhouse-Friderichsen syndrome. Commonly associated with meningococcal septicaemia, but may develop as a complication of any overwhelming infection. The patient suddenly becomes cyanotic and shocked. Skin haemorrhages are commonly present. The infant becomes rapidly moribund. Urgent resuscitation is required with adrenocortical hormone replacement. The extensive subcutaneous haemorrhages are seen in this infant who died from meningococcal septicaemia.

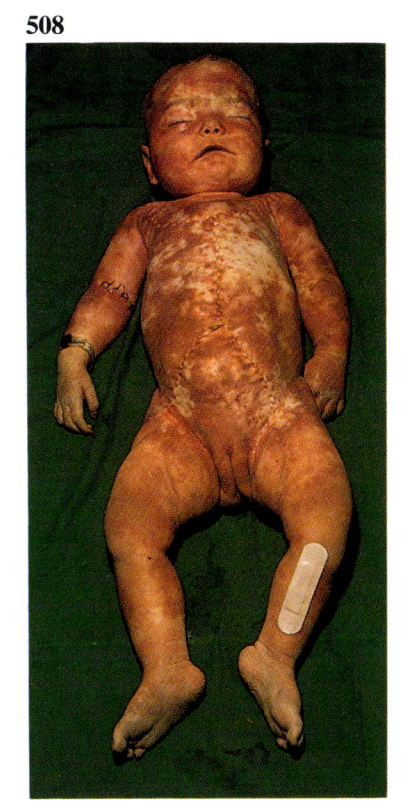

509 Waterhouse-Friderichsen syndrome. Acute adrenal deficiency arises as a result of haemorrhagic necrosis of the adrenal glands. The glands are enlarged and largely replaced by blood clots. The haemorrhage occurs primarily in the medulla and the cortical tissue is stretched out around the periphery.

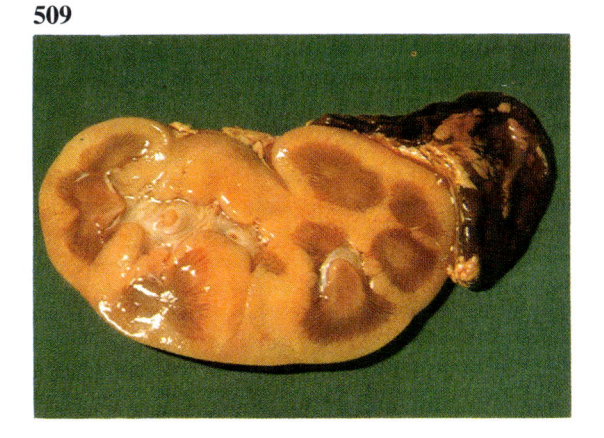

36 Retroperitoneal tumours

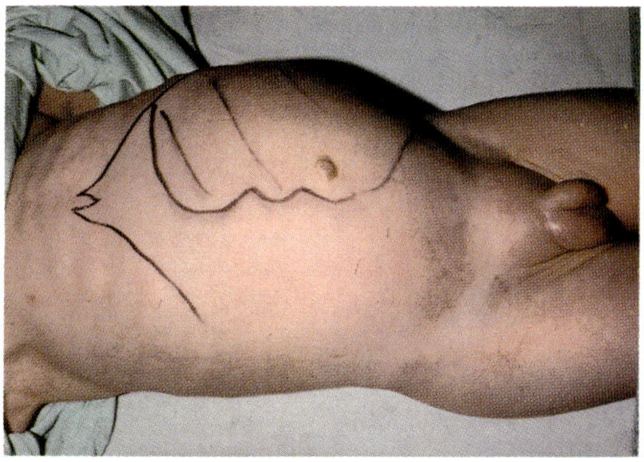

510 Nephroblastoma (Wilms' tumour). Most common intrarenal malignant tumour of childhood. Peak age of incidence is three to four years. Presenting symptom is most frequently an increase in the size of the abdomen or an abdominal mass found incidentally during bathing or on routine physical examination. The mass is firm and smooth and arises out of the flank, but may cross the midline.

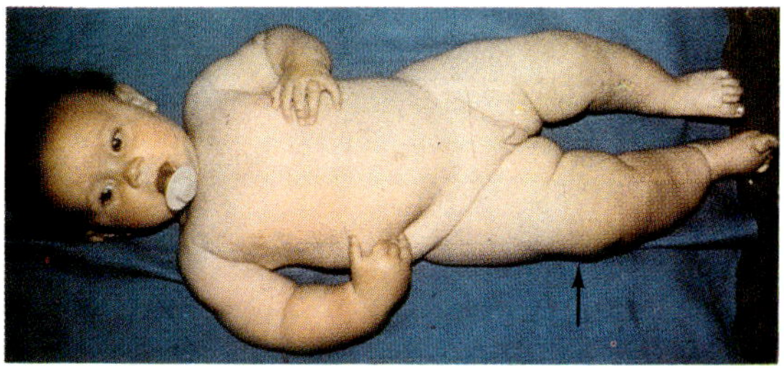

511 Hemihypertrophy. Congenital hemihypertrophy involving either the entire side of the body or confined to a single part (limb, face, tongue) is recognised to be associated with an increased incidence of Wilms' tumour.

512 Aniridia. The association between sporadic congenital aniridia (absence of the iris) and Wilms' tumour is well documented.

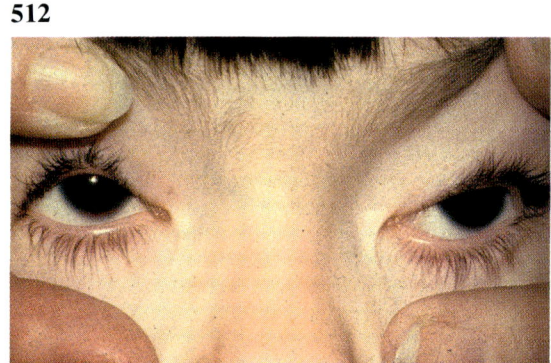

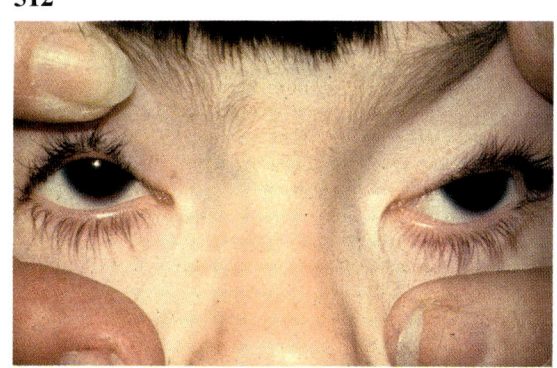

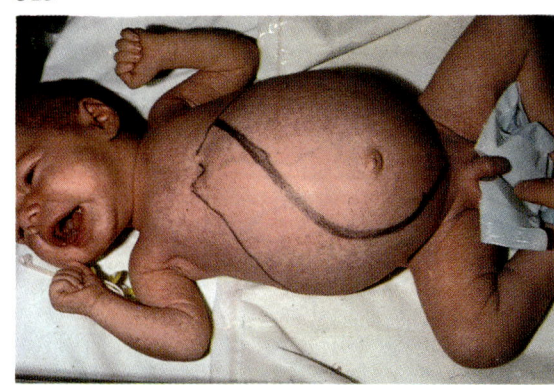

513 Neonatal nephroblastoma (mesoblastic nephroma or foetal renal hamartomas). Associated with an excellent prognosis. Differs from Wilms' tumour in absence of lobulation, necrosis or haemorrhage. Microscopically there is a preponderance of interlacing bundles of spindle cells.

514 Nephroblastoma. An excretory urogram in a child presenting with a large left flank mass. The calyceal pattern of the left kidney shows an intrarenal mass with stretching and distortion of the calyces. The contralateral kidney may also be involved (Stage V disease).

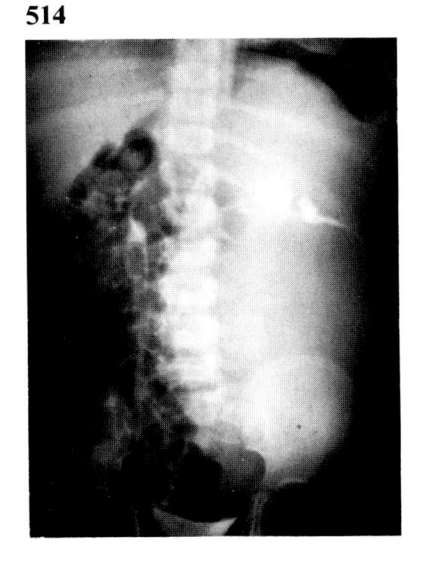

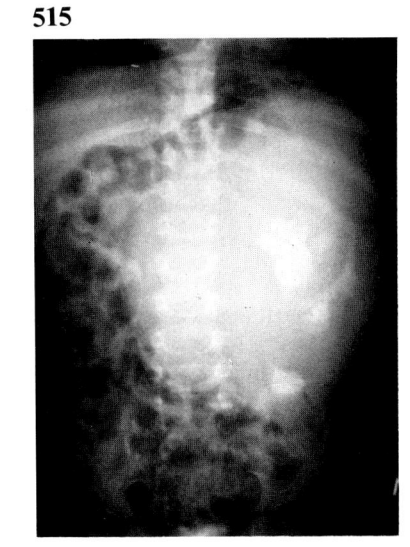

515 Nephroblastoma. The large radio-opaque left abdominal mass shows a completely distorted collecting system on excretory urography.

516 Nephroblastoma. If renal function is severely impaired no excretion may be evident on the involved side. Note the area of calcification in the non-opacified right renal mass.

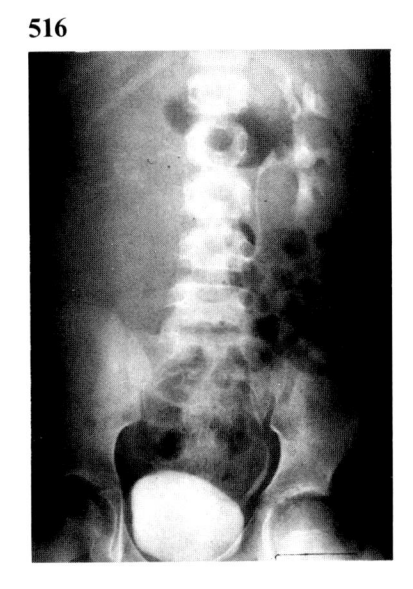

517 Wilms' tumour. Ultrasonogram of an abdominal mass showing areas of solid tumour tissue interspersed by cystic areas.

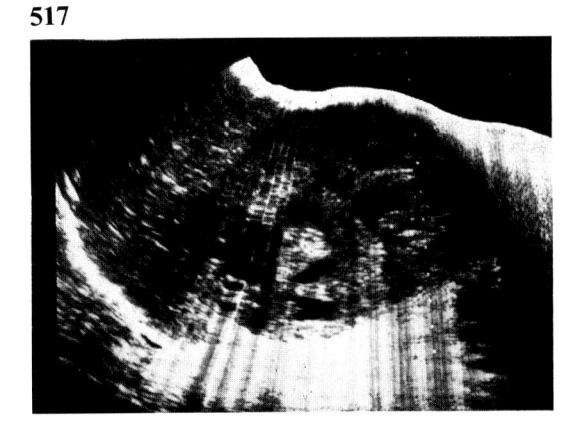

518 Selective renal angiography. Useful in selected cases where the diagnosis is in doubt on conventional studies. The right renal angiogram shows a filling defect in the upper lateral aspect of the kidney.

519 Pulmonary metastasis. Chest xray of a child presenting with an abdominal mass showing two discrete 'cannonball' metastases in the lungs – one in the right lower lobe and the second in the left midzone.

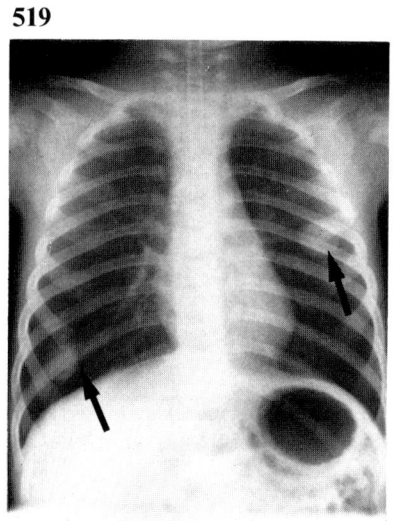

520 Pulmonary metastases. Chest xray in a child with an abdominal mass presenting with severe respiratory embarrassment. Both lung fields are extensively involved with metastatic tumour.

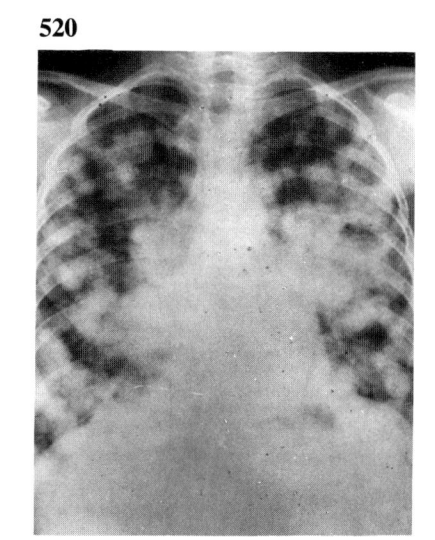

521 Recurrent nephroblastoma. Extensive intraperitoneal metastatic disease with massive ascites and numerous prominent superficial veins on the anterior abdominal wall indicating obstruction to the inferior vena cava.

522 Nephroblastoma. Resected specimen showing a large tumour with areas of haemorrhage and necrosis occupying the lower part of the kidney and separated by a fibrous pseudocapsule from the remaining normal rim of upper pole. Prognosis with surgery, radiotherapy and chemotherapy is relatively good.

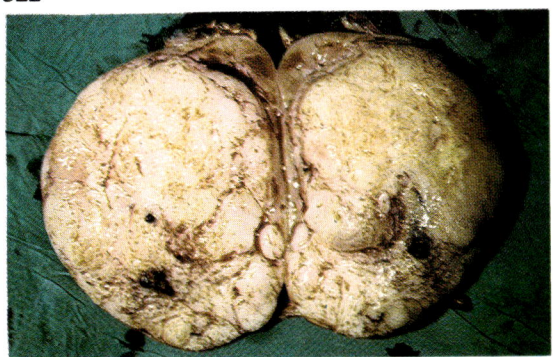

523 Nephroblastoma. Resected specimen showing extensive recent haemorrhage into the centre of the tumour. Gross haematuria is uncommon, but microscopic haematuria occurs in approximately 25 per cent of patients.

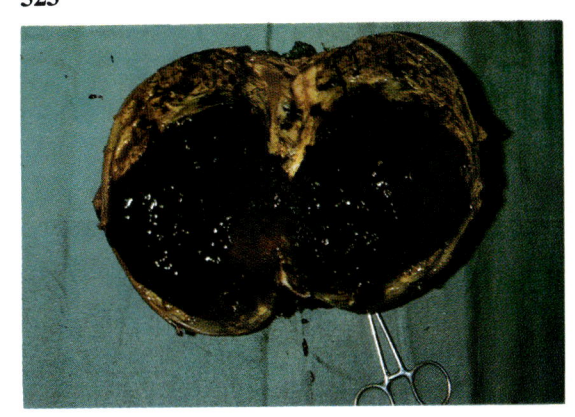

524 Nephroblastoma. Microscopic appearance of a tumour showing blastematous tissue with tubular and glomeruloid differentiation against a background of undifferentiated stoma (*H&E × 40*).

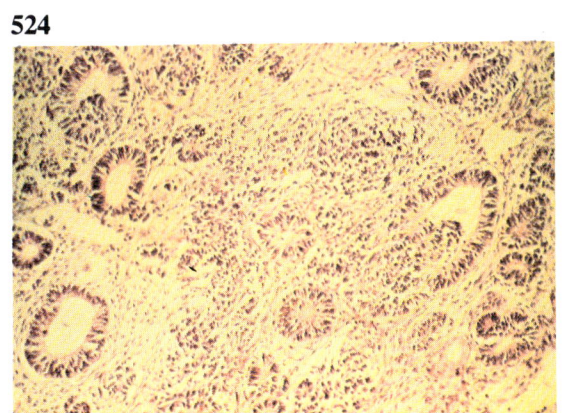

525 Neuroblastoma. Most cases present before five years of age, with peak incidence at two years. The tumour arises in sympathetic neural tissue – over 50 per cent occur in the retroperitoneal region (adrenal medulla or sympathetic ganglion). The tumour tends to be ill-defined, nodular, fixed to surrounding structures and often extends across the midline. Catecholamine excretion in the urine is elevated. (*VMA; HVA*).

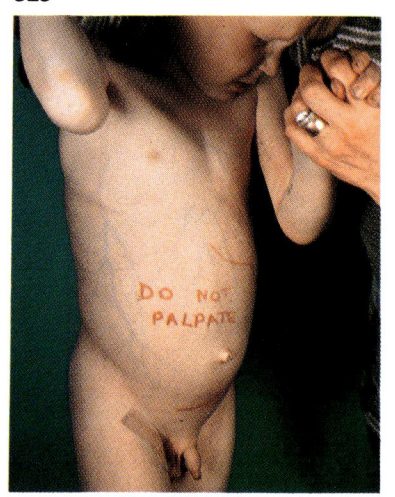

526 Infantile neuroblastoma. Stage IVS. The tumour is found in infants less than one year old in whom metastatic disease is confined to the liver, skin or bone marrow. The prognosis for these infants is excellent.

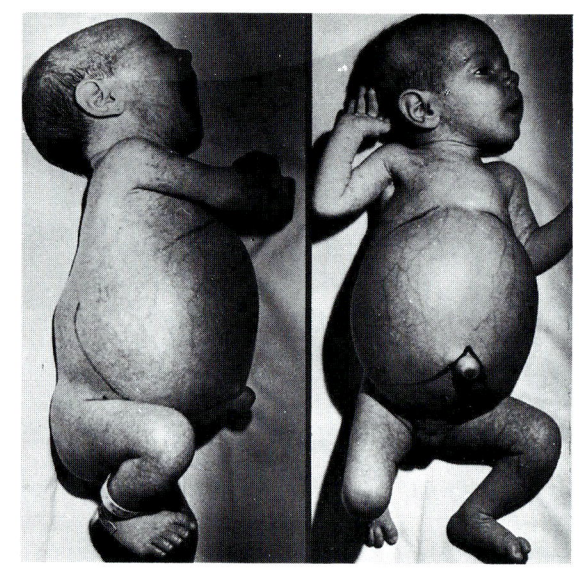

527 Neuroblastoma. Abdominal xray in a child presenting with a left flank mass showing fine stippled calcification in the left suprarenal region. Calcification occurs in about 50 per cent of neuroblastomas, but in less than 10 per cent of nephroblastomas.

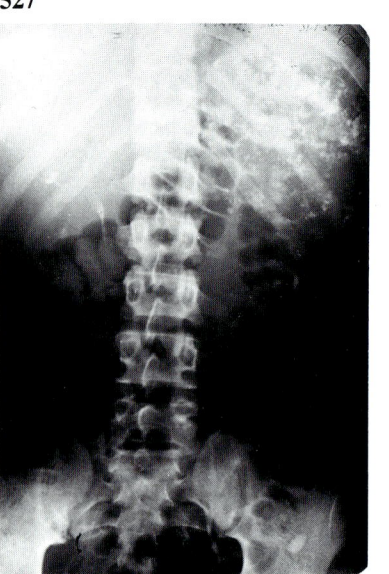

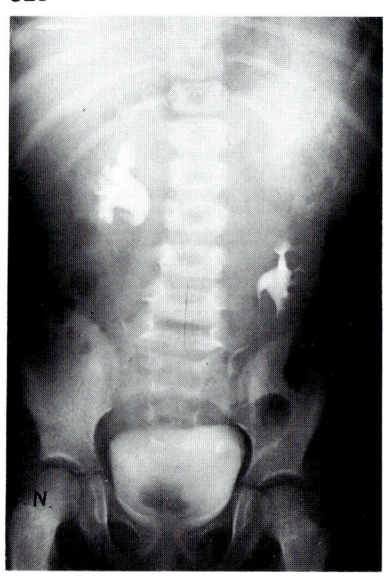

528 Neuroblastoma. An excretory urogram showing the presence of a finely calcified left suprarenal mass with inferior displacement of the left kidney.

529 Neuroblastoma. Operative view of a large adrenal tumour displacing the kidney inferiorly and laterally and causing superior and anterior displacement of the transverse colon.

530 Neuroblastoma. Resected specimen of a large adrenal tumour. Note irregular areas of haemorrhage and necrosis. Microscopically composed of small round cells with rosette formation and neurofibrils in well-differentiated cases.

531 Ganglioneuroma. More benign counterpart of the neuroblastoma and is composed largely of mature ganglion cells. May present with intractable diarrhoea caused by secretion of vasoactive intestinal peptides by the tumour.

532 Metastatic neuroblastoma. Skull xray showing punched out lytic areas in the frontal bone. Note also separation of sutures caused by metastatic disease.

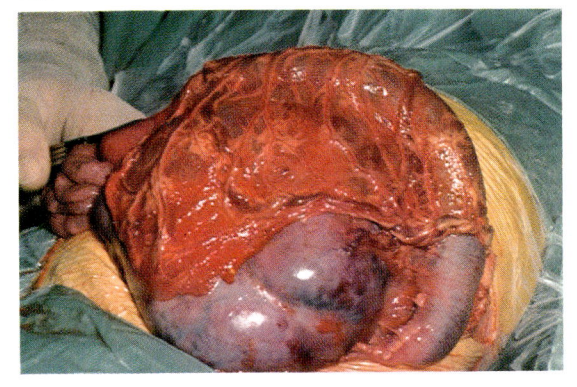

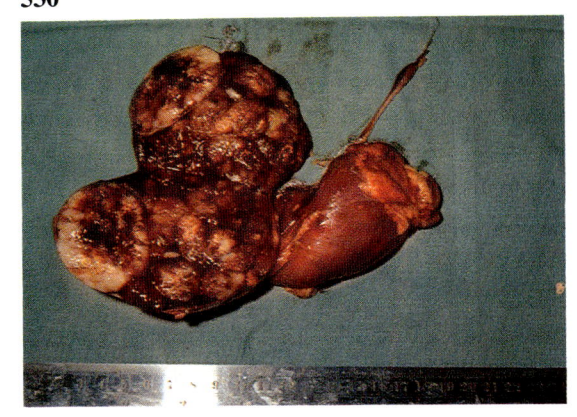

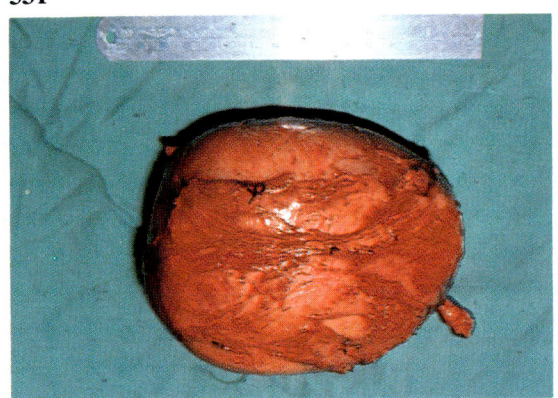

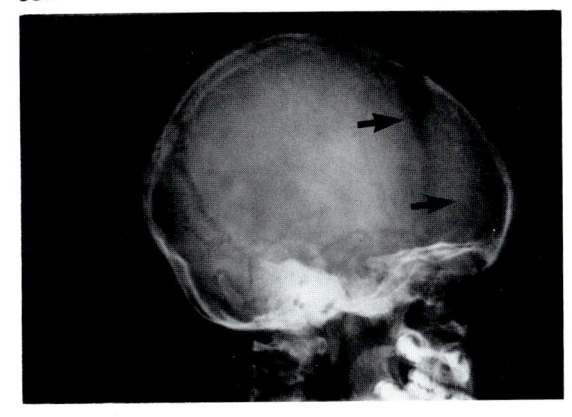

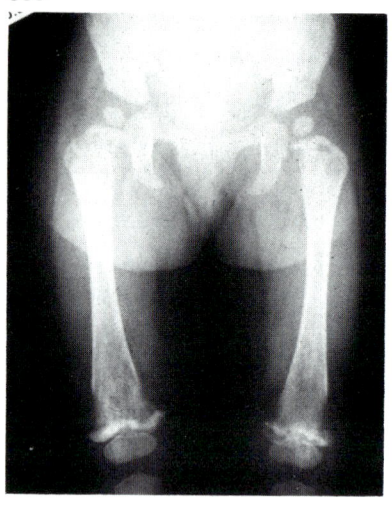

533 Bone metastases of neuroblastoma. Metastatic lesions usually occur in the diaphysial area and appear as lytic defects with irregular margins and some periosteal reaction. The lesions are frequently painful.

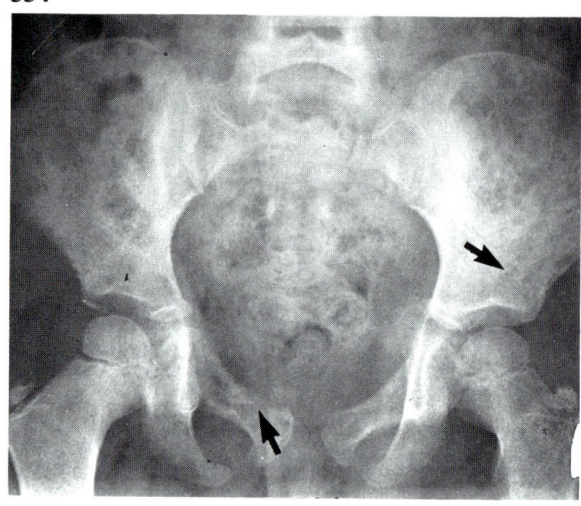

534 Metastatic neuroblastoma. The xray of the pelvis reveals an ill-defined patchy destruction of bone. This may be the only sign of widespread metastatic bony involvement. The child complained of generalised aches and pains.

535 Periorbital metastatic disease. The 'raccoon-like' appearance is caused by periorbital ecchymosis and is indicative of metastatic disease. Intracranial disease commonly involves the meninges but brain metastases are rare.

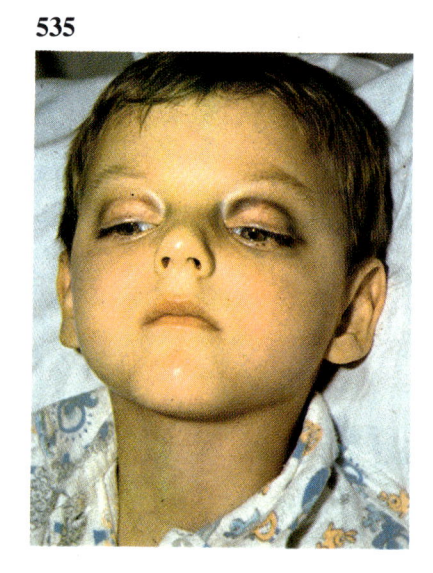

536 Neuroblastoma. Microscopic appearance of the tumour showing sheets of small round cells in a fibrillary stroma. Evidence of some degree of differentiation is proved by this stroma and the tendency of the cells to have vacuolated nuclei and prominent nucleoli. Rosette formation is also evident (*H&E × 40*).

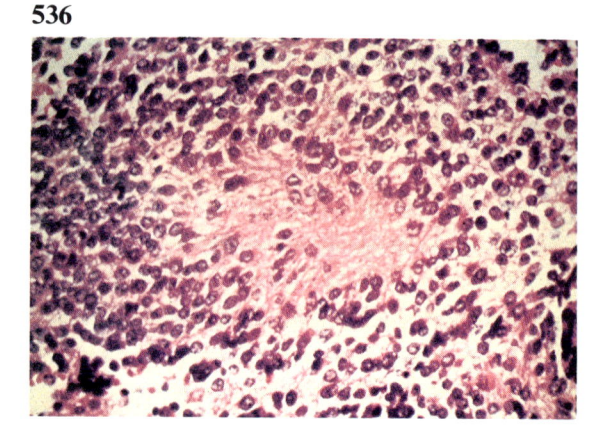

537 Retroperitoneal teratoma. Tend to be located in the retroperitoneal tissues. Present as an asymptomatic abdominal mass. The lateral view of the excretory urogram shows a large calcified retroperitoneal mass displacing the kidneys posteriorly.

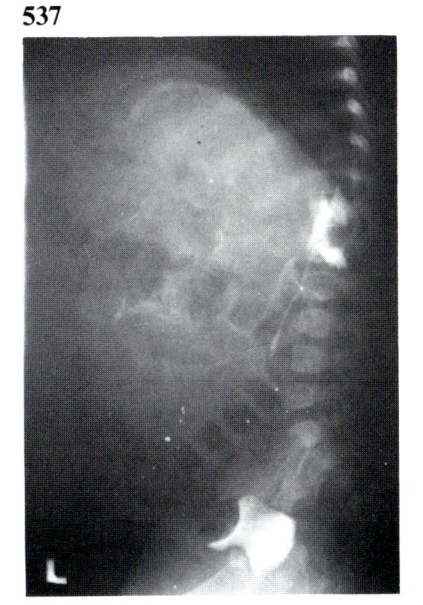

538 Retroperitoneal teratoma. Tumour found to be arising inferior to the left kidney in the retroperitoneal tissues. Tumour completely resected. Only about 10 per cent show malignant degeneration.

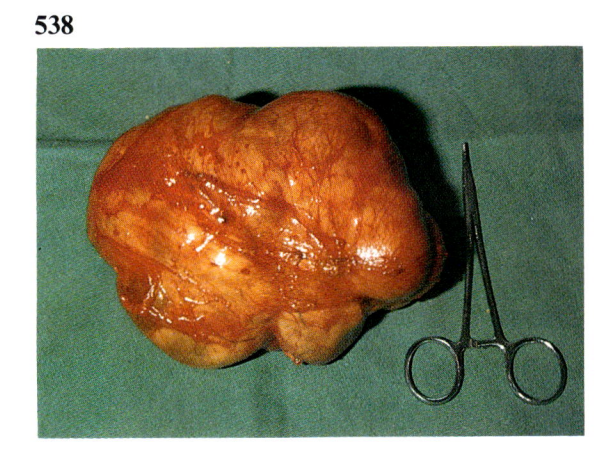

539 Retroperitoneal teratoma. The tumour has been opened to reveal multiplicity of tissue foreign to the anatomical region in which it was located. Brain, lung and intestine could be identified as well as cartilaginous tissue and muscle.

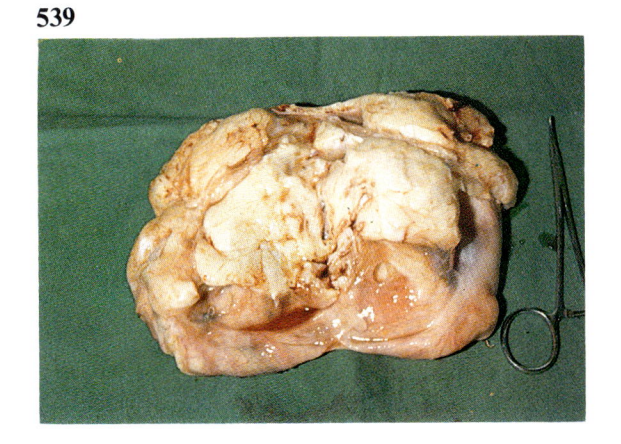

540 Sacrococcygeal teratoma. The infant is born with a mass of varying dimensions in the sacrococcygeal region of the spine. The tumour is usually midline and may extend into the pelvis displacing the anus anteriorly and palpable presacrally on rectal examination.

541 Sacrococcygeal teratoma. Huge sacrococcygeal teratoma in newborn infant. Contains tissue from all three germinal layers, but recognisable organs are rarely present. Seldom malignant in neonatal period but the incidence of malignant degeneration rises progressively to approximately 50 per cent after the age of one year. Serum alpha-foetoprotein levels may be increased (yolk-sac tumour).

542 Sacrococcygeal teratoma. Massive tumour with intrapelvic extension. Treatment consists of total excision including the entire coccyx (from which the tumour arises). The operation may involve combined abdomino-perineum approach.

543 Sacrococcygeal teratoma. Lateral pelvic xray showing the large mass with areas of calcification both in the tumour itself and in the presacral extension.

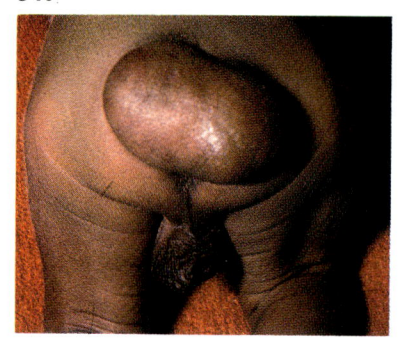

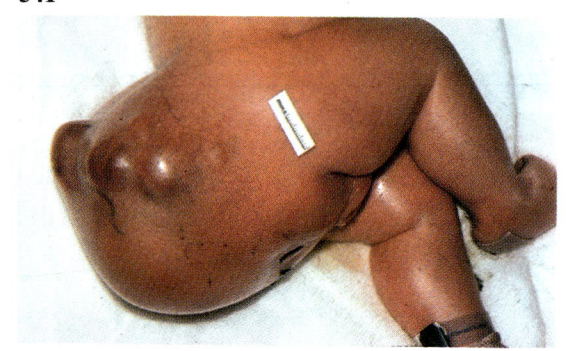

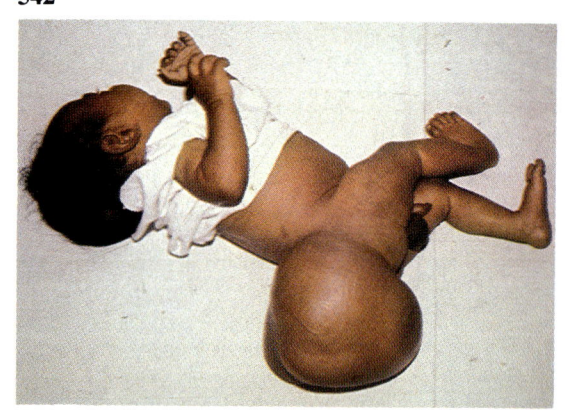

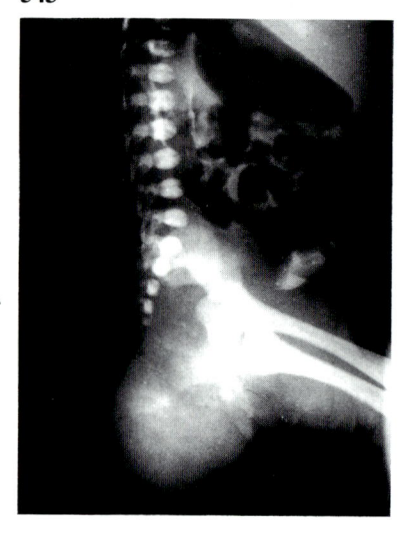

544 Chordoma. Arises from remnants of the notochord and is a very rare tumour of childhood. Most frequently encountered in the sacrococcygeal region. Radiologically there are areas of bone destruction, calcification and expansion of the sacrum. High incidence of malignant degeneration.

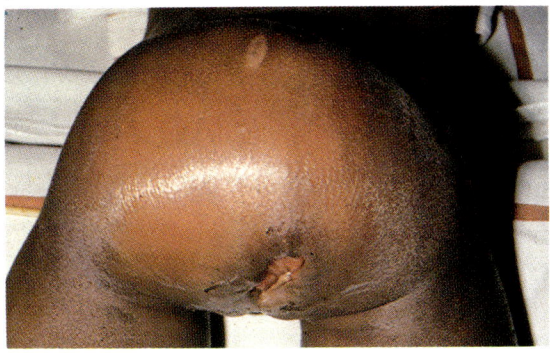

545 Neurofibroma. Massive lower abdominal and pelvic retroperitoneal tumour in an eight-year-old girl. The cut surface reveals a well-formed capsule and extensive areas of haemorrhage within the tumour mass. There were no features of von Recklinghausen's disease.

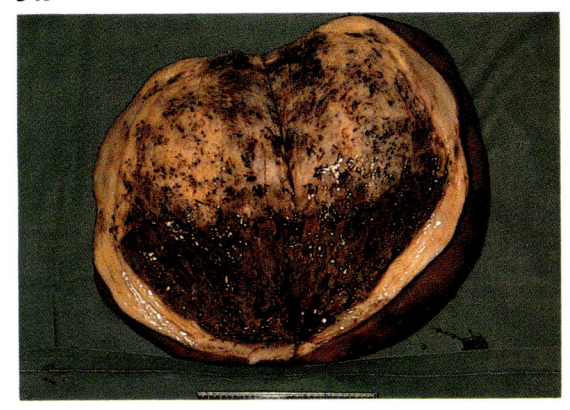

546 Von Recklinghausen's disease. Generalised neurofibromatosis with widespread thickening of nerves. Skin manifestations include coffee-coloured pigmentation (café-au-lait lesions) and/or elephantiasis. There is a large tumour (neurofibroma) in the left iliac fossa. Sarcomatous degeneration may be as high as 17 per cent.

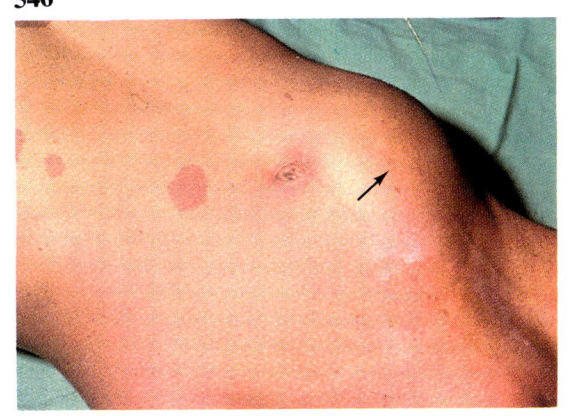

547 Birkitt's lymphoma. Non-Hodgkin's lymphoma frequently presents with abdominal disease with the tumour involving the retroperitoneal region, intestine, mesentery or ovary. Responds dramatically to combination chemotherapy but relapse rate is high.

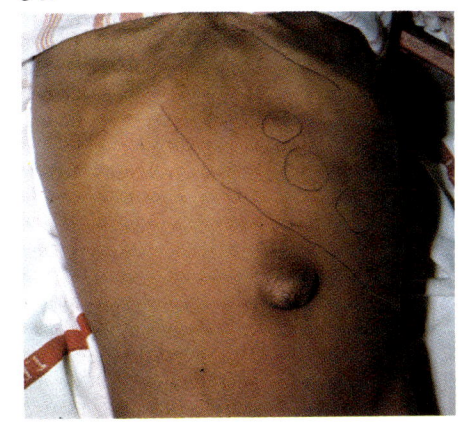

37 The kidney

548 Renal trauma. Usually sustained by blunt abdominal injury. Degree of haematuria does not necessarily correlate with the extent of kidney damage. Excretory urogram is essential. Minor extravasation of contrast from the right collecting system is evident. Conservative treatment is appropriate.

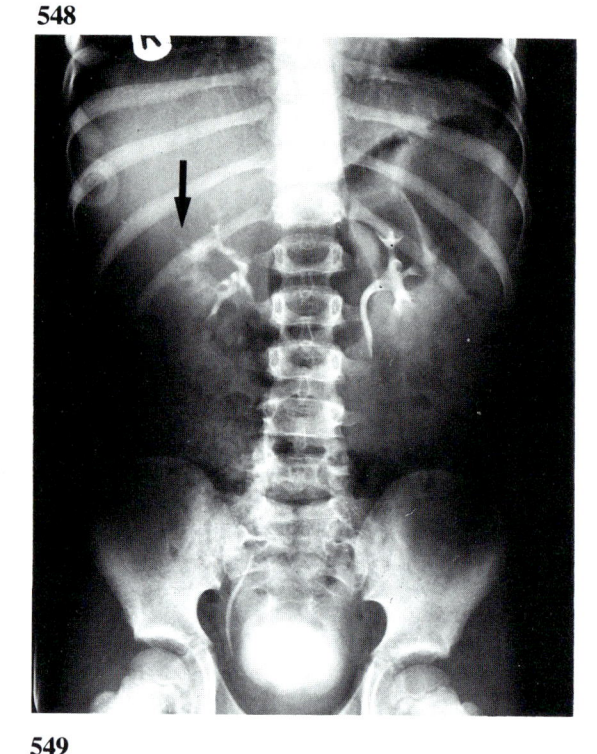

549 Renal trauma. Major extravasation of contrast from the right collecting system. There were signs of peritonitis and shock caused by extravasation of blood and urine into the peritoneal cavity. Surgical intervention is indicated in these cases.

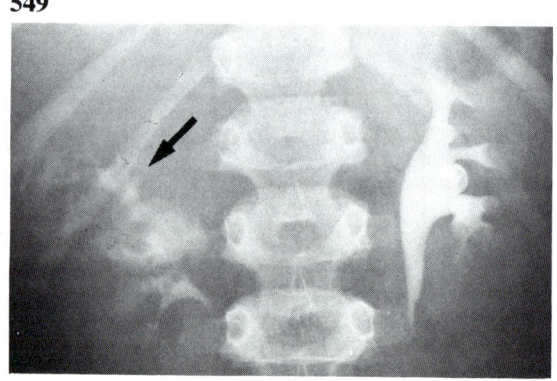

550 Ruptured kidney. Almost complete separation of the upper from the lower pole of the kidney. Conservative surgery, i.e. repair of the laceration or heminephrectomy should be considered. Nephrectomy may be life-saving but it is essential to establish function of the contralateral kidney.

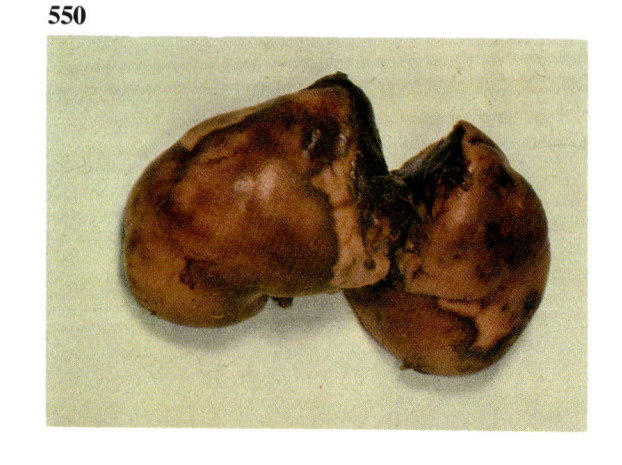

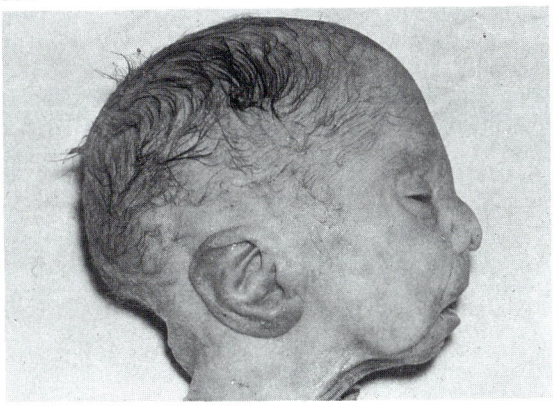

551 Renal agenesis. Complete absence of both kidneys associated with oligohydramnios. Characteristic Potter's facies with lowset ears, a broad flattened nasal bridge and eyes set widely apart. Incompatible with prolonged extrauterine survival.

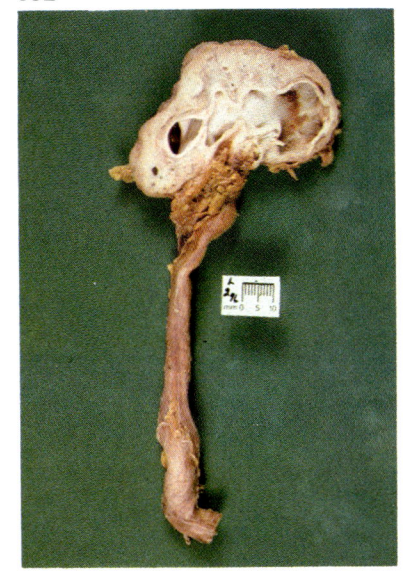

552 Cystic dysplastic kidney. The kidney is composed of primitive renal elements, cysts and foreign tissue, e.g. cartilage, muscle. The abnormal structure is prone to pyelonephritic changes and the abnormality manifests with recurrent attacks of urinary infection.

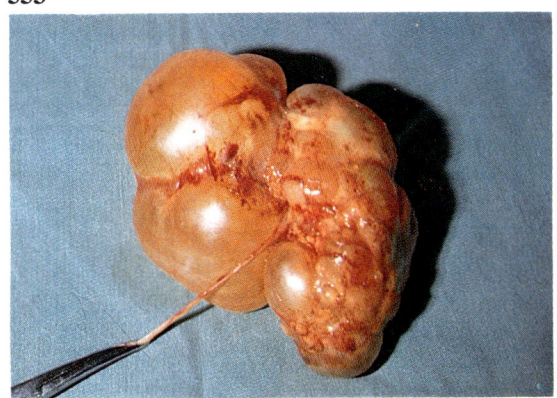

553 Multicystic kidney. Commonly presents as an asymptomatic lobulated flank mass in the newborn infant. Excretory urogram may reveal either non-excretion on the affected side or a 'soap bubble' appearance. The kidney is completely replaced by a number of cysts of varying size. The ureter is frequently atretic or represented by a thin strand of fibrous tissue. There is a high incidence of anomalies of the contra-lateral kidney, e.g. hydronephrosis.

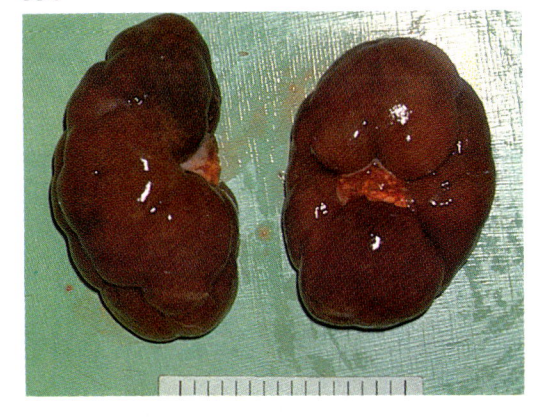

554 Infantile polycystic disease. Familial condition. Both kidneys affected. The kidneys are enlarged and have exaggerated foetal lobulations. Cut surface has honeycomb appearance caused by multiple radially arranged cystic spaces. Presents in neonatal period with loin masses and renal insufficiency. Associated cystic disease of liver, pancreas and lung may be present.

555 Crossed renal ectopia. Both kidneys sited on same side of the abdomen. The crossed kidney lies below and medial to the normally placed one. Ureteric openings are normally sited at either side of the trigone of the bladder. Usually presents as an asymptomatic mass but infection, hydronephrosis or calculi, may occur.

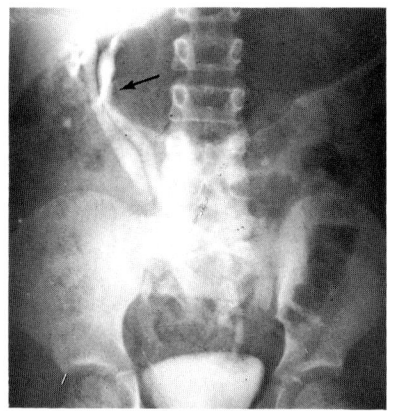

556 Horseshoe kidney. The lower poles of the kidneys are fused posterior to the ureters. Excretory urogram reveals inward rotation of the lower poles of the kidneys with anteriorly situated renal pelvices. Usually asymptomatic but may present with abdominal pain caused by obstruction or infection.

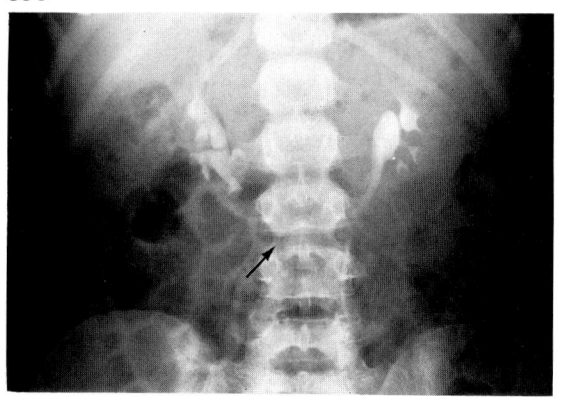

557 Pelvic ectopic kidney. Common anomaly. The ectopic organ may be palpable on abdominal examination and confused with a neoplasm. Blood supply arises from lower aorta or iliac artery. Excretory urogram is diagnostic. A filling defect may be visible on cystography.

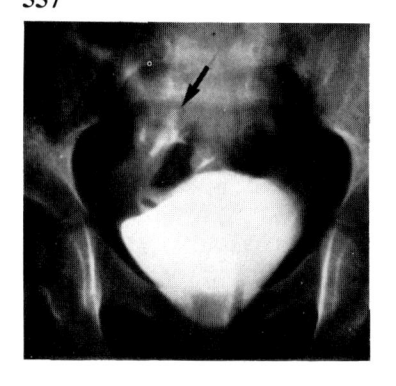

558 Hydronephrosis. Excretory urogram showing moderate degree of right-sided hydronephrosis and calyceal 'clubbing' caused by pelviureteric junction obstruction. Commonly presents with recurrent or chronic urinary infection with intermittent loin pain in the older child. Definite predisposition to calculus formation.

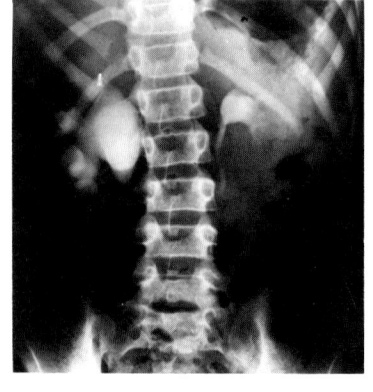

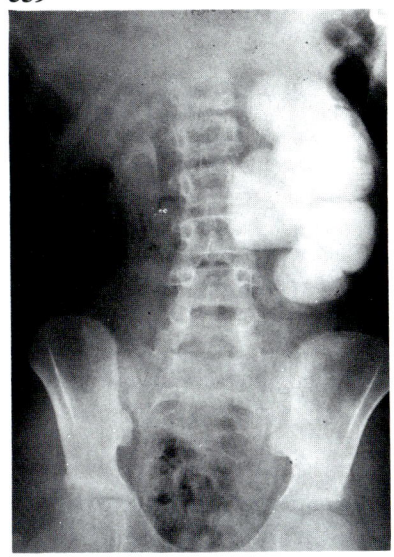

559 Hydronephrosis. Advanced degree of hydronephrosis secondary to pelviureteric junction obstruction. Haematuria may occur secondary to minor trauma or as a result of infection or calculus. Renal failure may occur as a complication of severe renal parenchymal thinning and compression.

560 Hydronephrosis. Ultrasonography showing the dilated renal pelvis and a thin rim of renal parenchymal tissue in an advanced degree of hydronephrosis.

561 Hydronephrosis. Operative view showing the dilated distended renal pelvis with lobulated renal parenchyma on the surface. Nephrectomy is only indicated in cases with complete parenchymal destruction. Treatment is by pyeloplasty with excision of the stenotic obstruction segment.

562 Pyonephrosis. Complication of chronic pelviureteric junction obstruction. The renal pelvis is tensely distended with pus. The patient presents with pyuria and a long history of ill-health. A tender mass in the loin may be present.

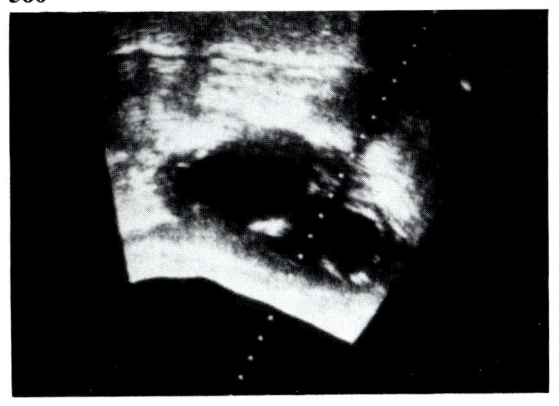

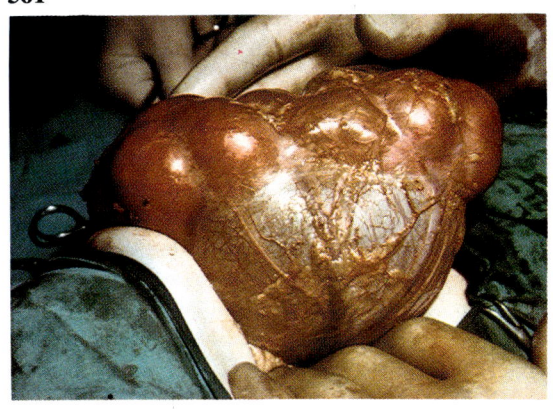

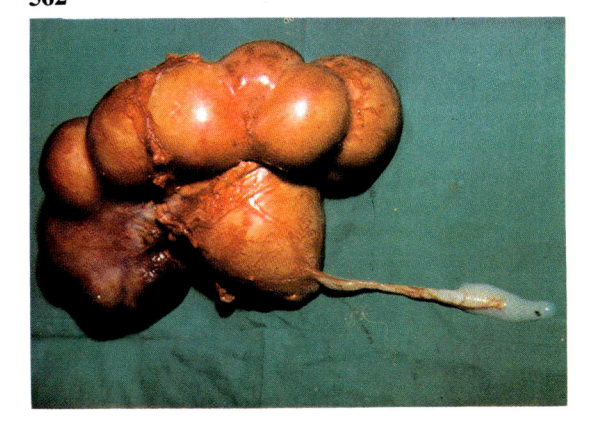

563 Duplex kidney. Incomplete duplication where the ureters draining the upper and lower poles of the left kidney unite just distal to the renal pelvis. Usually asymptomatic and an incidental finding during investigation for abdominal pain of undetermined origin.

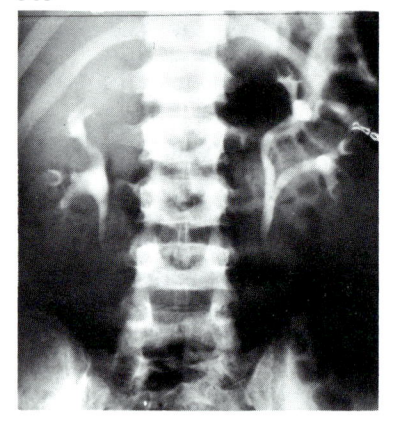

564 Complete ureteric duplication. The two ureters enter the bladder separately. The ureter draining the lower pole enters the bladder at the usual site, but has a short intramural course and is predisposed to reflux. The upper pole ureter drains into the bladder below and medial to the lower pole ureter.

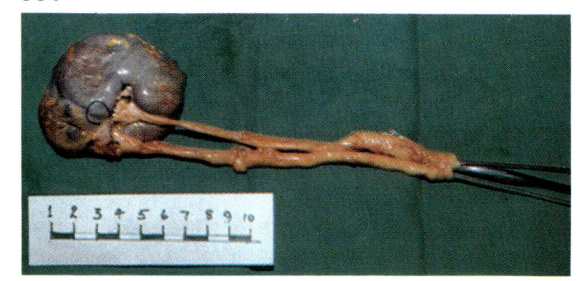

565 Duplex system with a hydronephrotic lower pole. The upper moiety of the left kidney appears normal while there is marked hydronephrosis of the lower moiety. This may be caused by reflux or obstruction by an ectopic ureterocoele. In this case the cause of obstruction was at the pelvi-uretoric junction. Treatment is by reimplantation of the ureters or heminephrectomy where indicated.

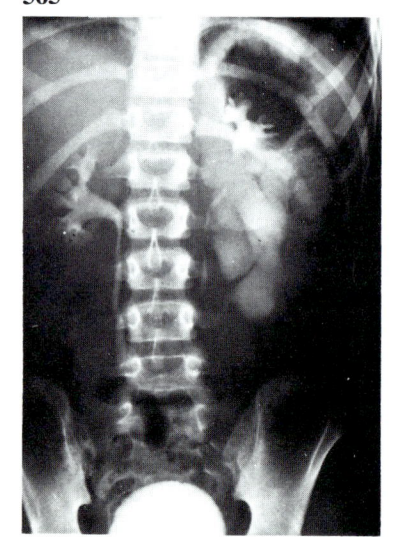

566 Ureteric duplication with hydronephrosis. There is dilatation of both ureters with advanced hydronephrosis. The kidney parenchyma has been completely destroyed and only a thin sac representing the kidney remains. Associated with ureterovesical obstruction, stenosis or ureterocoele.

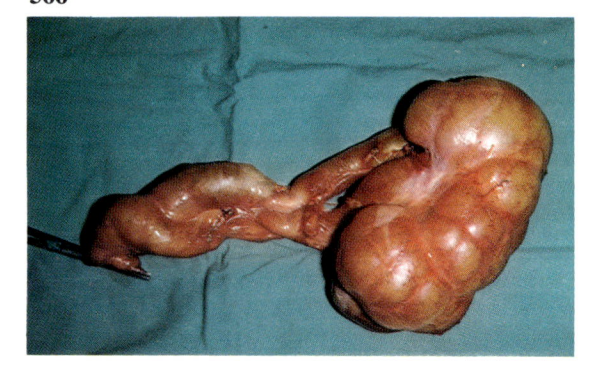

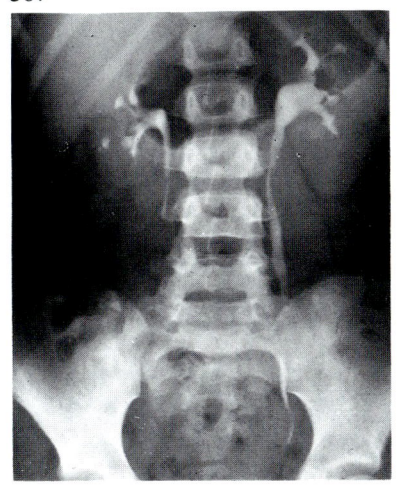

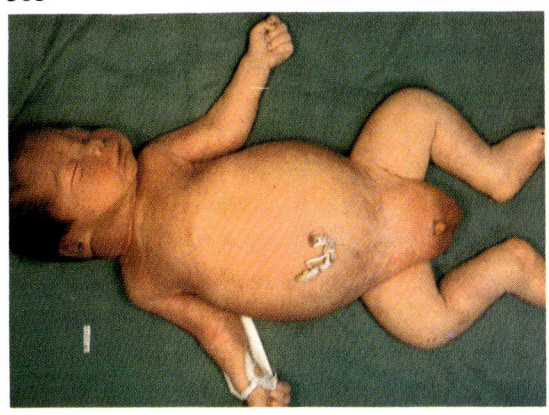

567 Pyelonephritis. Secondary to chronic reflux and urinary infection. The right kidney has an irregular surface and is contracted and scarred. The calyces are dilated. The left kidney shows evidence of compensatory hypertrophy.

568 Urinary ascites. Prenatal rupture of the urinary system with accumulation of urine in the peritoneal cavity. Most commonly occurs secondary to posterior urethral valves. Site of rupture may not be apparent at laparotomy.

569 Urinary calculi. May arise in the following circumstances:
a) endemic calculi, e.g. India, Philippines, Turkey, China.
b) stasis and infection – usually associated with an anatomical anomaly.
c) metabolic diseases, e.g. cystinuria, oxaluria, hypercalcaemia.
d) prolonged immobilisation.
e) foreign body, e.g. non-absorbable suture material.
f) idiopathic.
Excretory urogram shows calculi in the right kidney, lower ureter and bladder.

570 Staghorn calculus. There is a large conglomerate in the pelvis of the right kidney in association with other calculi in the substance of the right kidney and lower right ureter.

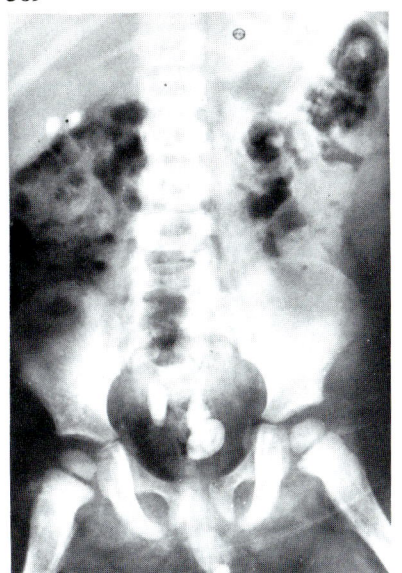

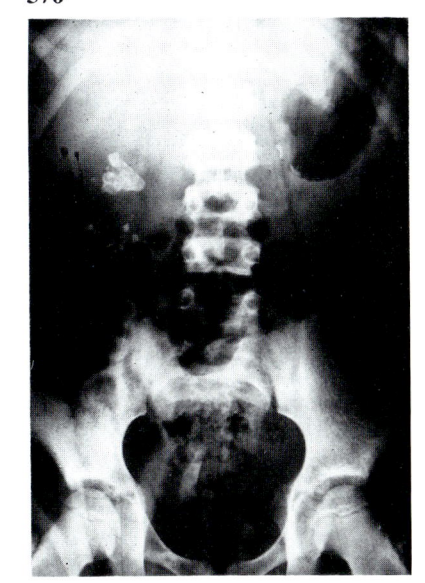

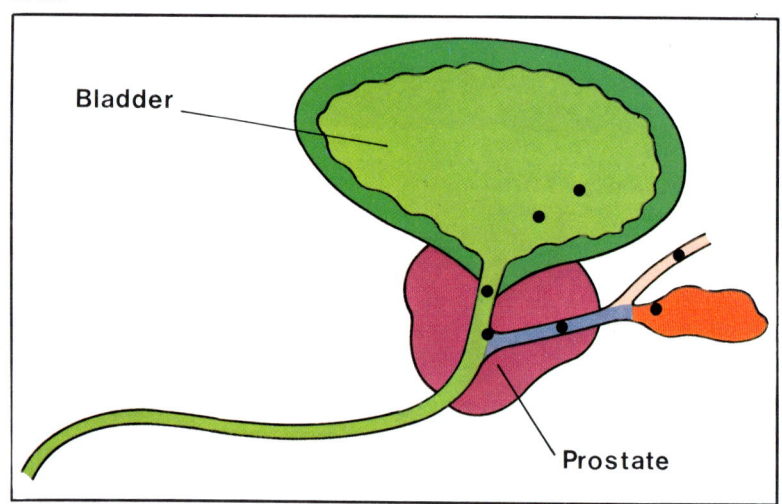

38 The ureter

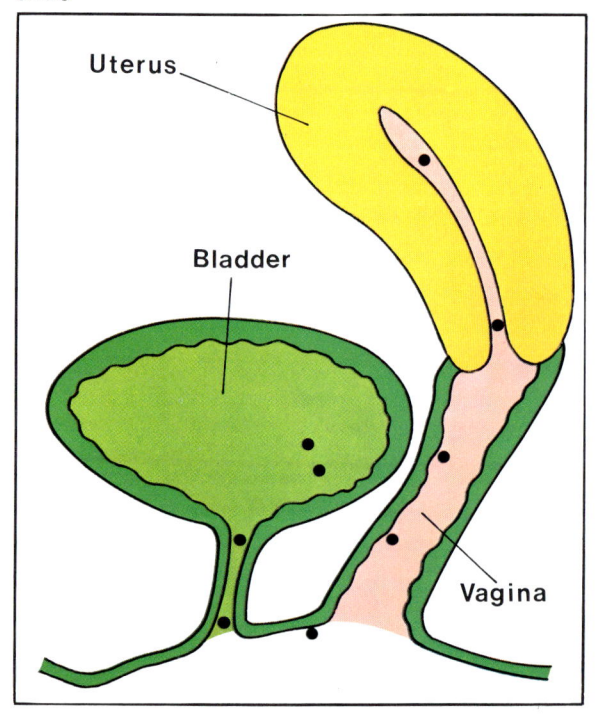

571 Ectopic ureter. The various anatomical sites at which the ectopic ureteric orifice may be found:
a) in the male
b) in the female.

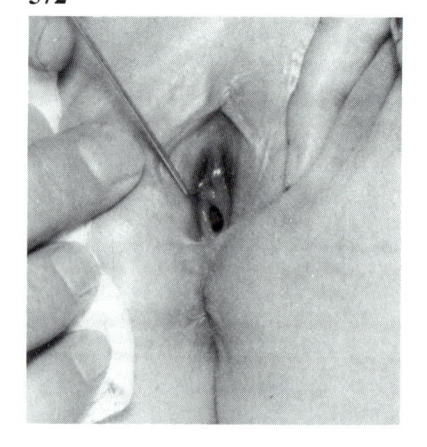

572 Ectopic ureter in the female. The site of the ectopic orifice just lateral to the normal urethra opening is shown. The patient presents with constant wetness (dribbling incontinence) but is able to void normally.

573 Single ectopic ureter. The excretory urogram shows non-functioning left kidney. Micturating cystourethrogram demonstrates massive reflux into a widely dilated left ureter. Urethroscopy confirmed the presence of an ectopic ureteric opening into the urethra.

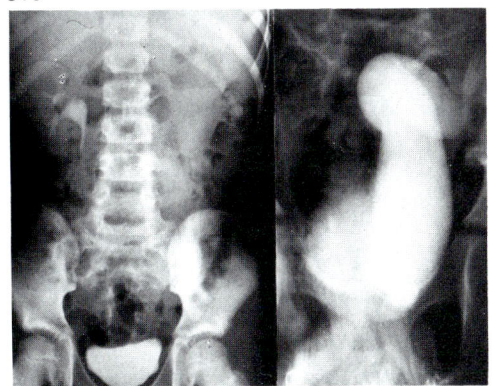

574 Ectopic ureterocoele. The cystic dilatation of the termination of the ectopic ureter in the urethra has prolapsed into the vulva. The ectopic ureterocoele is virtually confined to the upper pole ureter of a duplex system.

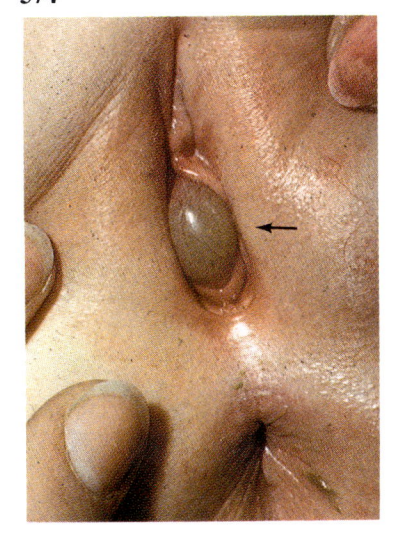

575 Ureterocoele. Cystic dilatation of the intravesical portion of the ureter. Arises secondary to stenosis of the ureteric orifice. May be unilateral or bilateral and may prolapse into the bladder neck causing outlet obstruction. There are bilateral filling defects in the bladder on cystography (characteristic halo effect).

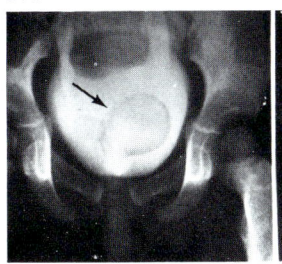

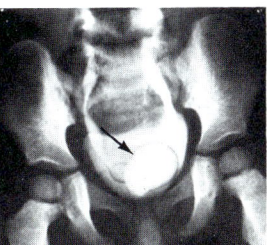

576 Ureterocoele. Operative view on opening the bladder showing the pale cystic swelling inside the bladder. Treatment consists of excision of the ureterocoele and reimplantation of the ureter.

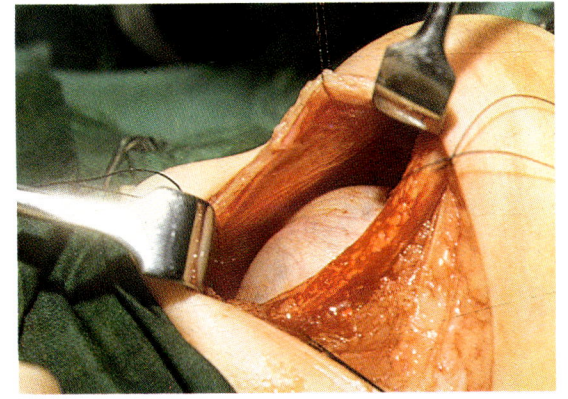

577–580 Vesicoureteric reflux. May be primary as a result of an anomalous ureterovesical junction or secondary to an infravesical obstruction, neurological lesion or infection.

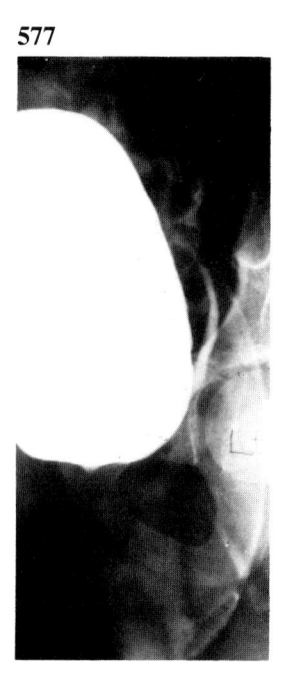

577 Grade I: minimal vesicoureteric reflux with filling of a normal calibre lower ureter only on cystography.

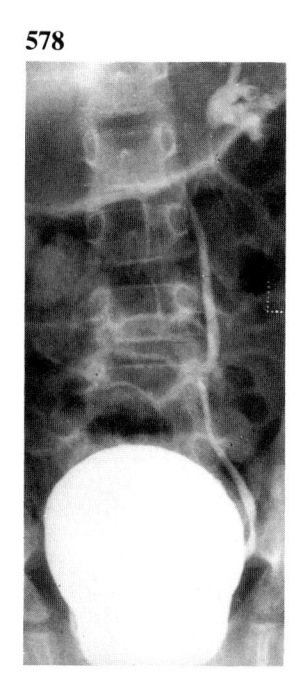

578 Grade II: moderate vesicoureteric reflux. The contrast has reflux into the pelvicalyceal system but calyceal damage has not occurred.

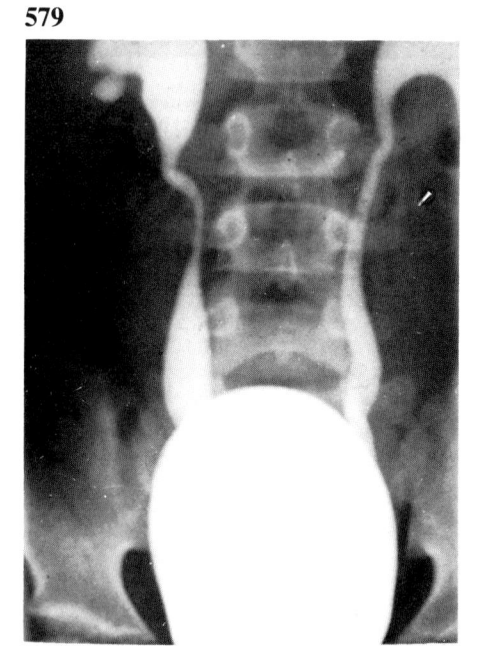

579 Grade III: severe vesicoureteric reflux. There is reflux of contrast into a dilated system including clubbing of the calyces.

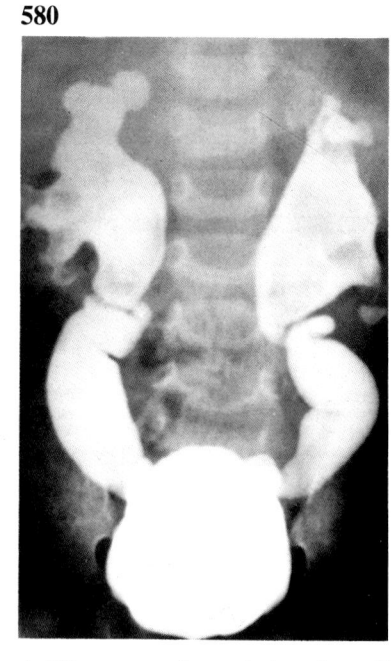

580 Grade IV: gross vesicoureteric reflux with severe dilatation of the upper urinary tract with intrarenal backflow.

581 Primary obstructive megaureter. There is a functional obstruction at the vesicoureteric junction with dilatation of varying degree of the upper urinary tract. In severe cases the ureter is lengthened and tortuous in addition to the dilatation.

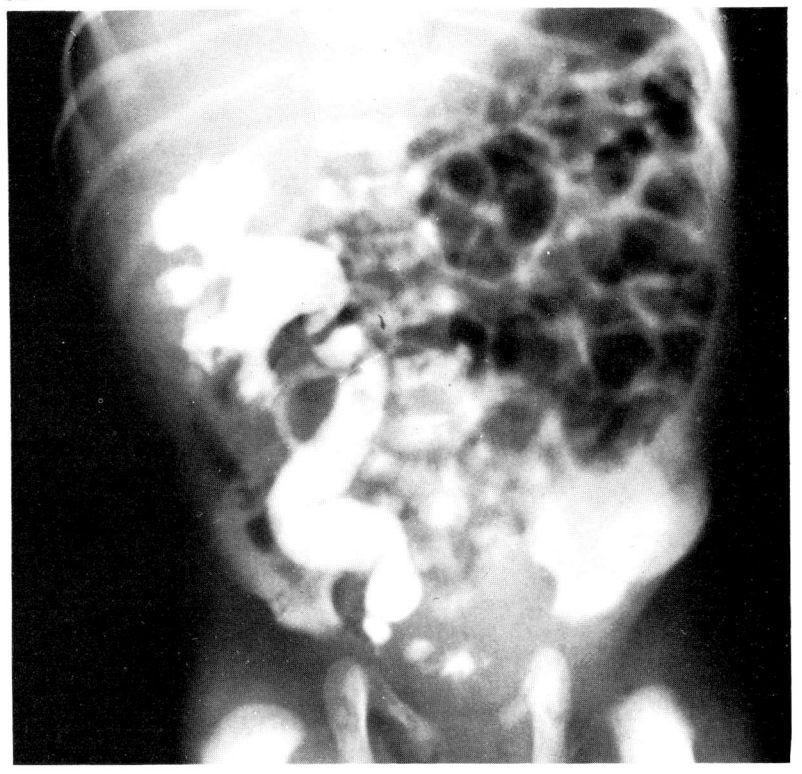

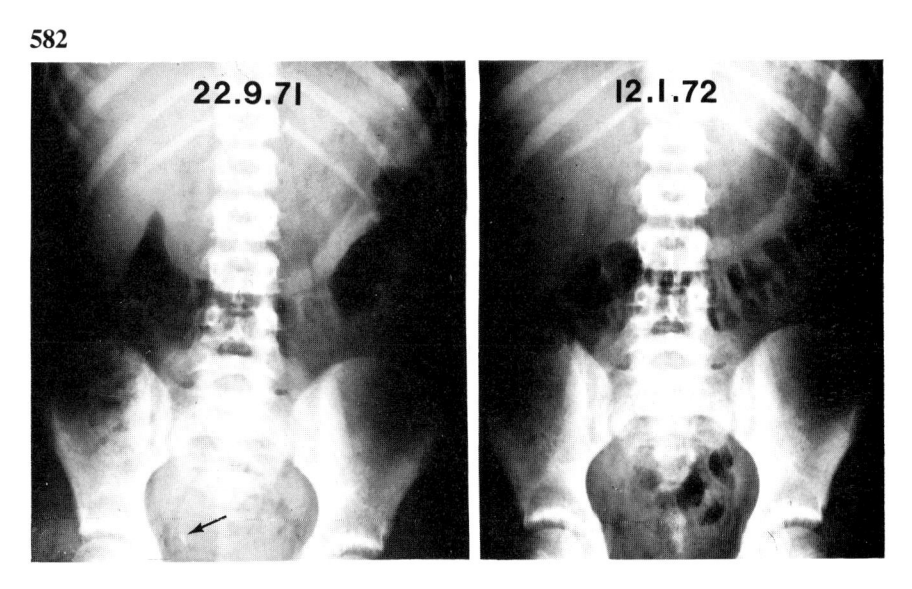

582 Ureteric calculus. Classically presents with acute abdominal pain which in the older child follows the typical ureteric colic distribution. Past history of recurrent urinary tract infections is common. Haematuria frequently occurs.

39 The bladder

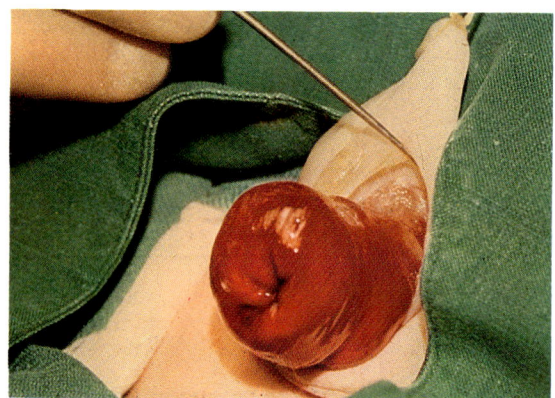

583 **Urachal fistula.** Failure of the urachus to obliterate completely results in a persistent urinary leak at a slightly abnormal looking umbilicus. In the absence of a bladder outlet obstruction, simple extraperitoneal excision of the fistula and the urachus is advisable.

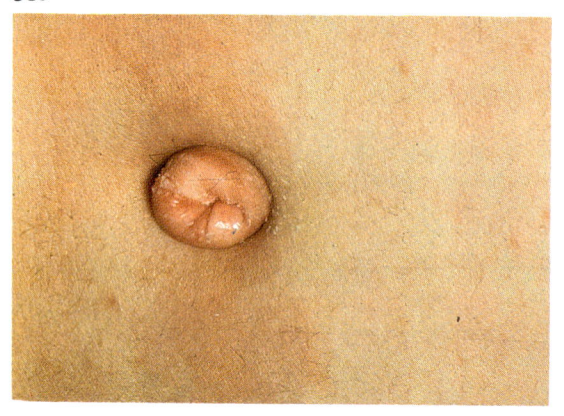

584 **Patent urachus.** In the neonate it is almost invariably associated with bladder outlet obstruction, e.g. posterior urethral valves, congenital deficiency of abdominal musculature. The anomaly shown was associated with a minor exomphalos.

585 **Urachal diverticulum.** A micturating cystogram reveals a bladder diverticulum at the apex of the bladder caused by enlargement of a pre-formed urachal diverticulum. There is also moderate distension of the urethra in this female child.

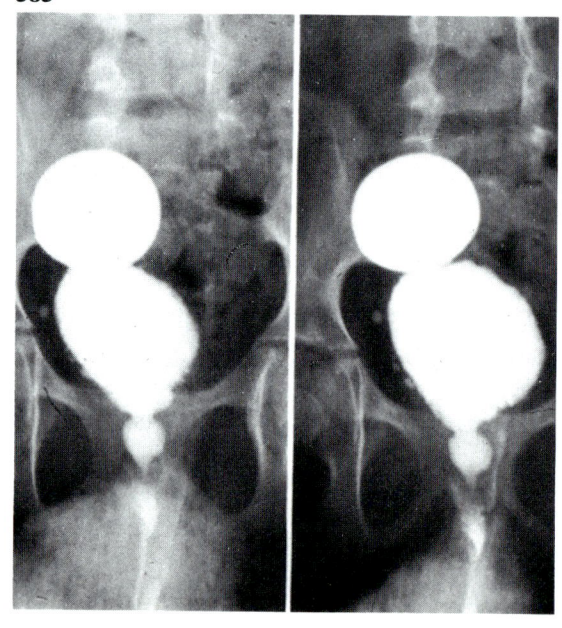

586 **Duplications of the bladder.** In complete duplications there are completely separate bladders supplied by individual ureters and draining by separate urethras. Associated anomalies of the large bowel and rectum are common. Obstruction may be present in one of the bladders leading to gross hydroureter and hydronephrosis.

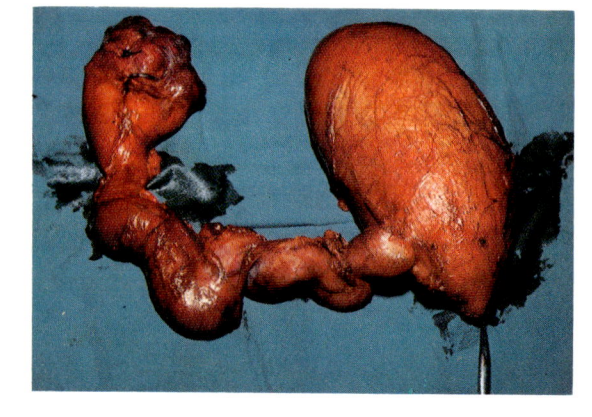

587 Bladder diverticulum. These are herniations of the bladder mucosa through a weak point in the detrusor muscle. May be associated with bladder outlet obstruction, e.g. posterior urethral valves or neuropathic bladder, e.g. spina bifida. Present with recurrent urinary tract infections. Note multiple succulations in addition to the large left diverticulum in a girl with myelomeningocoele.

588 Bladder exstrophy. The bladder lies open and everted on the surface of the lower abdominal wall. The exposed mucosa is continuous peripherally with the skin. There is complete epispadias and wide separation of the symphysis pubis. Treatment consists of either primary reconstruction or urinary diversion.

589 Exstrophy with rectal prolapse. Associated with bladder exstrophy there is frequently laxity of the pelvic floor and anal sphincters. This allows complete prolapse of the rectum to occur and precludes ureterosigmodostomy as a possible method of urinary diversion.

590 Vesicointestinal fissure (exstrophy of the cloaca). This complex anomaly of development of the lower half of the anterior abdominal wall consists of: a) exomphalos; b) bladder exstrophy in which the two hemibladders are separated in the midline by c) an exposed everted loop of intestine – ileocaecal region – through which the distal ileum commonly prolapses; d) anorectal agenesis with a short blind ending colon and e) wide diastasis of the symphysis pubis.

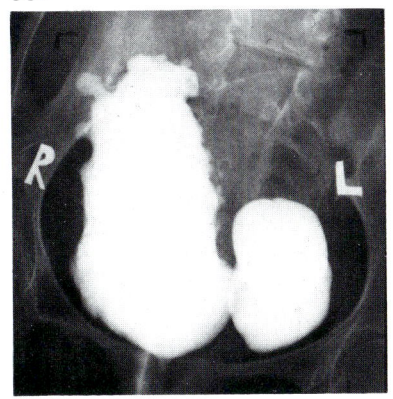

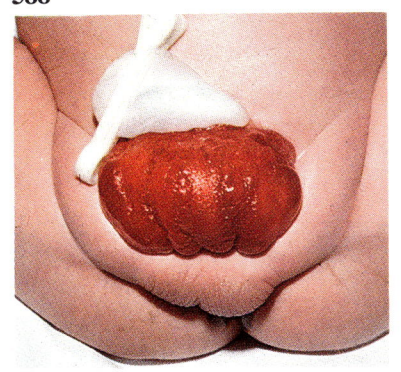

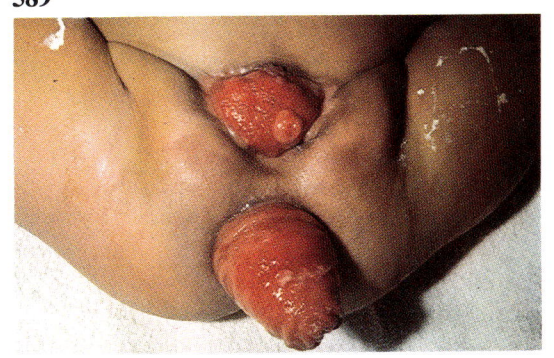

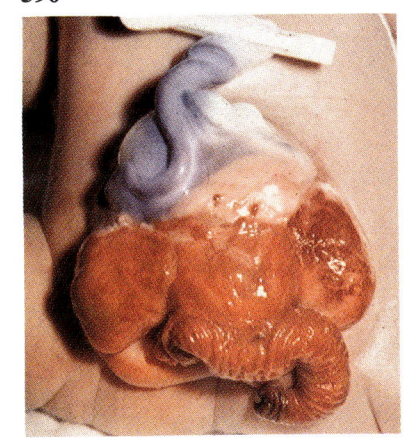

591 Prune belly syndrome (agenesis of the abdominal muscles). There is absence or hypoplasia of the abdominal musculature. Condition virtually confined to males. There are severe associated urogenital anomalies, i.e. hypertrophy of the bladder and hydroureter and hydronephrosis. The testes are usually intra-abdominal.

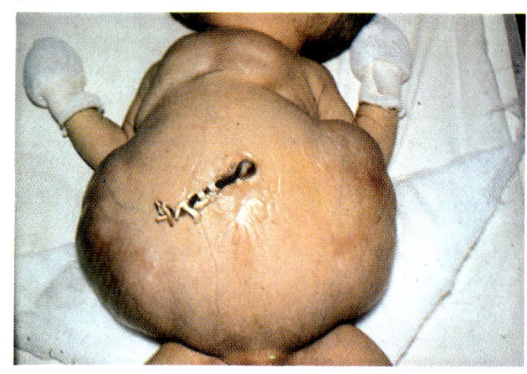

592 Prune belly syndrome. A less dramatic example of the syndrome in an older child. Management should be concerned with maintaining renal function and avoiding unnecessary surgical procedures on the abnormal urinary system. Constipation may be a difficult problem to manage.

593 Prune belly syndrome. An excretory urogram showing bilateral hydronephrosis and the dilated tortuous ureters. The large capacity bladder can be seen filling the pelvis and lower abdomen.

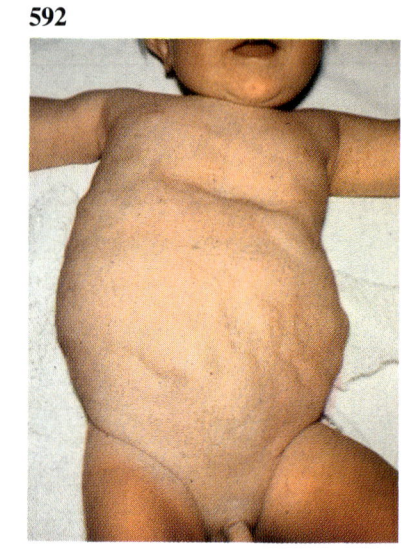

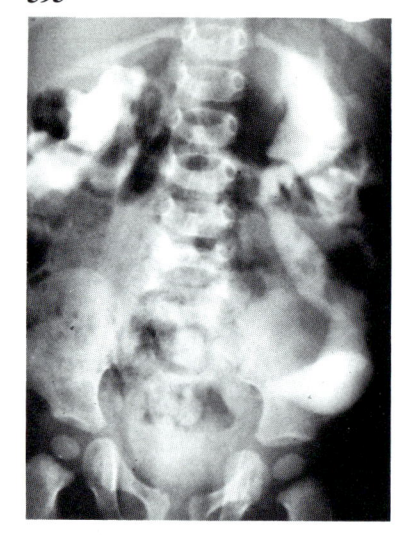

594 Neuropathic bladder. Most commonly seen in children with myelomeningocoele (note the abnormally wide lumbosacral canal), but may also occur in sacral agenesis, spinal dysraphism, traumatic paraplegia. The cystogram shows a narrow elongated trabulated bladder with numerous diverticuli. Stasis with resultant infection or bladder outlet obstruction causing back-pressure effects on the kidney are the major problems.

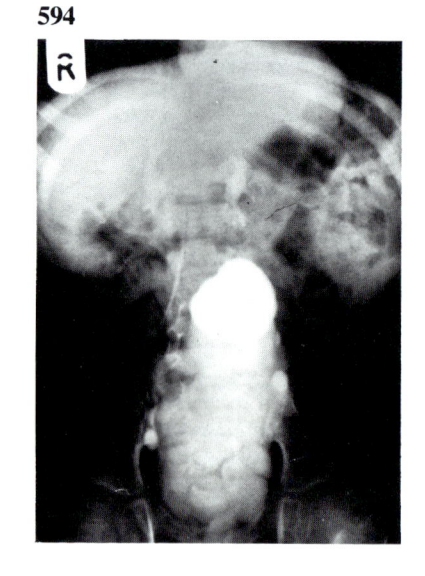

595 Rhabdomyosarcoma of bladder. Malignancy which arises from embryonal mesenchyme which gives rise to striated muscle. The tumour originates in the submucosal and superficial muscular layers of the base of the bladder and tends to fungate into the lumen of the bladder. Presents with urinary obstruction or haematuria.

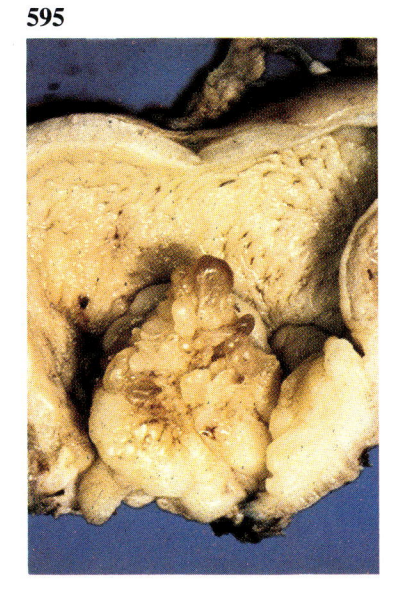

596 Rhabdomyosarcoma of the bladder. The excretory urogram reveals irregular filling defects in the base of the bladder with early evidence of obstruction to the left upper tract. Diagnosis is confirmed on endoscopic biopsy.

597 Rhabdomyosarcoma of the vagina. Sarcoma botryoides is term used to describe the characteristic grape-like lobules of tumour which appear at the vulva. This is usually the first sign of disease. Rapid growth with involvement of the bladder commonly occurs.

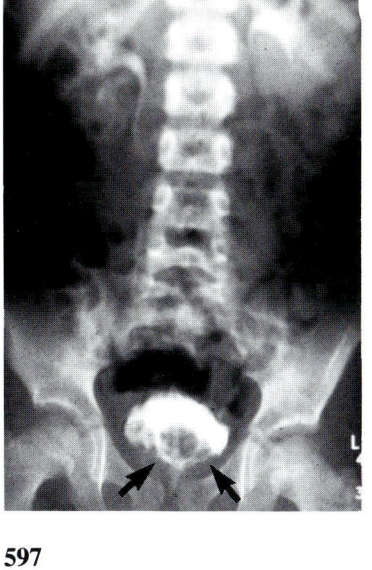

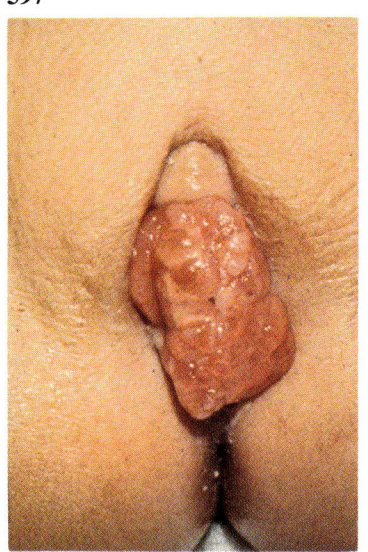

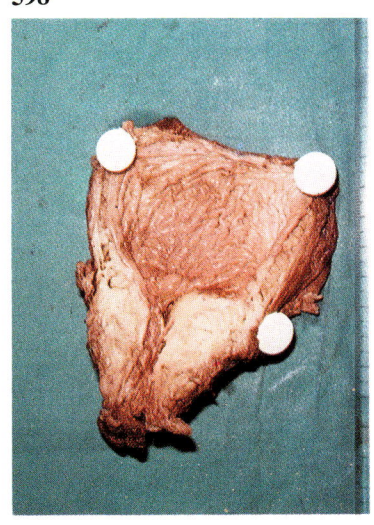

598 Rhabdomyosarcoma of the prostate. The tumour displaces the bladder upwards and stretches the urethra producing outflow obstruction and urinary retention. The base of the bladder is infiltrated. The tumour is palpable on rectal examination. Needle biopsy will confirm the diagnosis.

40 The urethra

599 Posterior urethral valves. Necropsy specimen of the opened out bladder and urethra showing the mucosal folds extending downwards from the lower end of the verumontanum to meet in an anterior commissure at the lower end of the prostatic urethra. There are non-obstructive folds extending upwards from the verumontanum to the prominent bladder neck. Note the extremely thick bladder wall.

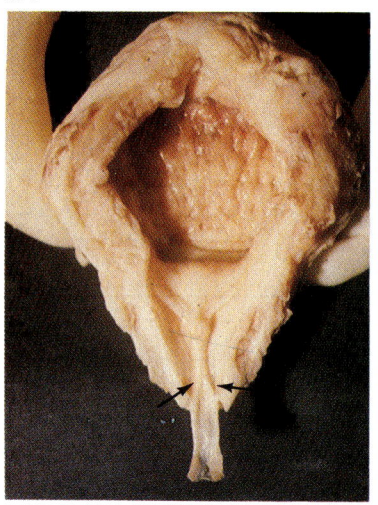

600 Posterior urethral valves. Usually presents in neonatal period with renal failure or with inability or difficulty to pass urine. The hypertrophied bladder is palpable as a hard suprapubic mass. A micturating cystourethrogram shows gross dilatation of the posterior urethra, a prominent bladder neck and reflux into a dilated left upper tract.

601 Duplication of the urethra. Usually associated with complete duplication of the urinary system, but occasionally occurs as an isolated anomaly. The accessory urethra may extend as far back as the base of the penis or enter into the bladder. Presents with either purulent discharge or symptoms of obstruction.

602 Anterior urethral diverticulum. Wide-mouthed diverticulum in the bulb of the urethra. The sac may be large enough to present as a swelling in the scrotal region particularly during micturition. Pressure on the swelling may produce urine at the external meatus.

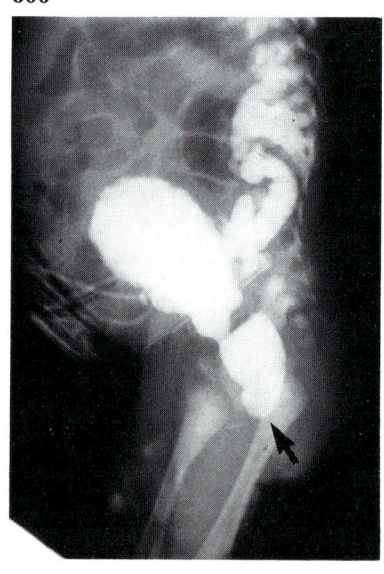

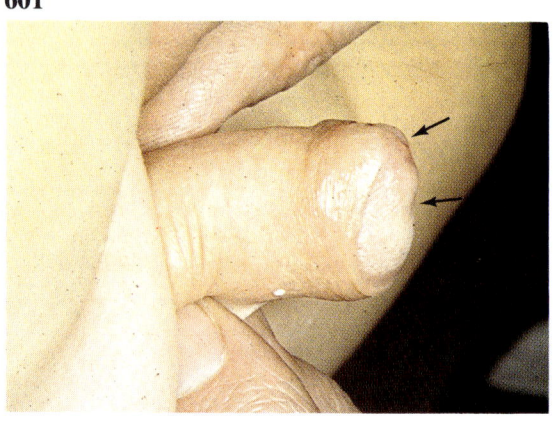

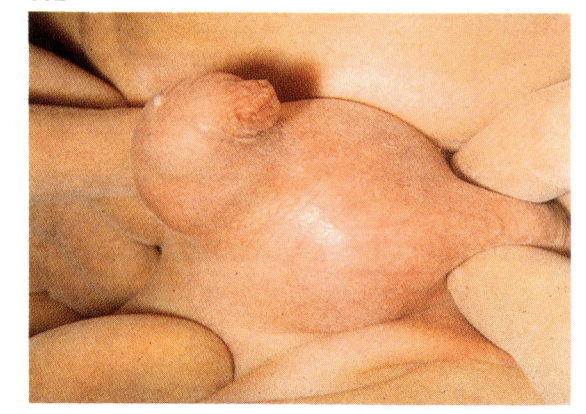

603 Anterior urethral diverticulum. Micturating cysto-urethrogram showing a narrow-necked anterior urethral diverticulum. There is no outflow obstruction but stasis leads to recurrent infection and predisposes to calculus formation.

604 Rupture of the bulbar urethra. Occurs in males as a result of straddle injury or kick in the perineum which compresses the urethra against the pubic arch. If the child micturates after the injury, urinary extravasation into the penis occurs.

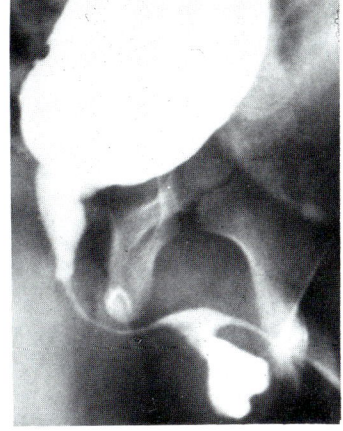

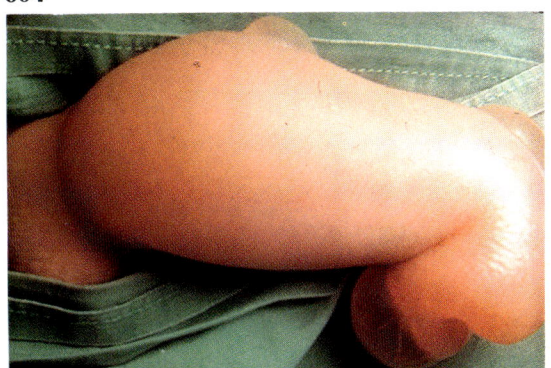

605 Teratoma of the urethra. Extremely rare tumour presenting at the vulva and arising from the wall of the urethra.

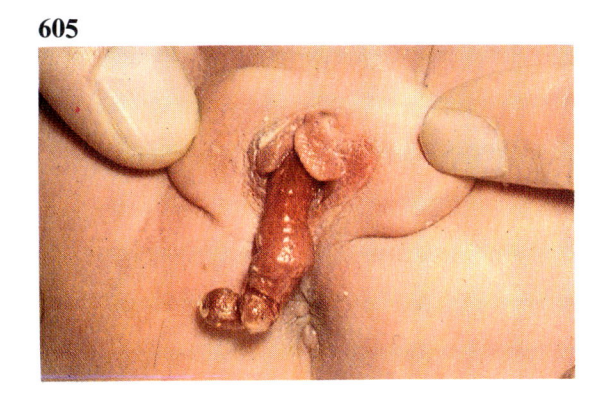

606 Female epispadias. The urethra appears as a broad transverse slit in the flattened pubic region. The clitoris is split into two separate bodies which are displaced laterally. There is almost complete urinary incontinence.

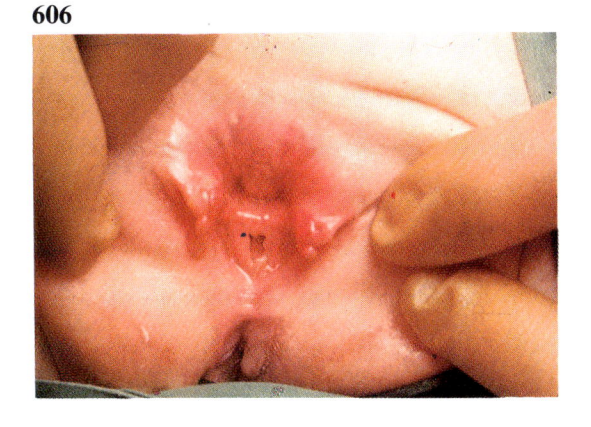

41 Penile disorders

607 Congenital absence of the penis. The phallus is entirely absent and the scrotum bifid. The urethra may either open on the perineum or in the rectum.

608 Micropenis. Most commonly caused by burying of the penis in an enlarged suprapubic pad of fat. True micropenis at puberty with bilaterally descended testes.

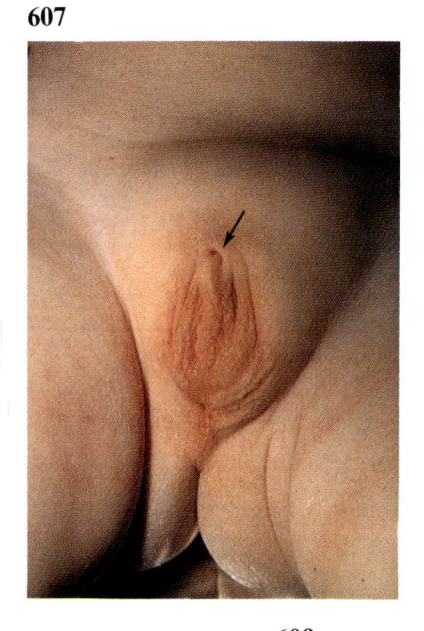

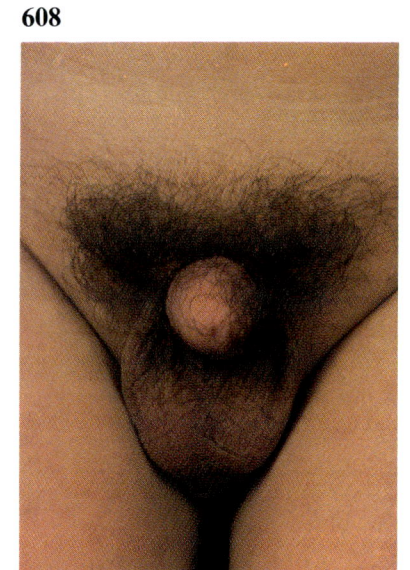

609 Megalopenis. Occurs in association with megalourethra. The penis is enlarged and lax. Appears to be due to a defect in the cavernous tissue. Other urinary anomalies are frequently present. May occur in association with congenital lymphoedema.

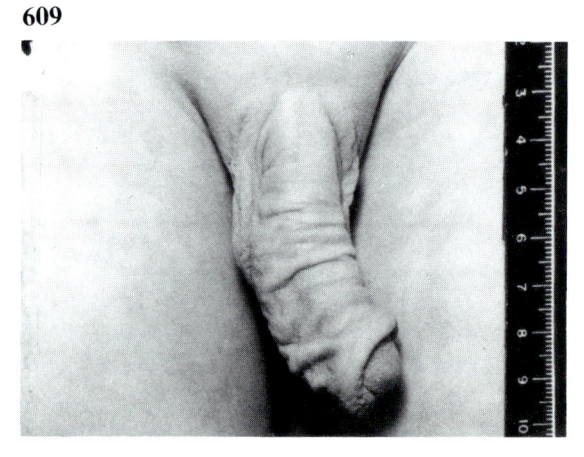

610 Balanoposthitis. Inflammation of the glans of the penis and foreskin extending into the shaft of the penis. Caused by retained smegma and infection.

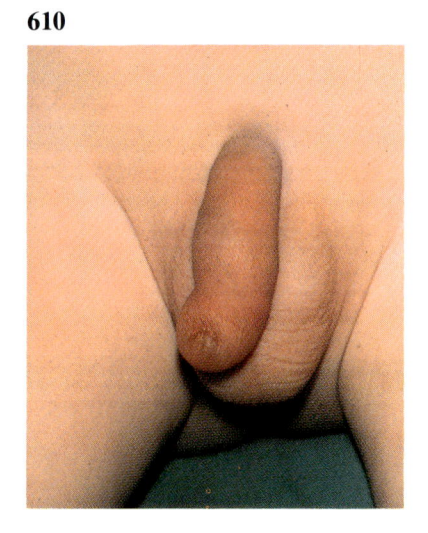

611 Retained smegma ('smegmal cyst'). Presents as a swelling on either side of the glans beneath the prepuce. Often confused with a cyst or tumour. The retained smegma can easily be removed once all the preputial adhesions have been released and the foreskin fully retracted.

612 Phimosis. The preputial orifice is narrowed and scarred by fibrous tissue. Usually follows repeated attempts at retraction by medical attendant or parents. The trauma causes splitting of the foreskin and subsequent healing occurs by fibrosis. Rare in boys under 5 to 6 years of age. Definite indication for circumcision.

613 Ammoniacal dermatitis (nappy rash). Caused by the presence of ammonia released by action of bacteria on the urea contained in the urine. Always involves the tip of the prepuce (posthitis), but widespread involvement of perineum and thighs can occur. Absolute contraindication to circumcision.

614 Meatal ulcer. Shallow red painful ulcer at the external urethral meatus. Caused by ammoniacal dermatitis and virtually confined to circumcised infants. May heal by cicatrisation and result in a meatal stenosis.

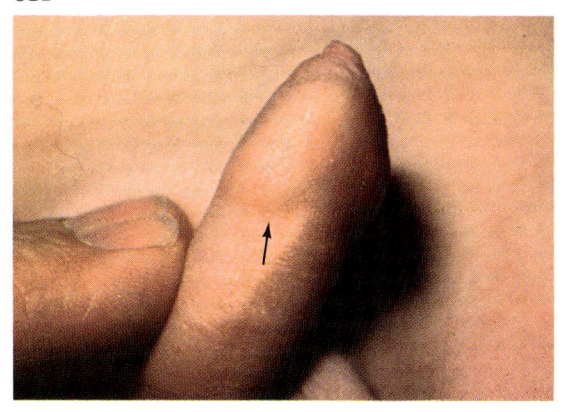

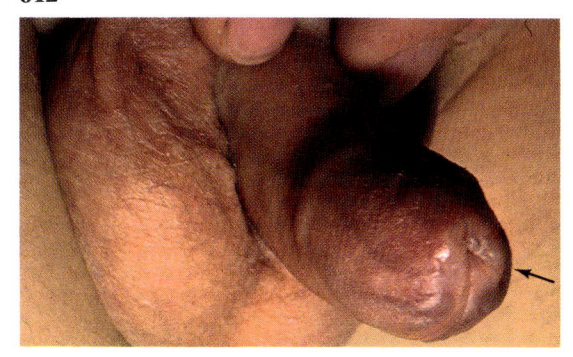

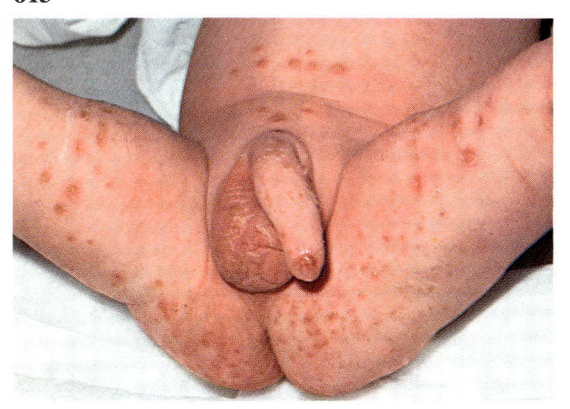

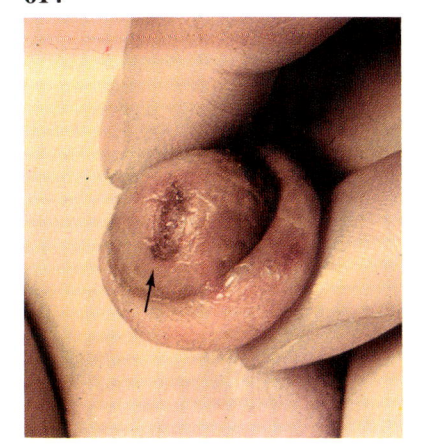

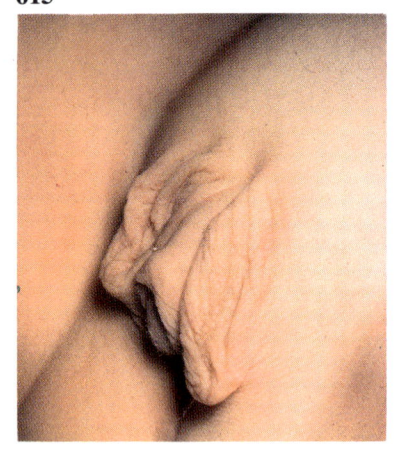

615 Hypospadias. Caused by failure of closure of the urethral groove as a consequence of which the urethral opening lies on the ventral aspect of the penis. The anomaly is classified according to the site of opening of the urethra – glandular, penile, penoscrotal and perineal. An example of perineal hypospadias associated with a bifid scrotum. Each hemi-scrotum contained a testis.

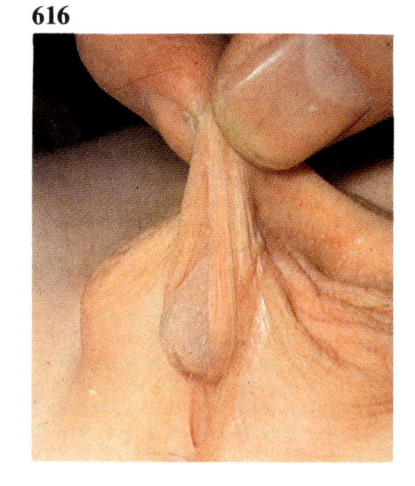

616 Hypospadias. The redundant foreskin on the dorsal aspect of the penis characteristically forms a 'hood'. This is a constant feature of all hypospadias. The redundant foreskin is used in the repair of the anomaly. Circumcision is absolutely contraindicated in the presence of hypospadias.

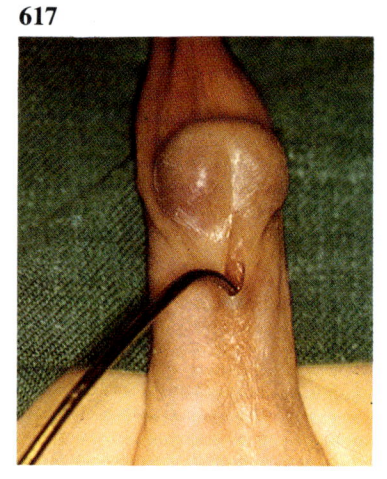

617 Penile hypospadias. The urethral opening on the ventral aspect of the shaft of the penis is demonstrated. The meatus is seldom stenotic but it is impossible to direct the stream of urine forward.

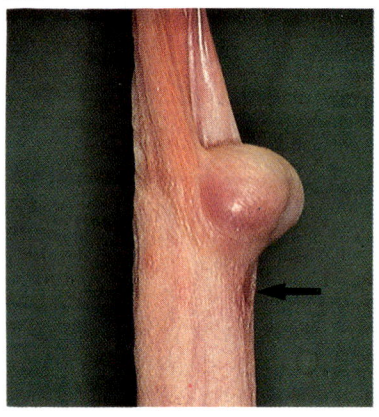

618 Penile hypospadias with chorde. Note the 'hooded' foreskin and the obvious ventral curvature of the glans of the penis caused by a relative deficiency of tissue between the meatus and the glans.

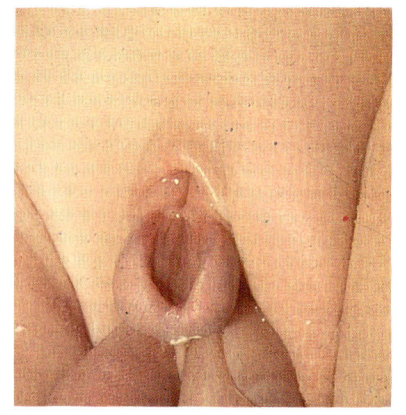

619 Epispadias. The urethra presents as an opened strip of exposed mucosa on the dorsal aspect of the penis. Distally it broadens out onto the flattened glans. With the exception of the mildest cases, there are associated anomalies of the bladder neck and sphincter mechanism and diastasis of the symphysis pubis.

42 Testis and scrotum

620 Maldescent of the testis.
Retractile testis is caused by elevation of the testis out of the scrotum and into the inguinal region by the action of the cremaster muscle.
Ectopic testis where the testis has emerged through the inguinal canal but has become lodged in an abnormal site, e.g. superficial inguinal pouch, perineum, prepubic, femoral regions (on the left groin in the diagram).
Undescended testis is caused by an arrest of testicular descent along a normal pathway from the site of development in the urogenital ridges of the retroperitoneum to the scrotum (on the right groin in the diagram).

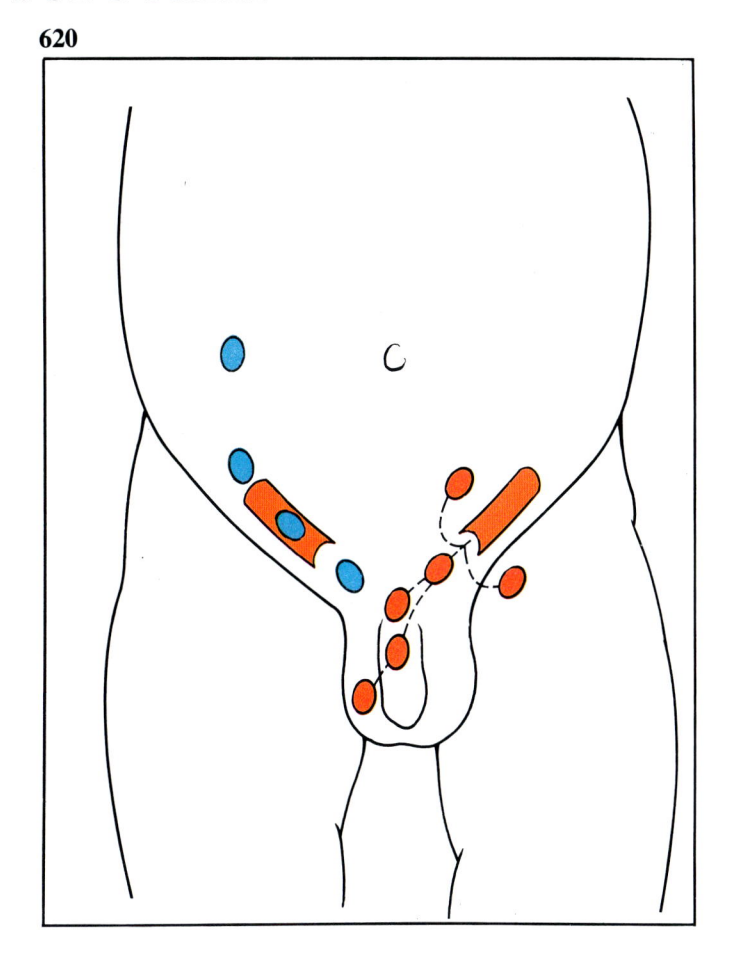

621 Undescended testis. The left testis is visible in the scrotum while the right hemi-scrotum is empty. The testis is palpable in the superficial inguinal pouch. Almost all undescended testes and at least half of the ectopic testes have an associated indirect inguinal hernia.

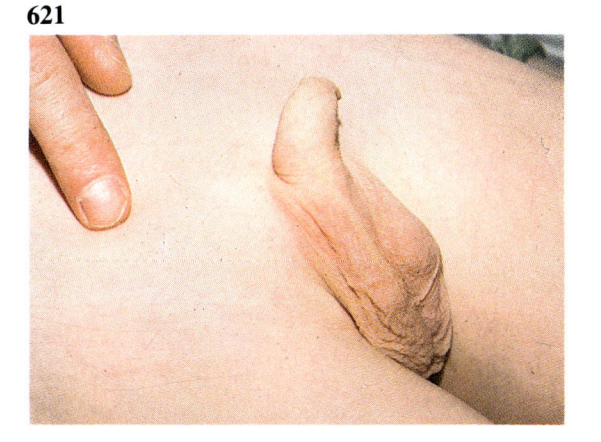

622 Idiopathic scrotal oedema. Acute oedematous swelling of the scrotum of rapid onset. Usually bilateral and extends into the perineum. Little or no associated pain. The testes are scrotal in position and not tender on palpation.

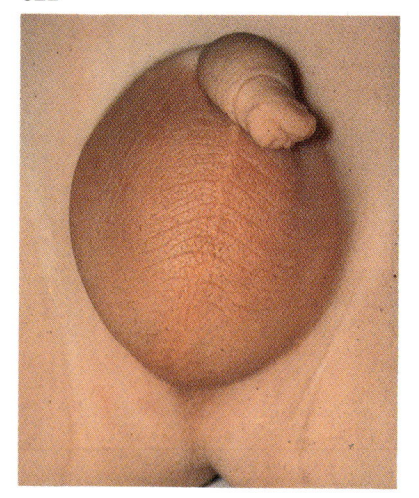

623 Torsion of the testis. May be supravaginal where the entire cord undergoes torsion or intravaginal as a result of an abnormal insertion of the spermatic cord (horizontal testis). Classically presents with acute onset of excruciating pain in the involved side of the scrotum. Surgical exploration as an emergency should be undertaken. It is essential to fix the contralateral testis prophylactically.

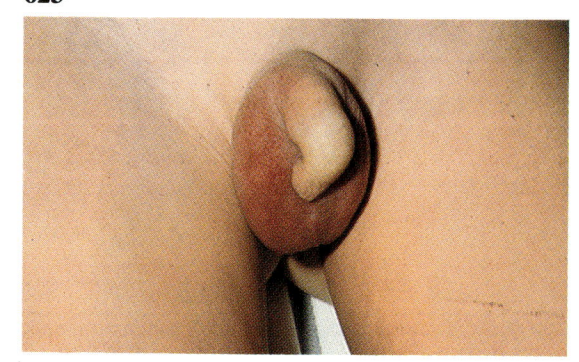

624 Torsion of the testis. Intravaginal torsion of the testis exposed at exploration showing the swollen cyanotic testis as a result of vascular insufficiency. Orchidectomy should not be performed as the Leydig cells withstand ischaemia better than the seminiferous tubules and may help to contribute to hormonal function.

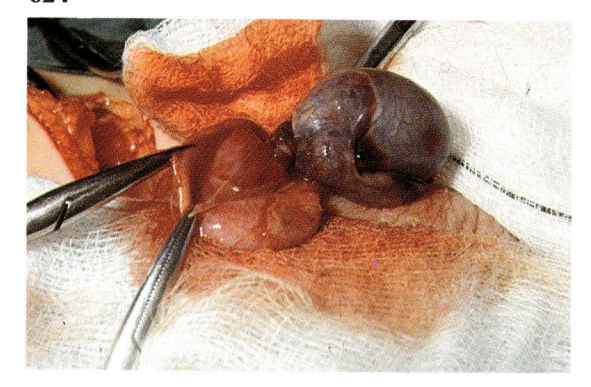

625 Torsion of the hydatid of Morgagni. Torsion of the appendix testis or epididymis may be clinically undistinguishable from torsion of the testis. Urgent surgical exploration should be carried out and the necrotic appendage excised.

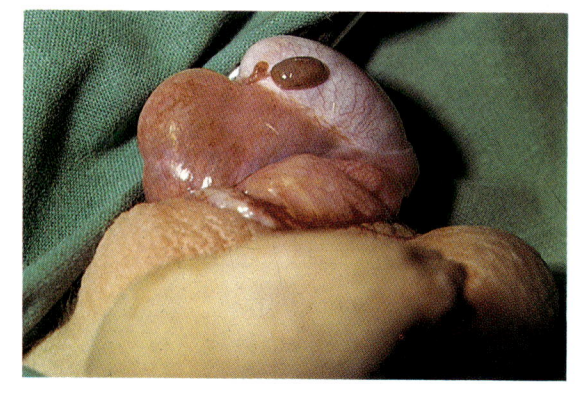

626 Epididymo-orchitis. Rare in infancy and childhood. Occurs mainly as a consequence of an acute urinary infection and is usually unilateral. Clinically it may be impossible to distinguish it from testicular torsion. If in doubt about the diagnosis, exploration should be undertaken.

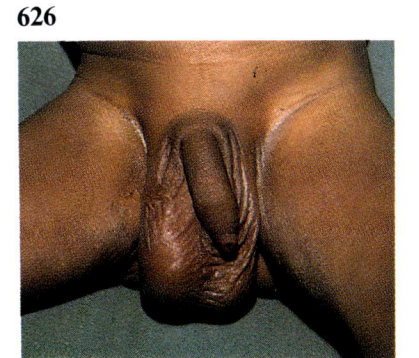

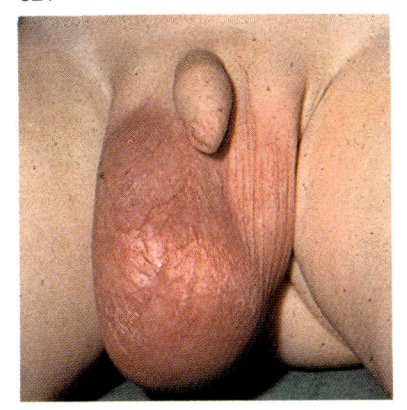

627 Orchioblastoma. Classically presents in the child under three years of age with gradual appearance of a painless swelling in the testis. The testis is firm and does not transilluminate. Treatment is by radical orchidectomy. Prognosis is good.

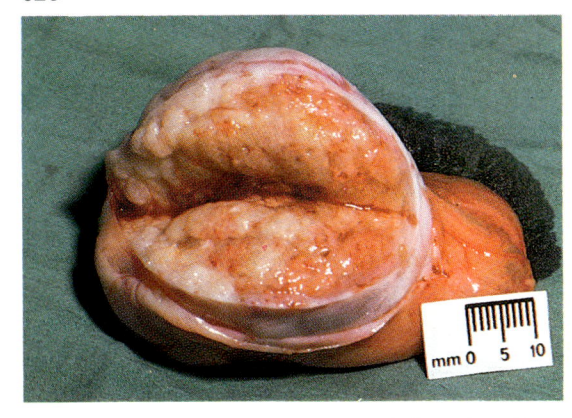

628 Orchioblastoma. The entire testis is replaced by a solid tumour which on section reveals irregular areas of haemorrhage and necrosis.

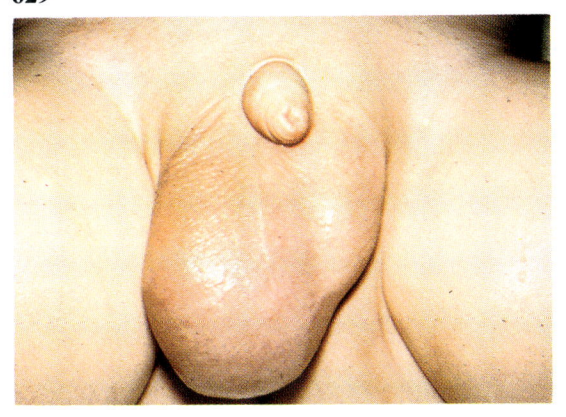

629 Teratoma of the testis. Presents with a non-inflammatory swelling of the involved side of the scrotum. Seminoma, more common in the undescended testis, rarely occurs before puberty.

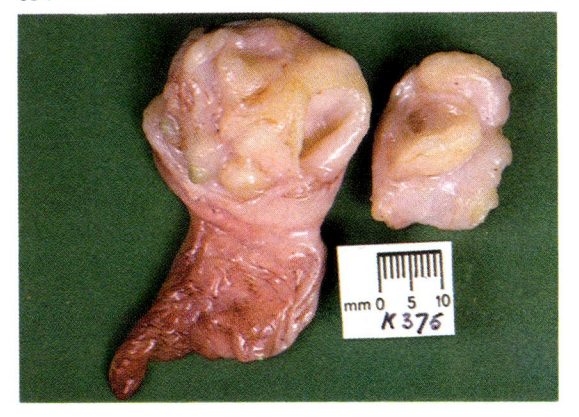

630 Teratoma of the testis. Section of the excised testis reveals the presence of foreign tissue and organs, e.g. intestine, cartilage. The tumour is invariably benign in the young infant, but at a later age it is often malignant.

631 Bifid scrotum. The scrotum is split into two halves each containing a gonad. Commonly associated with a severe degree of hypospadias or an anorectal anomaly.

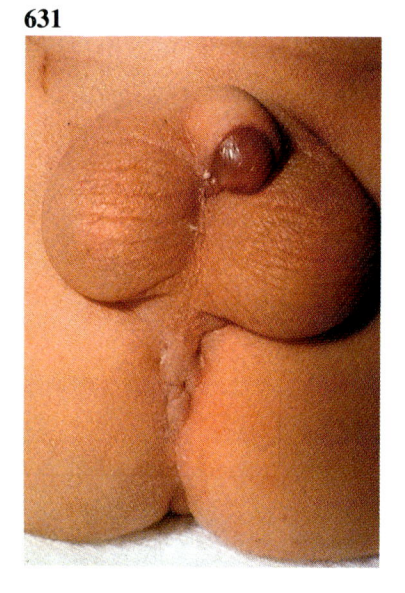

632 Perineal defect. Unusual malformation in which the left half of the perineum has failed to develop and the rectal mucosa has prolapsed into the deficient area. Note the widely split scrotum. There was also a perineal hypospadias.

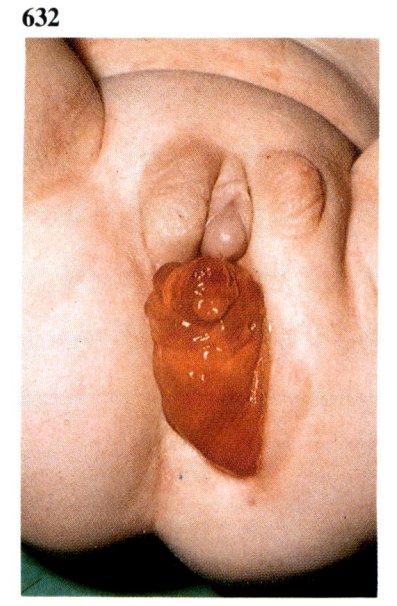

633 Perineal hernia. There is a herniation of the rectum through a defect in the attachment of the pelvic floor.

634 Perineal haematoma. Commonly occurs after a straddle injury. The haematoma has spread from the perineum to the base of the scrotum. It is important to exclude an associated urethral injury.

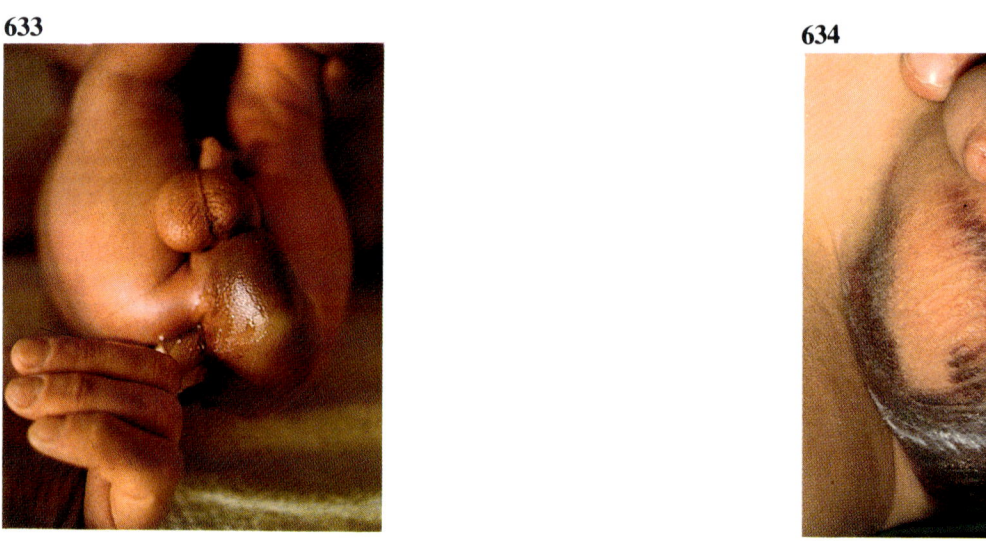

43 Female genital organs

635 Ovarian cyst. In children most ovarian tumours are of the germ-cell origin (teratoma, dysgerminoma, embryonal carcinoma, yolk-sac tumour, etc). They usually present as asymptomatic abdominal masses or with acute abdominal pain caused by torsion.

636 Ovarian teratoma. Plain xray of the abdomen shows an ovoid radio-opaque mass filling the lower abdomen and pelvis. An area of dense calcification is present in the left upper part of the mass. This is characteristic of a teratoma.

637 Ovarian teratoma. Ultrasonography shows a cystic mass with an area of calcification in the anteroinferior aspect.

638 Ovarian teratoma (dermoid). Operative view showing a large cystic ovarian mass. Most of these tumours are benign. Treatment consists of excision with conservation of the remaining ovarian tissue where possible. The contralateral ovary should always be inspected.

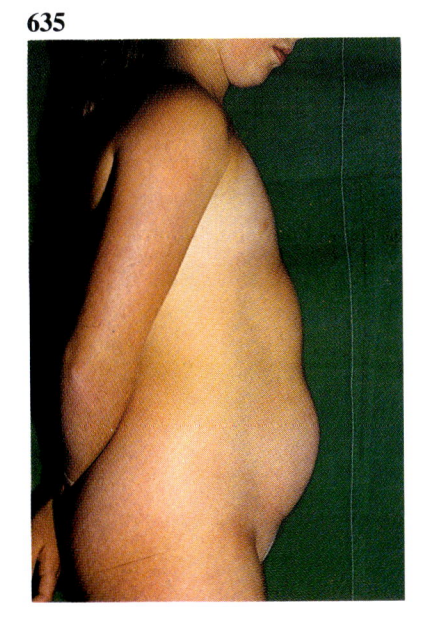

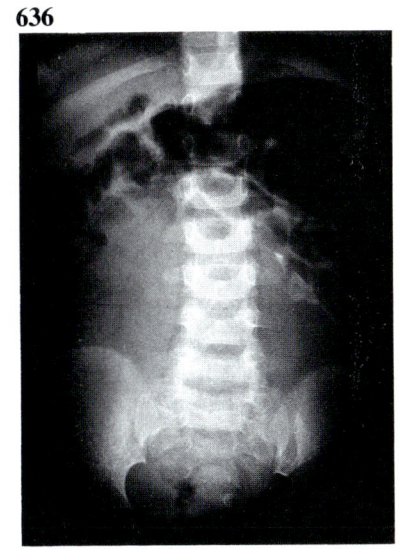

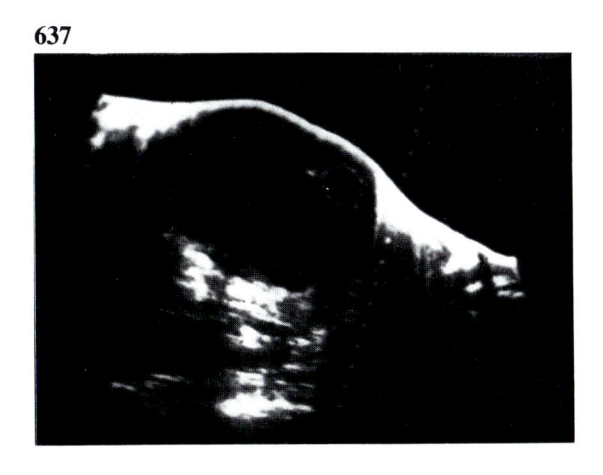

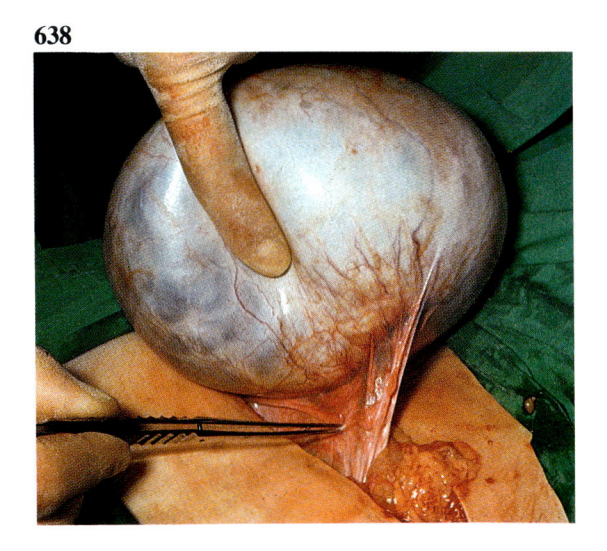

639 Endodermal sinus (yolk-sac) tumour. Most common extraembryonal germ cell tumour of the ovary. These tumours grow rapidly and may present with extensive intra-abdominal and intrapelvic spread. Alpha-foetoprotein levels are frequently elevated.

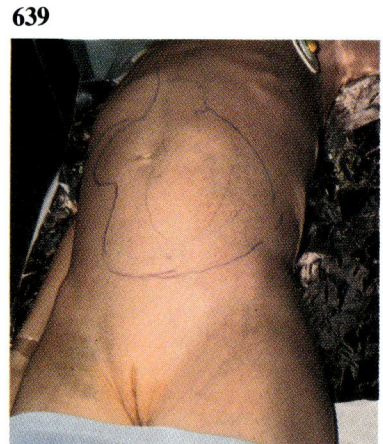

640 Yolk-sac tumour of the ovary. Excised specimen shows a large non-encapsulated tumour with areas of haemorrhage and necrosis. Excision was incomplete and recurrence developed within a short period.

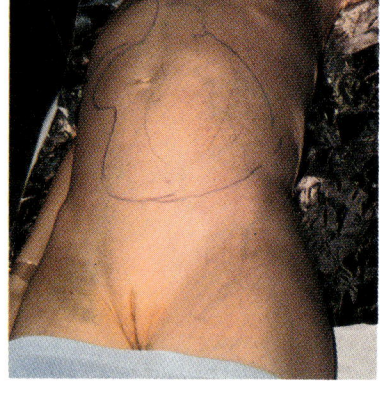

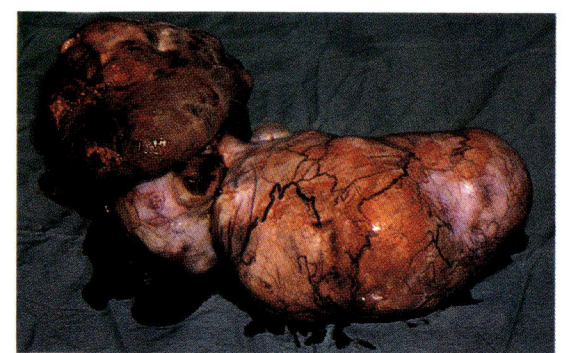

641 Hydrocolpos. Visible lower abdominal mass in an infant with hydrocolpos. Part of the mass is caused by a distended bladder as a result of urethral obstruction from the distended vagina. Note the discoloration and oedema of the lower abdominal wall.

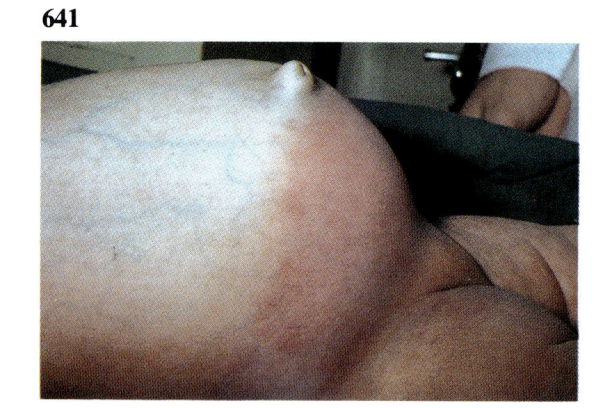

642 Hydrocolpos. The most common cause of hydrocolpos is a membranous obstruction in the region of the hymen. The bulging membrane in the perineum is well shown. Treatment is by simple incision of the membrane.

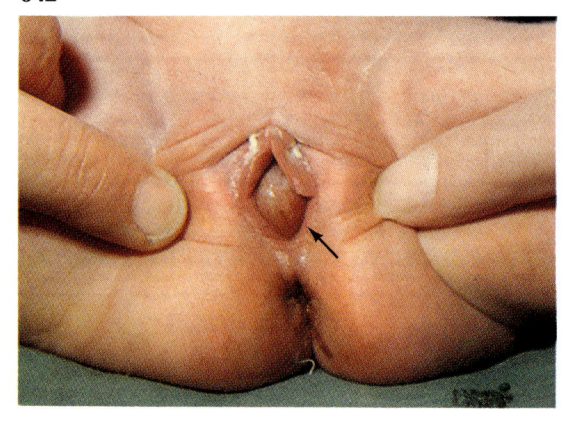

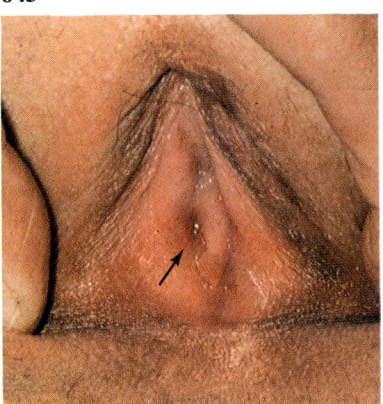

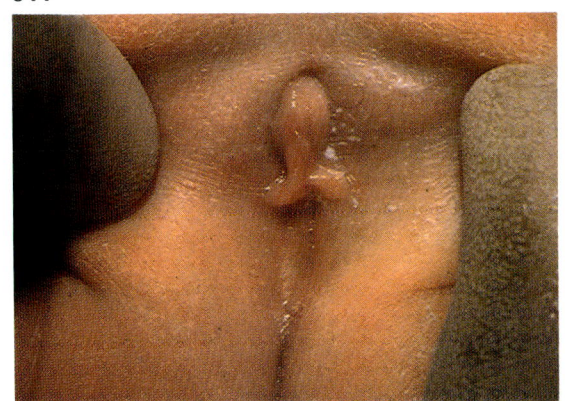

643 Vaginal atresia. Usually involves the lower third of the vagina; the upper part becomes distended with blood during menstruation (haematocolpos). The patient presents after puberty with periodic menstrual pain and amenorrhoea. Later urinary symptoms as a result of obstruction may occur.

644 Labial adhesions. The labia minora are fused in the midline by flimsy adhesions leaving only a small opening anteriorly for the urethral orifice. The adhesions can be lysed by gentle traction on the labia with or without the aid of a probe.

645 Vaginal discharge. A purulent vaginal discharge in a young child is frequently caused by a retained foreign body in the vagina. Urinary tract infection or threadworm infestation may also be responsible. Vaginoscopy is required to exclude a foreign body.

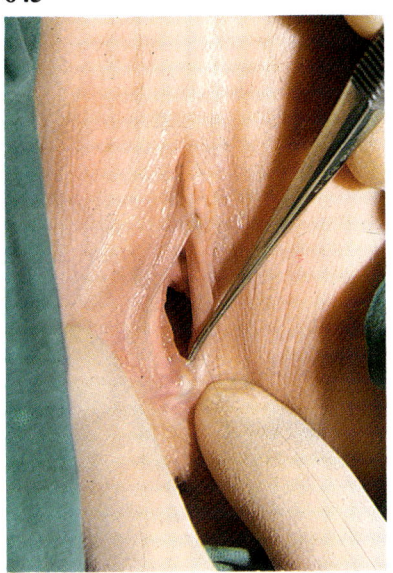

646 Hamartoma of the vulva. A rare pedunculated 'tumour' or malformation arising from the posterior wall of the vulva and presenting at birth. No malignant potential. Treatment consists of simple excision.

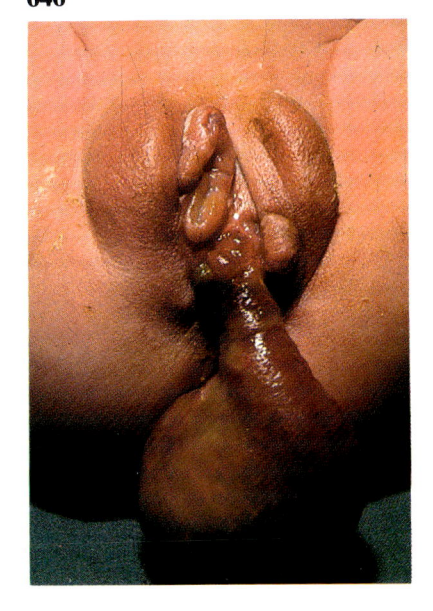

44 Intersex

Classification of abnormal sexual development is as follows:
1. Abnormal gonadal development, i.e. true hermaphrodite.
2. Abnormal genital development in the presence of normal ovarian tissue, i.e. female pseudohermaphrodite.
3. Abnormal genital development in the presence of normal testicular tissue, i.e. male pseudohermaphrodite.

647 True hermaphrodite. The penis is well developed but with a severe degree of perineal hypospadias. The gonads contain both ovarian and testicular elements. Most cases are chromatin-positive and have a 46XX karyotype.

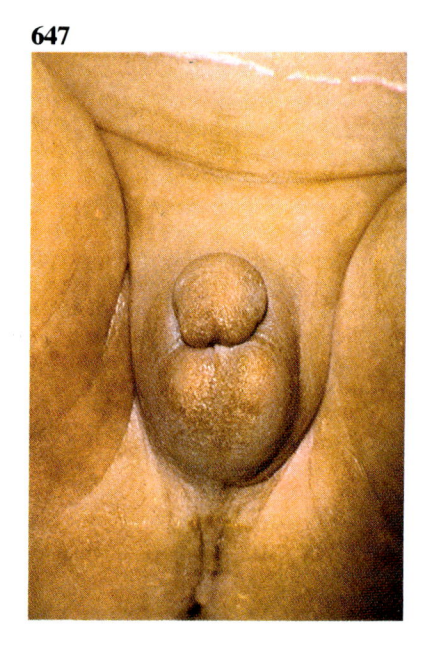

648 True hermaphrodite. At puberty, breast development occurs and menstruation begins. The latter may be mistaken for haematuria where there is a complete male type of urethra. The phallus also enlarges and pubic and facial hair appears.

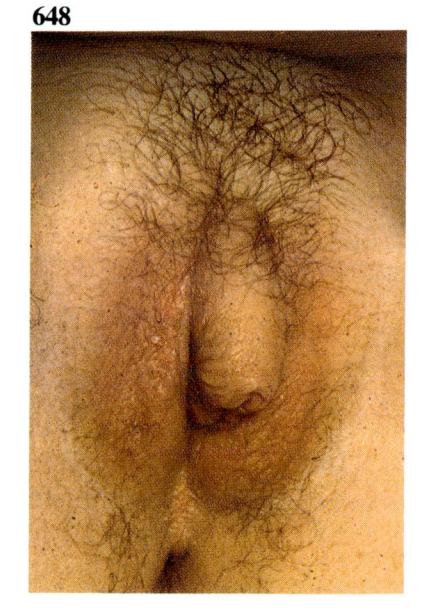

649 Female pseudohermaphrodite. Masculinisation of the female (XX karyotype and normal ovaries) caused by excessive androgen production. Fusion of the labia with enlargement of the clitorus is evident. The adrenogenital syndrome is the most common cause of virilisation in the female.

650 Ambiguous genitalia. The phallus is well developed but the labioscrotal folds are separated by a funnel-shaped urogenital sinus.

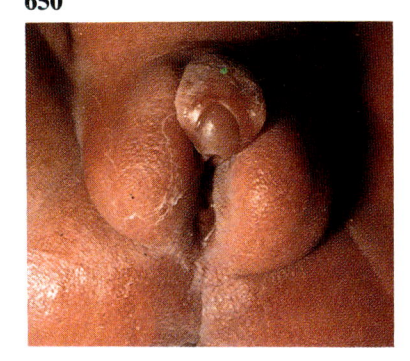

651 Adrenogenital syndrome. Urogenital sinogram showing a normal urethra anteriorly with a posterior located normal vagina, cervix, appearing as a W-shaped indentation in the vagina and a large uterus. This indicates that the patient is female.

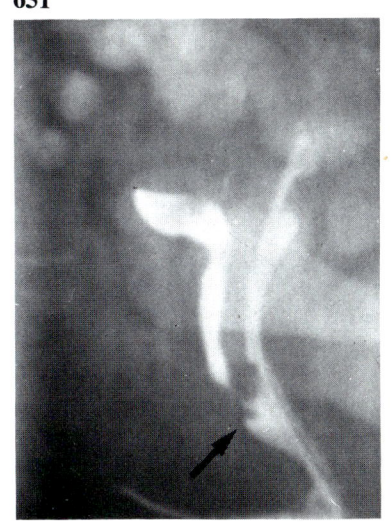

652 Male pseudohermaphrodite – testicular feminisation syndrome. External genitalia are those of a normal female. The child presents with an inguinal hernia (usually bilateral) which contains a gonad. Approximately one per cent of girls with bilateral inguinal hernia have the testicular feminisation syndrome. Chromosomal studies should be carried out on all girls with bilateral inguinal hernia. Gonadal biopsy should be taken from a gonad which appears abnormal.

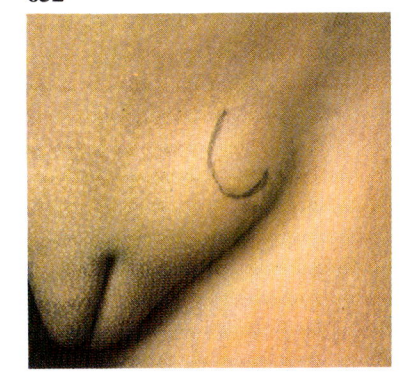

45 Central nervous system

Spina bifida. Results from a developmental anomaly in the formation of the spinal cord and/or vertebral column. The degree of spinal dysraphism varies from:
i) spina bifida occulta where there is merely a gap in the vertebral arch,
ii) meningocoele where only the meninges are involved; may be entirely skin covered,
iii) myelomeningocoele where the neural tissue and membranes are involved, to
iv) rachischisis where the neural tube lies wide-open and exposed on the surface of the lesion.

653 Spina bifida occulta. May be an incidental finding on xray in 10 to 20 per cent of normal individuals. The lesion may be associated with overlying skin anomalies such as a hairy patch, naevus, haemangioma, dermal sinus.

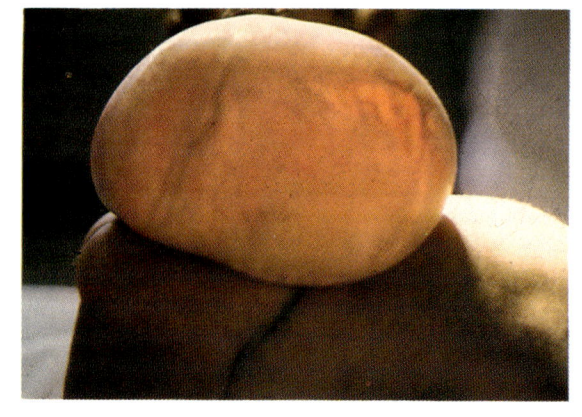

654 and 655 Meningocoele. The cystic lesion in the sacral region of the spine contains cerebrospinal fluid only and no nervous tissue (**654**). The lesion is skin covered and brilliantly transilluminable (**655**).

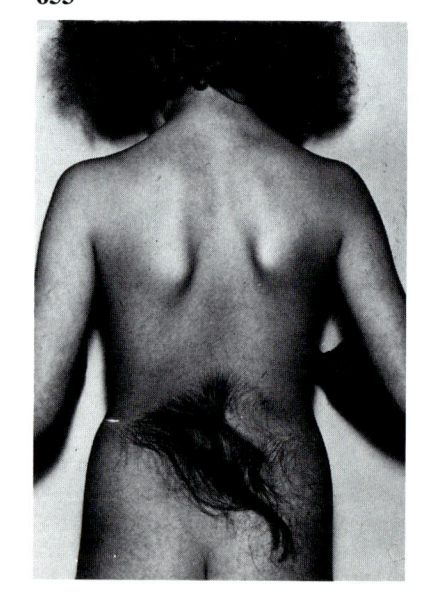

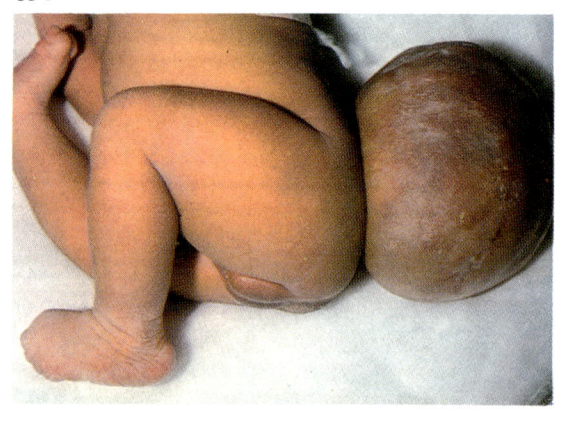

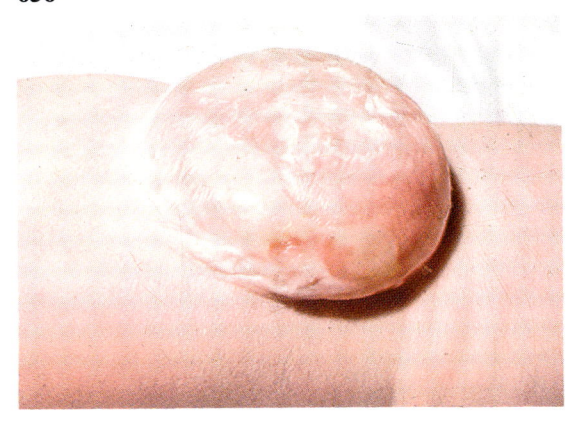

656 Meningocoele. The cystic lesion in the lower lumbar region is covered by skin around the periphery and by meninges over the dome of the swelling.

657 Myelomeningocoele. The neural component occupies the central strip of the lesion. Laterally the opened out meninges merge with the skin around the periphery of the defect. Leakage of cerebrospinal fluid is almost invariably present.

658 Myelomeningocoele. Thoracolumbar myelomenginocoele of severe proportions. There is complete flaccid paralysis of the lower extremities, neuropathic bladder and incontinence of urine and faeces. Hydrocephalus is almost always present in these cases.

659 Rachischisis. The neural tissue in the centre of the lumbosacral myelomeningocoele represents the opened spinal canal. The neural groove in the midline is evident. Nervous function distal to the lesion is severely affected.

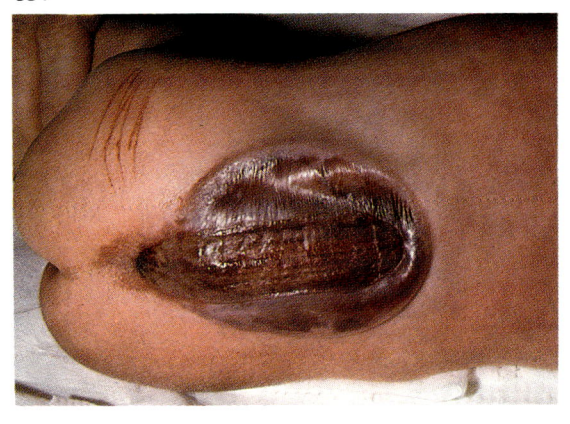

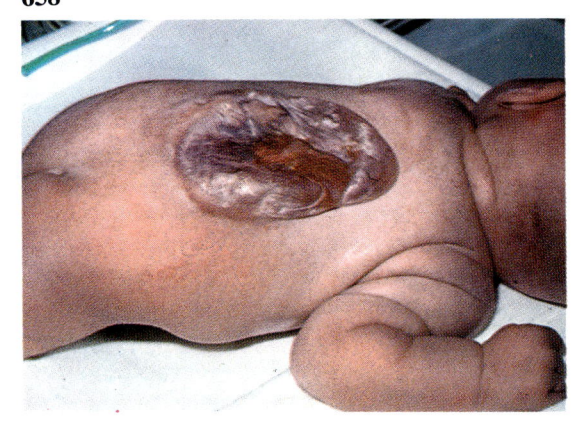

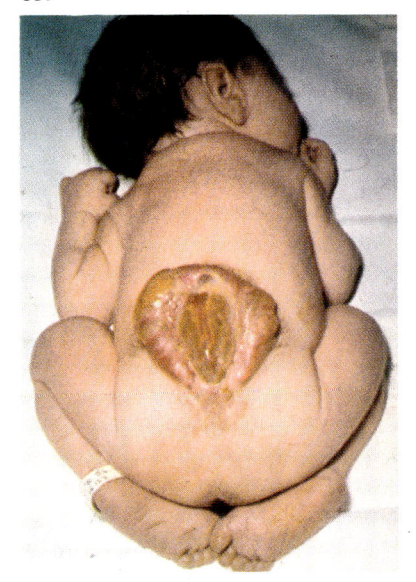

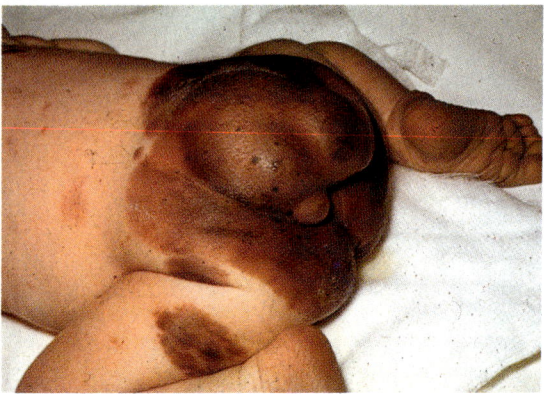

660 Myelodysplasia. The sacral meningocoele (skin covered) is associated with extensive pigmentation of the surrounding skin and with an underlying lipoma.

661 Sacral sinus. Sinuses overlying the sacrum may communicate with the spinal canal. If the base of the lesion cannot be visualised, excision is recommended. Injection of contrast material or probing of the sinus is strictly contraindicated because of the risk of introducing infection.

662 Congenital dermal sinus. The sinus is sited in the midline of the neck. It is deep and narrow and should be excised as it probably communicates with the spinal canal. Meningitis is a risk, if left untreated.

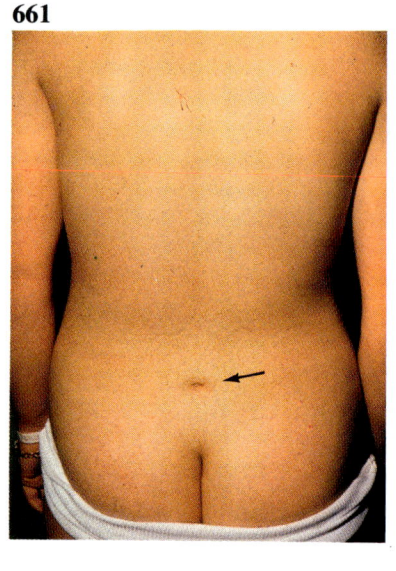

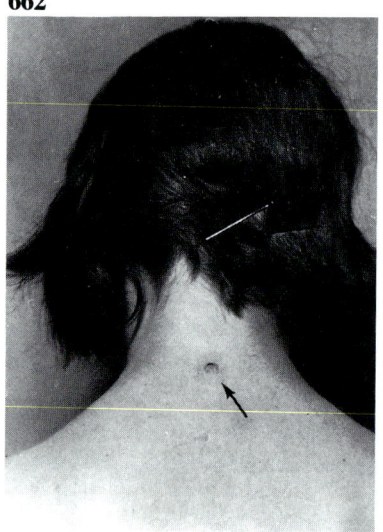

663 Spinal dermoid cyst. The cyst is present over the mid-sacrum and may communicate through a defect in the vertebral arch with a similar lesion within the spinal theca. Pressure symptoms caused by the intraspinal dermoid may be the first signs of the lesion.

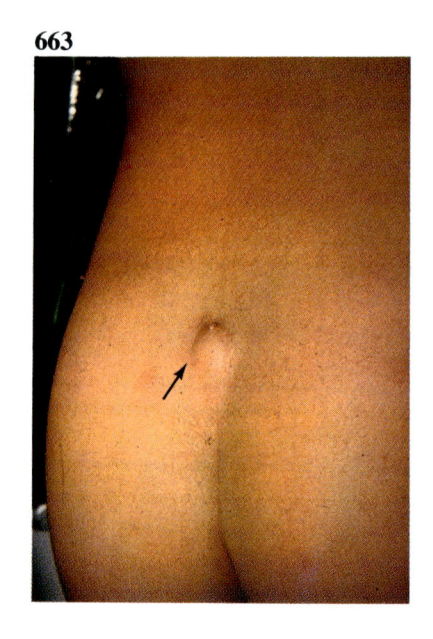

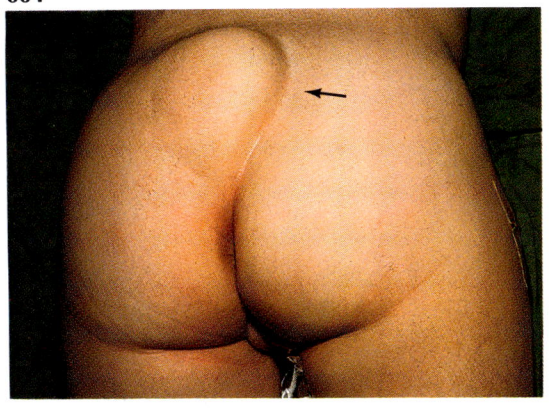

664 Lipoma of the cauda equina. Superficial fatty tumour in the lumbosacral region often displaced to one side of the midline. May be associated with a spina bifida occulta, naevus or sinus. Frequently extends into spinal canal and is connected to the spinal cord, filum terminale or cauda equina. May present with neurological deficit, e.g. urinary incontinence, lower limb neuropathy.

665 Cervical meningocoele. Situated in the upper cervical spine. Often confused with an encephalocoele. Skin covered and rarely associated with any neurological deficit.

666 Sincipital encephalocoele. Common in south-east Asia. Nasofrontal meningocoele which is skin covered and contains only cerebrospinal fluid. Repair should include covering of the bony defect to prevent recurrence of the herniation.

667 Sincipital encephalocoele. Fronto-ethmoid encephalocoele of enormous proportion containing a major part of the frontal lobes of the brain. Associated with hydrocephalus. High incidence of mental retardation.

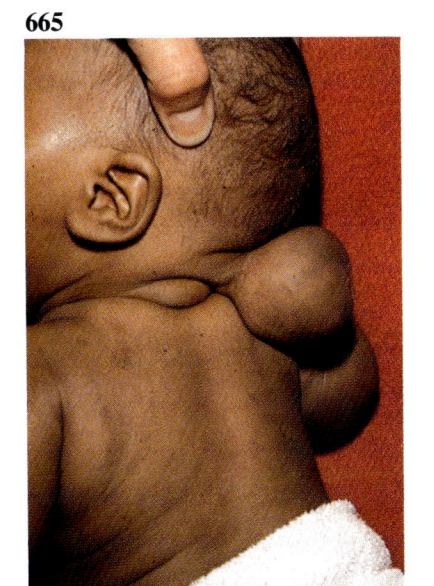

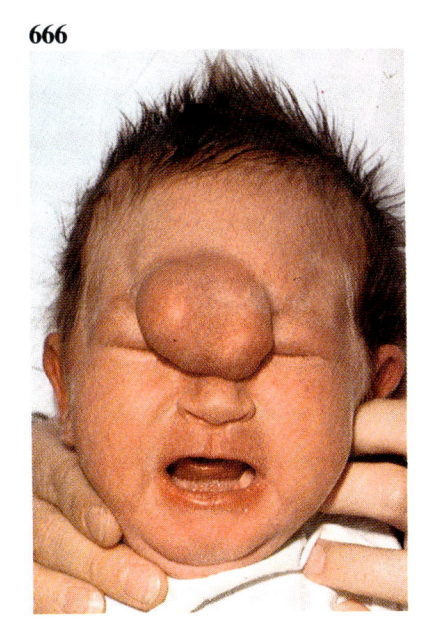

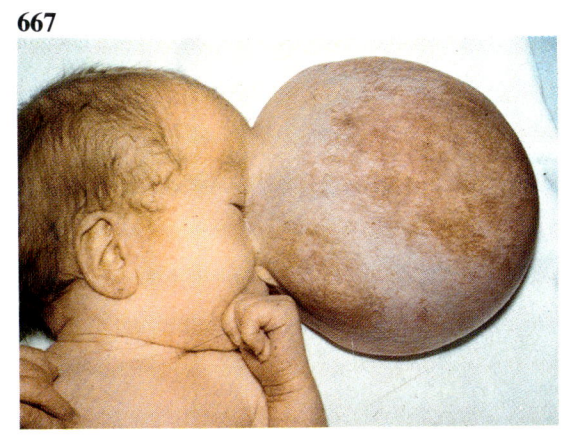

668 Frontal encephalocoele. There is a bulging of the entire forehead through an extensive defect in the frontal bone. The sac contains a major part of the frontal lobes.

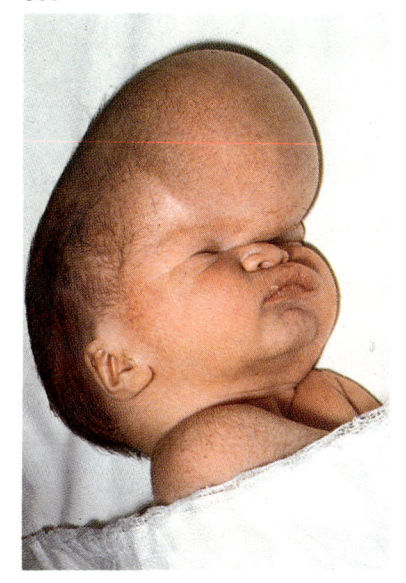

669 Parietal encephalocoele. The large lesion contains a major portion of the cerebral cortex and is associated with microcephaly.

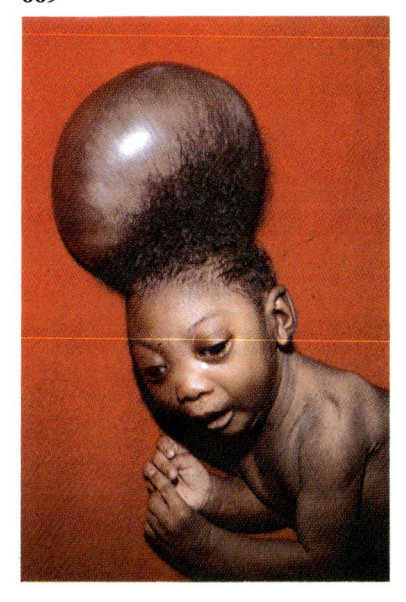

670 Occipital encephalocoele. The bony defect may be confined to the occipital bone or may extend into the foramen magnum. The hernial sac contains parts of the occipital lobes and occasionally cerebellum and brainstem. Associated microcephaly is frequently present as is hydrocephalus.

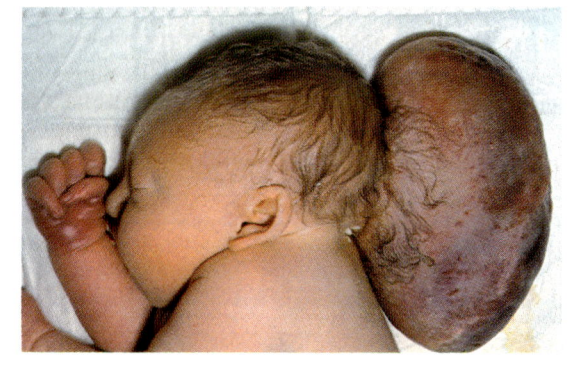

671 Hydrocephalus. Abnormal enlargement of the cranium as a result of an interference with the circulation of cerebrospinal fluid. May be 'internal' (obstructive) or 'external' (communicating). The head is obviously enlarged and prominent subcutaneous scalp veins are visible. The eyes are displaced downwards ('setting sun' sign) so that the upper sclera is visible. Cranial sutures are widely splayed.

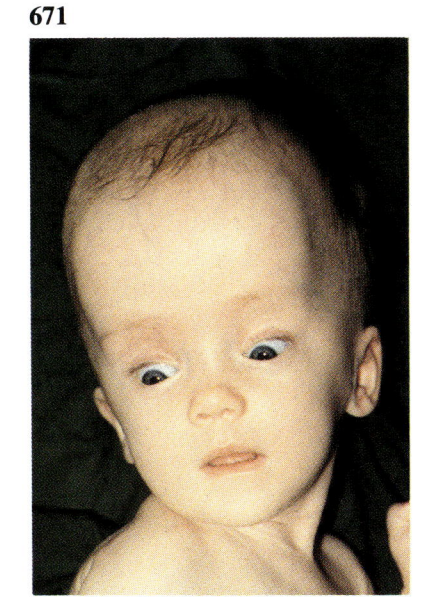

672 Hydrocephalus. The skull is transilluminable in severe cases of hydrocephalus with marked thinning of the cerebral cortex or in cases of hydrencephaly.

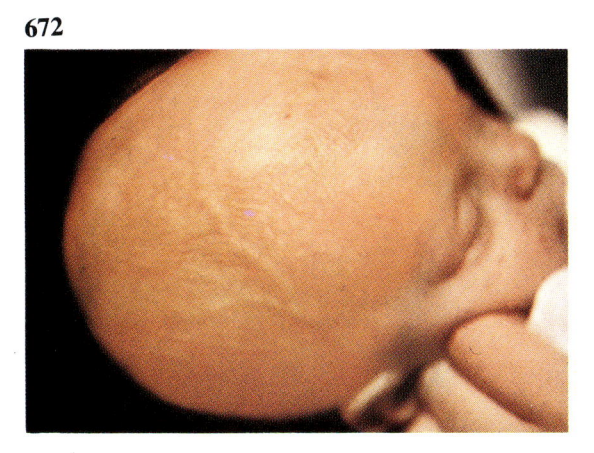

673 Papilloedema. Usually bilateral and results from raised intracranial pressure. The margin of the optic disc is obscured. The retinal veins are distended and tortuous and can be seen to course over the bulging optic disc. Retinal haemorrhages occur at an advanced stage.

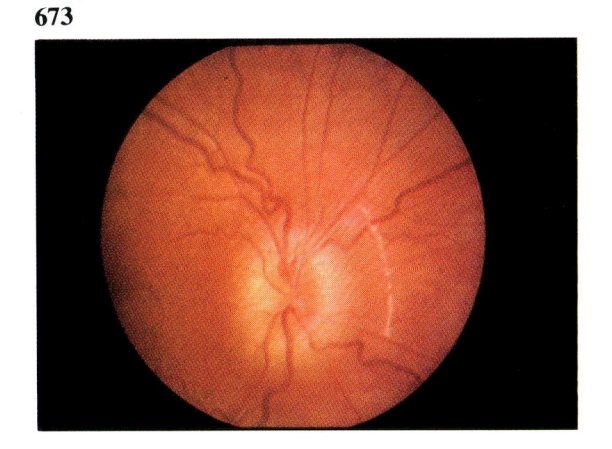

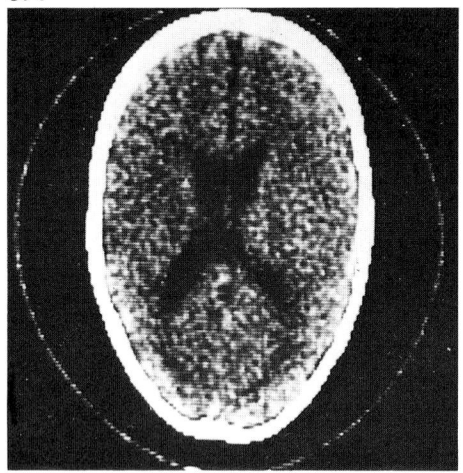

674 Mild hydrocephalus. Computerised axial tomography (CT) shows mild dilatation of the lateral ventricles.

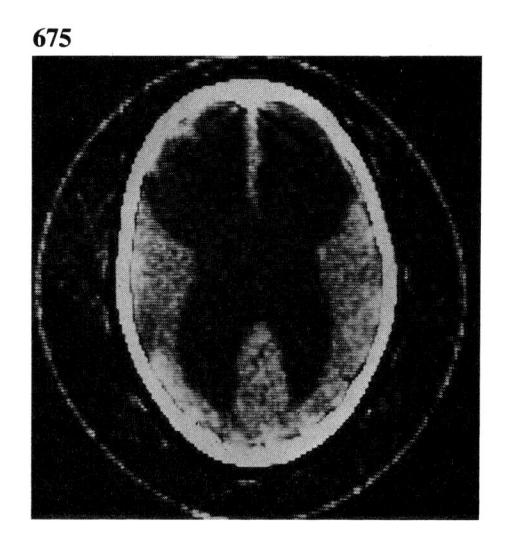

675 Severe hydrocephalus. CT scan shows marked dilatation of the ventricular system with peripheral compression of the cerebral cortex.

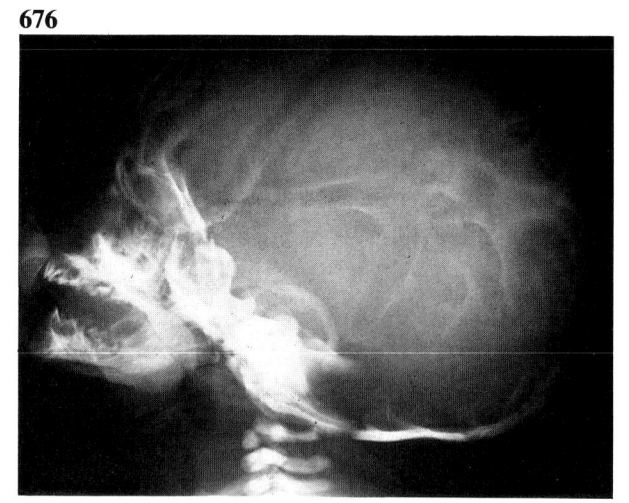

676 'Lacunar' skull. The presence of craniolacunae on the lateral skull xray in an infant with myelomeningocoele. This feature is apparent at birth and has a high association with hydrocephalus.

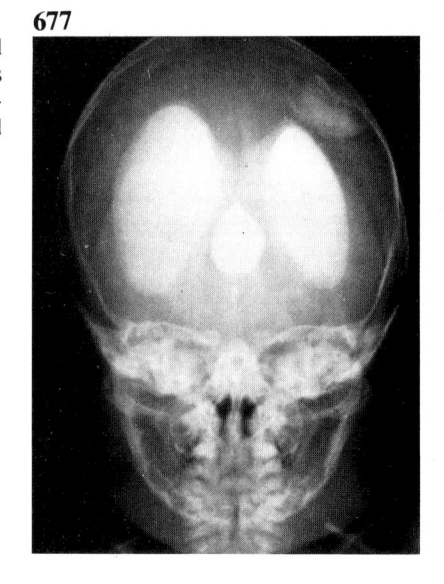

677 Contrast ventriculogram. Contrast material has been introduced into the lateral ventricles via ventricular puncture. The contrast outlines the dilated lateral and third ventricles. The extent of cerebral compression can also be assessed. The examination has been largely superseded by computerised tomography.

678 Hydrocephalus. Sagittal section through the brain showing the marked degree of ventricular dilatation.

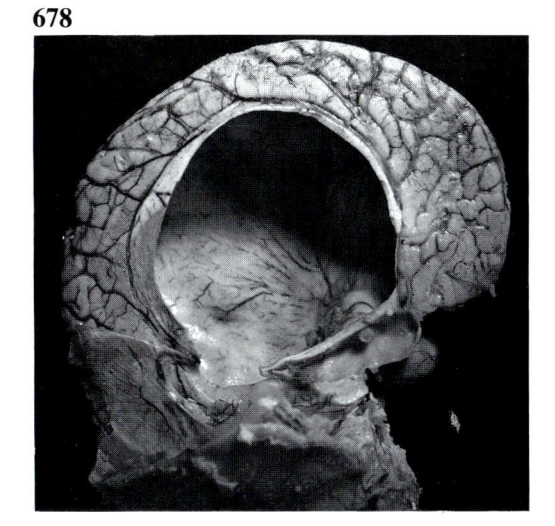

Craniosynostosis. Premature closure of the cranial sutures leads to craniosynostosis:
679 premature closure of the sagittal suture – scaphocephaly. The head is elongated and narrow.
680 premature closure of the coronal suture – brachycephaly. The head is high, broad and short. Surgical treatment should be carried out before three months of age for maximum cosmetic benefit.

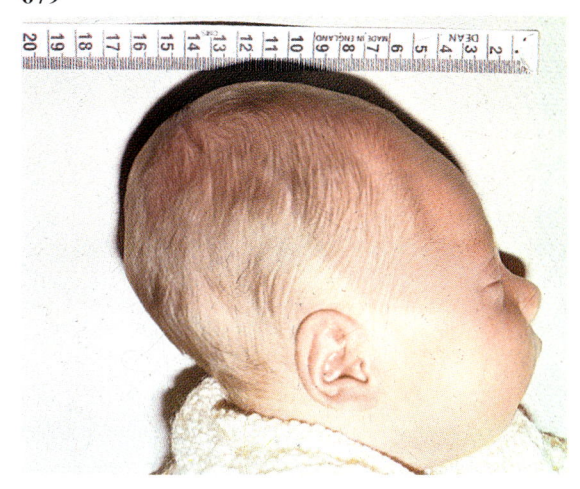

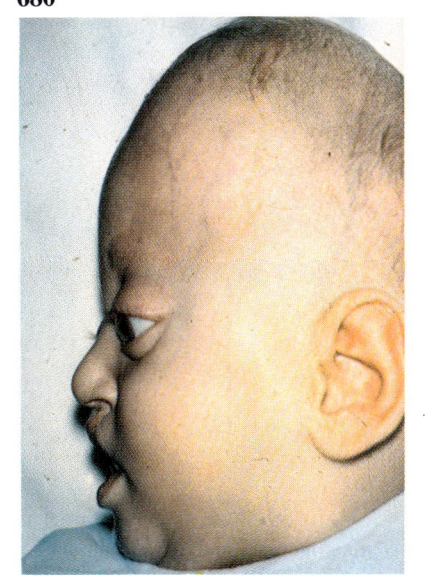

Brain tumours. Classification of the common brain tumours in childhood according to site and pathological type:

A Infratentorial
   cerebellar astrocytoma
   medulloblastoma
   ependymoma
   brain stem glioma (astrocytoma)

B Supratentorial
   astrocytoma
   ependymoma
   optic nerve glioma
   craniopharyngioma

Cause clinical symptoms by obstruction of cerebrospinal fluid circulation and consequent raised intracranial pressure. Symptoms include headache, irritability, vomiting.

Physical findings may include a large head and bulging fontanelle (in young infants) or papilloedema. Visual defects also occur, e.g. sixth nerve palsy.

681 Cerebellar astrocytoma. Computerised tomographic scan (CT scan) showing an oval area of low attenuation in the left cerebellar hemisphere. The fourth ventricle is displaced forwards and to the right.

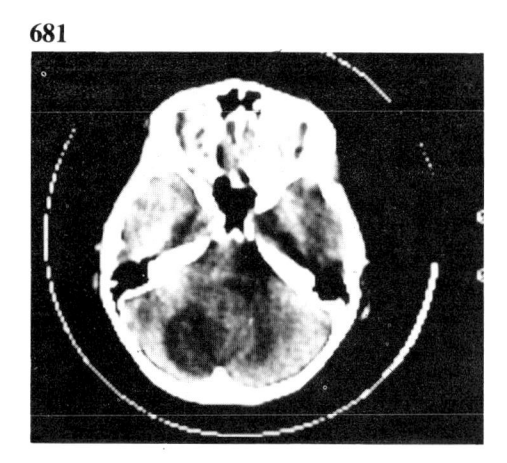

682 Ependymoma. CT scan combined with injection of contrast medium. There is a mass of high attenuation in the midline of the posterior fossa which has filled and enlarged the fourth ventricle. The low attenuation within the mass represents small cysts or necrotic tissue.

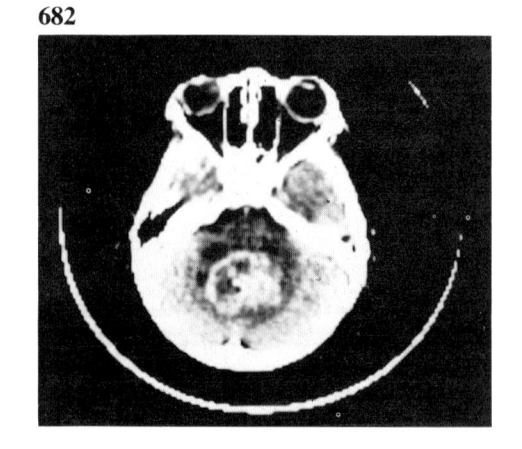

683 Medulloblastoma. CT scan after introduction of contrast medium. The tumour in the fourth ventricle shows dense enhancement and a lobulated surface. Medulloblastomas are highly malignant tumours with a poor prognosis.

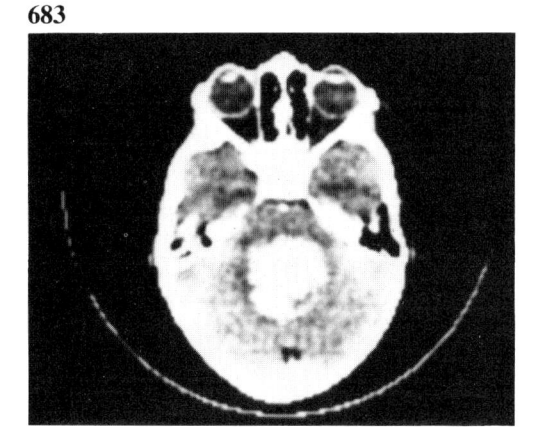

684 Craniopharyngioma. Calcifying cystic lesion in the supracellar region on CT scan. The cyst fluid is rich in cholesterol and its density is less than that of cerebrospinal fluid. The tumour arises from the remnants of Rathke's pouch. Tissues are not usually malignant. Symptoms are produced by blockage of CSF circulation causing increased intracranial pressure and by inducing visual defects.

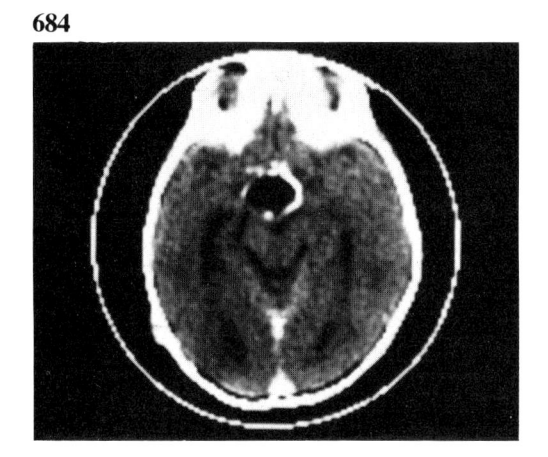

685 Temporal astrocytoma. Left temporal astrocytoma shown on common carotid angiogram. There is elevation of the branches of the middle cerebral artery in the Sylvian fissure, maximum in the posterior temporal region. The tumour is avascular.

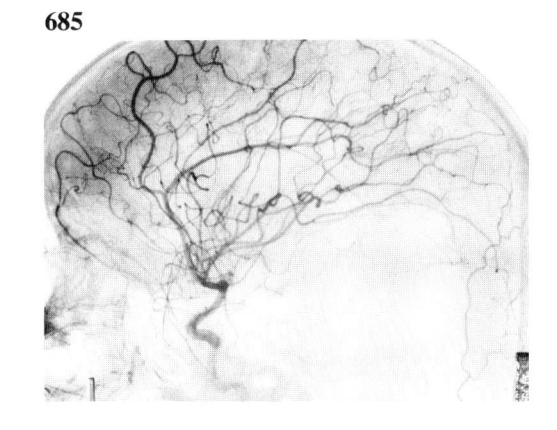

46 Skin and subcutaneous tissue

686 Naevus. Pigmented naevi rarely show malignant change before puberty. Only aim of surgical treatment in childhood is cosmetic.

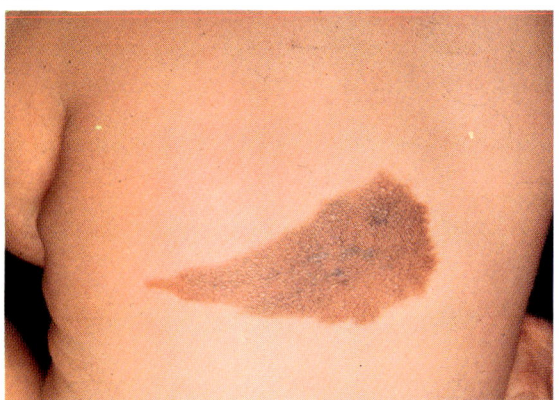

687 Hairy naevus. The lesion occupies the posterior aspect of the thigh and consists of a pigmented area covered by dark fine hair. Numerous raised black areas are visible within the pigmented lesion. Treatment consists of excision and skin grafting as there is a definite increased risk of malignancy.

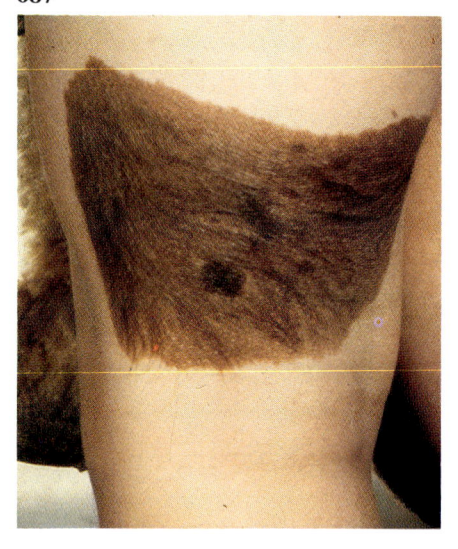

688 Giant hairy naevus. The lesion covers most of the trunk or an extremity. Considerable increased risk of malignant transformation before puberty. Treatment consists of excision and skin grafting where feasible. Shaving off the superficial layer is beneficial particularly where the surface is nodular. It also results in reduced pigmentation.

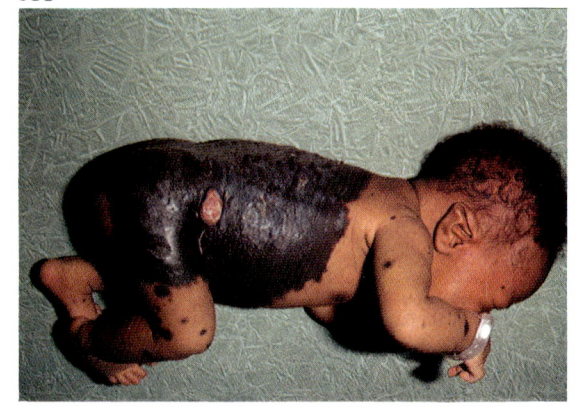

Haemangiomata. Malformation of blood vessels. May be classified into:
a) capillary – port wine stain
b) cavernous:
   i) superficial – 'strawberry mark'
   ii) deep
   iii) mixed (most common)
c) arteriovenous

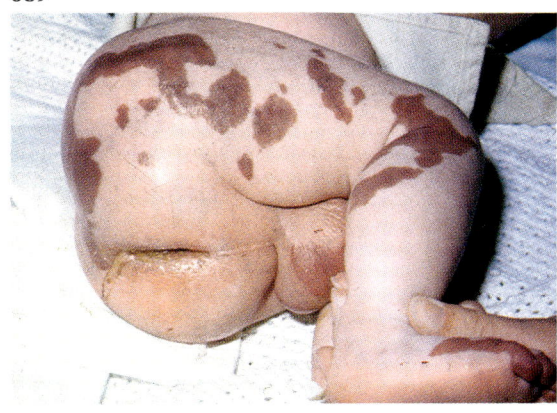

689 Capillary haemangioma. Lies in or immediately under the dermal layer of the skin and appears as a well demarcated purplish lesion which projects only slightly above the level of the skin.

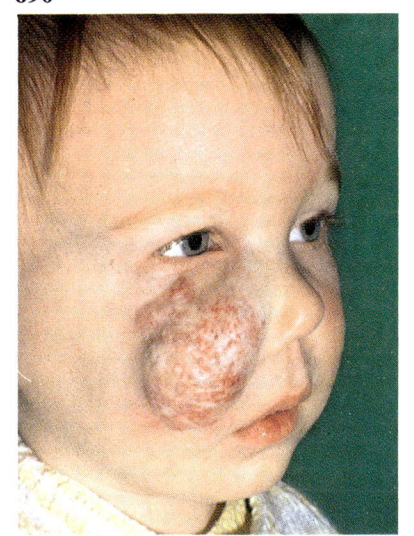

690 'Strawberry mark'. Commences soon after birth as a tiny red spot which rapidly enlarges over a few weeks. Growth ceases at about six months and the raised lobulated swelling persists for two to three years. It then regresses spontaneously over three to five years.

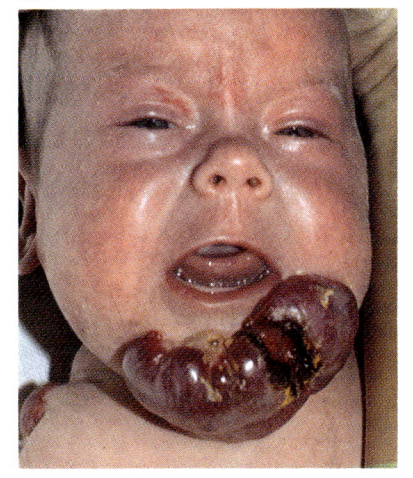

691 Cavernous haemangioma. Extensive raised lobulated and partially ulcerated lesion involving the chin. Excision was required because of repeated episodes of haemorrhage from the ulcerated portion.

692 Cavernous haemangioma. Regression may be accelerated by injection of sclerosing agents. Extensive lesions may be complicated by thrombocytopenia (Kasabach-Merritt syndrome).

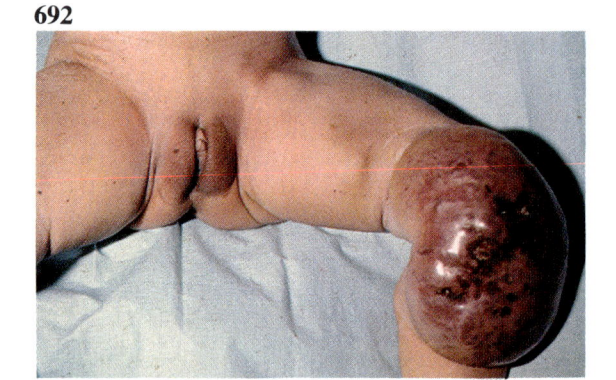

693 Involuting haemangioma. Ulceration has occurred in the centre of the lesion but areas of decreased vascularity are evident.

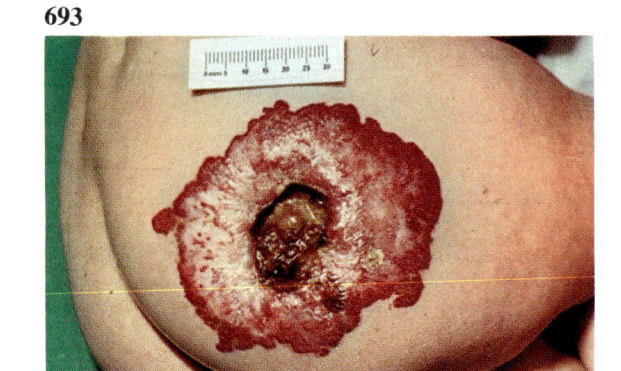

694 Arteriovenous malformation. In simple form resembles a cavernous haemangioma, but may be associated with local hypertrophy of the extremity or part involved.
Numerous superficial vessels may be visible and bruits are audible over the entire length of the part involved.

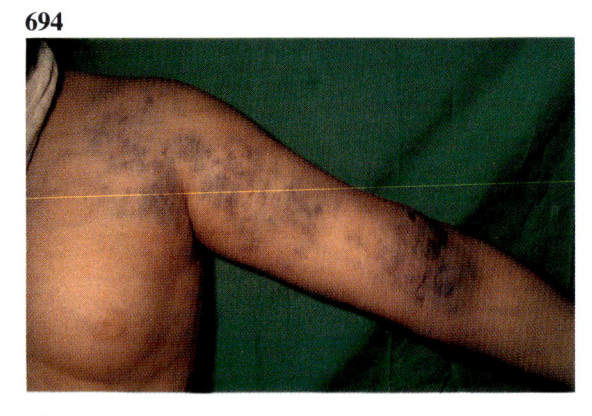

695 Arteriovenous aneurysm. Rare lesion. Presented as a pulsatile localised swelling in the left side of the neck. There were no associated circulatory problems (i.e. hyperdynamic circulation) or congestive cardiac failure.

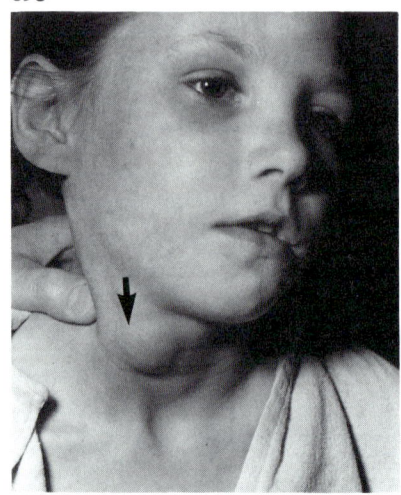

Lymphangioma. Malformation of lymphatic vessels. More commonly a hamartomatous lesion. Rarely undergoes spontaneous regression. Most common in neck (cystic hygroma) but can occur at any site where lymphatics are normally present. The lesions are soft, fluctuant, non-tender and transilluminate brilliantly.

696 **Extensive lymphangioma** of the right chest wall causing respiratory embarrassment.

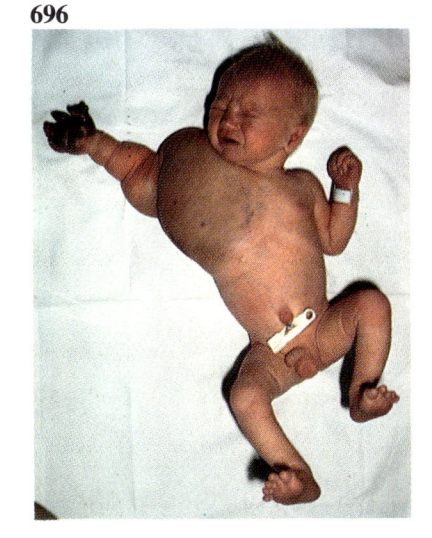

697 **Localised lymphangioma** of the dorsum of the foot.

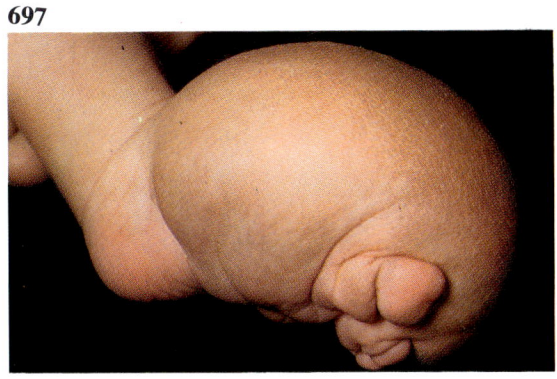

698 **Elephantiasis.** Massive swelling of the lower limb caused by a hamartomatous malformation of blood vessels, lymphatics and subcutaneous tissue.

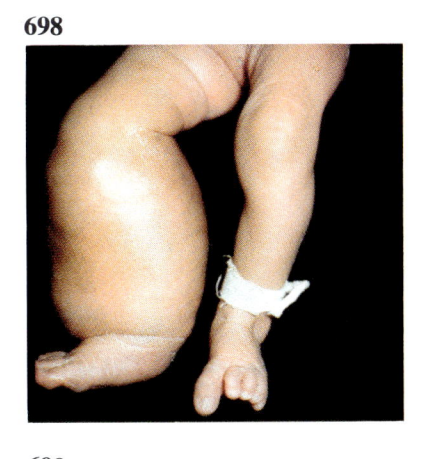

699 **Frostbite.** Late phase with partial skinloss and ulceration, areas of blister formation and hyperaemia of the surrounding skin.

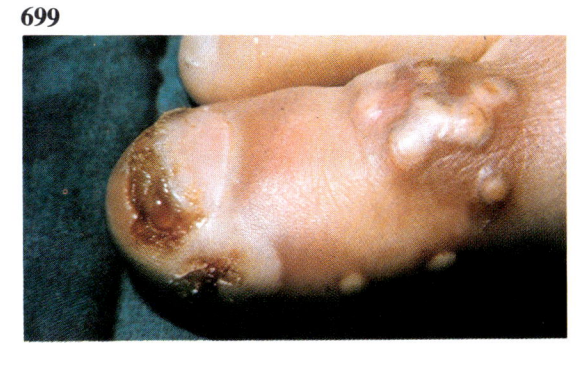

Gangrene of the extremities. More commonly affects the lower extremity. Arterial occlusion may be caused by:
a) sepsis and dehydration
b) thermal factors – either prolonged untreated pyrexia or hypothermia
c) thrombosis or embolism
d) anaphylactoid purpura
e) steroid therapy
f) polyarteritis nodosa
g) intravascular procedures – IV therapy (especially parenteral nutrition), cannulation, e.g. areteriography, chemotherapy
h) traumatic
i) idiopathic

700 Gangrene of the finger tips caused by non-accidental severance of the brachial artery.

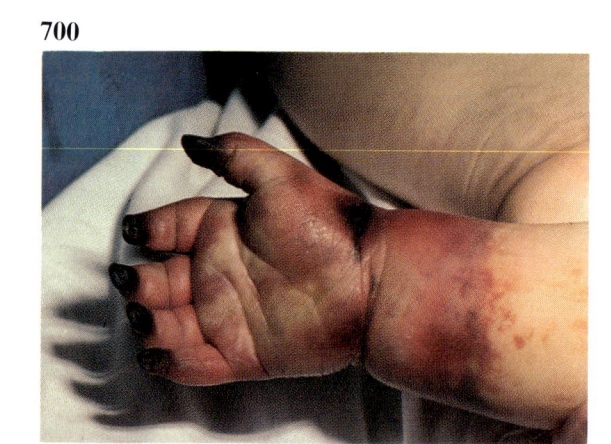

701 Lower limb gangrene from prolonged umbilical arterial pressure monitoring.

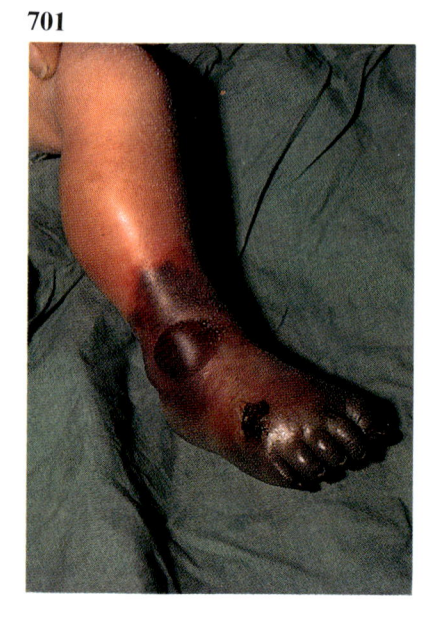

702 Bilateral forearm gangrene in an infant after severe dehydration and shock during an episode of gastroenteritis.

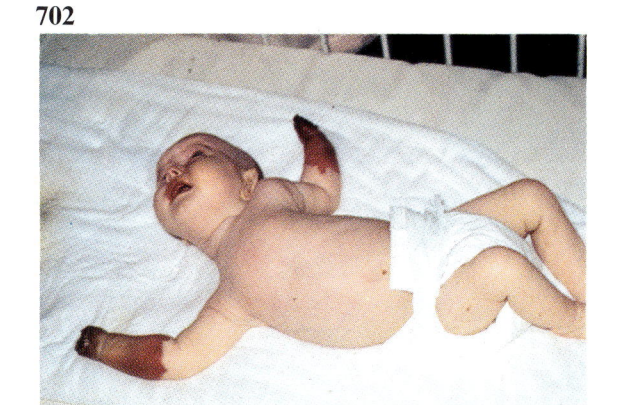

703 Toxic epidermal necrolysis. Caused by staphylococcal skin infection. The ill-defined patchy red areas of skin rapidly become denuded of superficial epidermis, leaving raw areas resembling scalds. Face and trunk most commonly affected. May also be caused by drug eruptions, e.g. sulphonamides, barbiturates, etc.

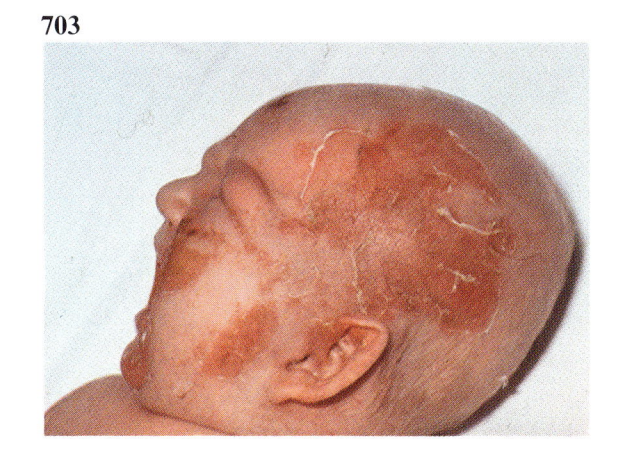

704 Lipoma of the thigh. Soft tissue subcutaneous mass in the mid-thigh. Painless swelling the surface of which is lobulated. May demonstrate the 'slipping' sign, i.e. if the edge of the lump is pressed, the swelling slips beneath the finger.

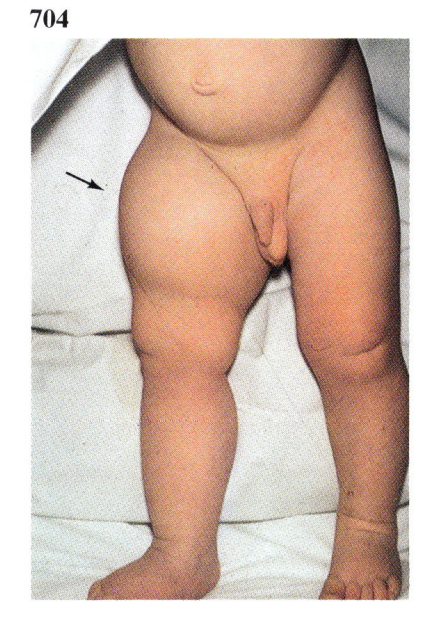

47 Musculoskeletal system

Hand deformities

705 Syndactyly. Complete syndactyly involving the middle and ring fingers. Surgical separation, which always involves the use of split skin grafts, should be carried out at four to five years of age. For optimal functional improvement, the child should be able to co-operate in carrying out exercises postoperatively.

706 Polydactyly. Duplication of the thumb. Considered to be an inherited malformation and is frequently associated with other anomalies. In uncomplicated polydactyly the accessory digit should be amputated. In more complex varieties it may be necessary to perform partial wedge excisions from both elements.

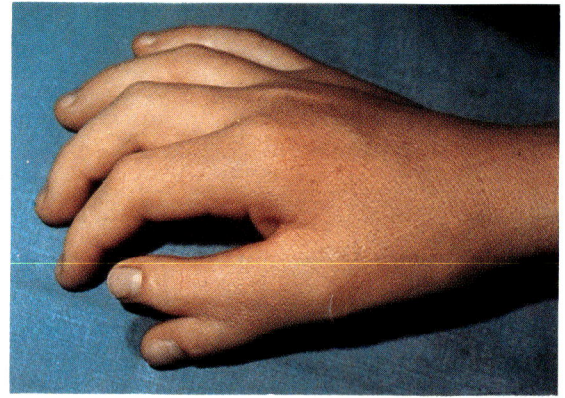

707 Polydactyly. The duplication involves a supernumerary little finger. Treatment consists of excision of the accessory little finger with possible reconstruction of the remaining fifth digit.

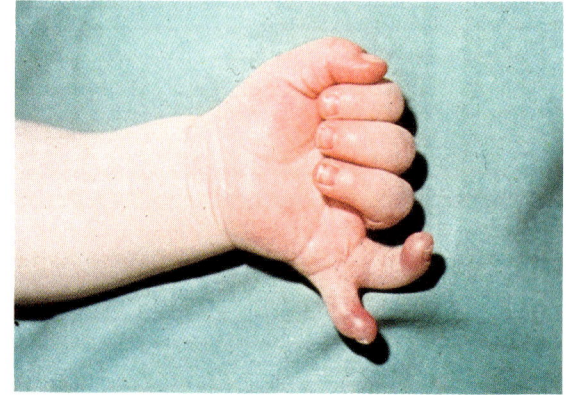

708 Ectrodactyly. i.e. absence of part or all of a digit. One or more digits may be involved. The thumb is normally formed in this example. In planning reconstructive surgery retention of function is essential. Parts should not be ablated unless it is certain that they cannot be used.

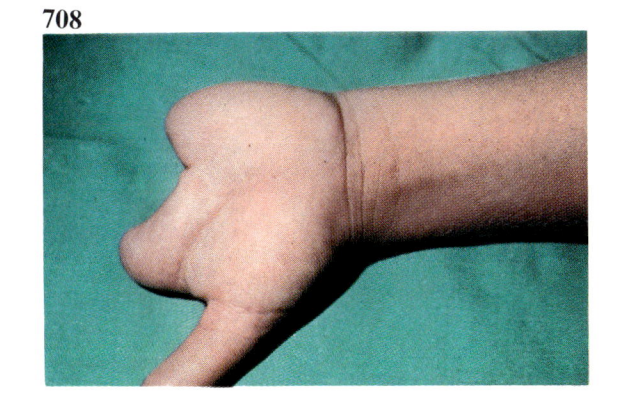

709 Lobster-claw hand. The index and middle rays are suppressed. It is a form of ectrodactyly. Characterised by a deep V-shaped defect in the central part of the hand. Treatment varies with the type of anomaly and the functional impairment. In most cases no specific treatment is required.

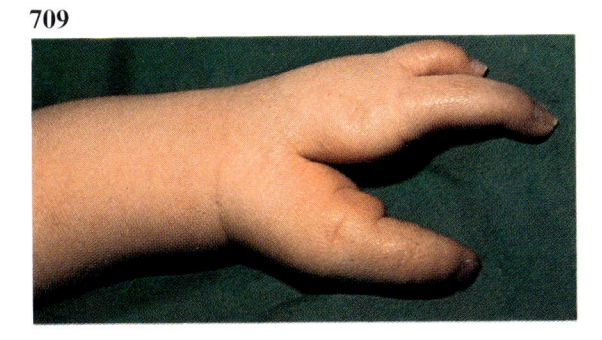

710 Floating thumb. The phalanges are present but the metacarpal is absent and the thenar muscles and long flexors and extensors of the thumb are missing. The thumb is displaced distally and no opposition is possible. In severe cases the thumb should be excised and replaced by pollicisation of the index finger, providing the index finger has not taken over the role of the thumb.

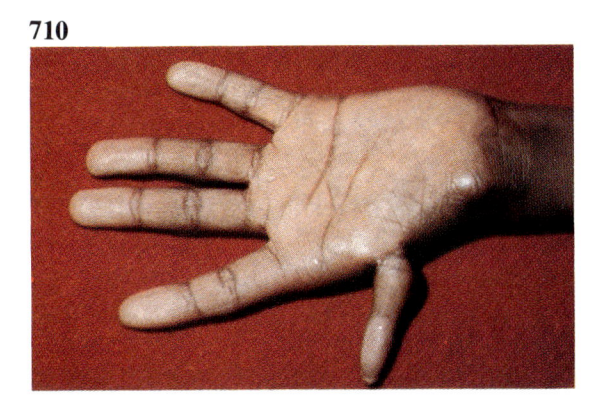

Upper extremity

711 Congenital amputation of the forearm (transverse hemimelia). May be associated with deep congenital annular constriction rings. The stump is usually well healed at birth. There is no tendency for bone overgrowth. Early fitting of a prosthesis is essential.

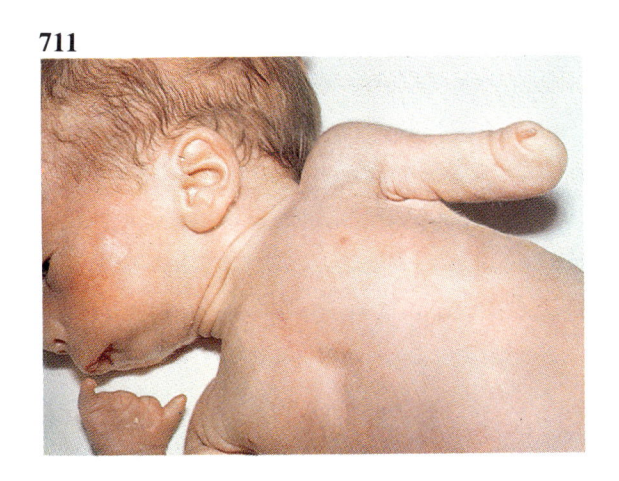

712 Congenital absence of the radius. There is a severe radial club hand. May be found in association with vertebral anomalies, anorectal malformation, oesophageal atresia with or without tracheo-oesophageal fistula and renal anomalies (Vater association). There is severe hypoplasia of the thumb.

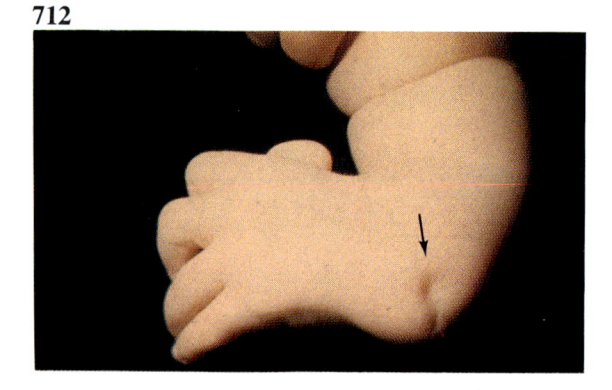

713 Severe ectromelia of upper limb. There is an almost complete absence of the humerus and the forearm is represented by one triangular bone. The hand is only partially formed with a reduced number of digits.

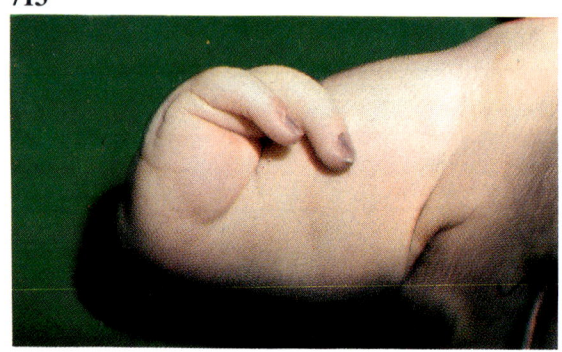

714 Congenital constriction rings (Streeter's dysplasia). The condition varies from a simple constriction ring affecting the skin and subcutaneous tissue to severe deep constriction rings with loss of brachial vessels and median and ulnar nerves or complete loss of limb. Treatment consists of staged excision of the constriction rings to restore venous and lymphatic drainage.

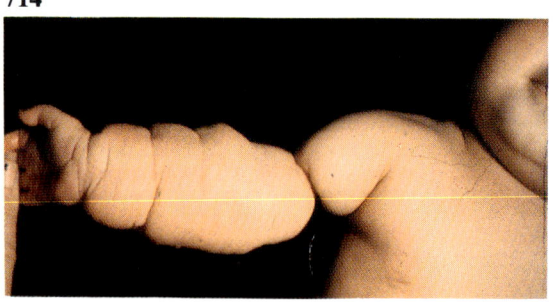

715 Congenital absence of pectoralis major. Usually well compensated by other muscles but does produce a cosmetic deformity of the upper chest wall. In this example the absence affects the costal part of pectoralis major only. May be associated with syndactyly in Poland's syndrome. Treatment is rarely necessary.

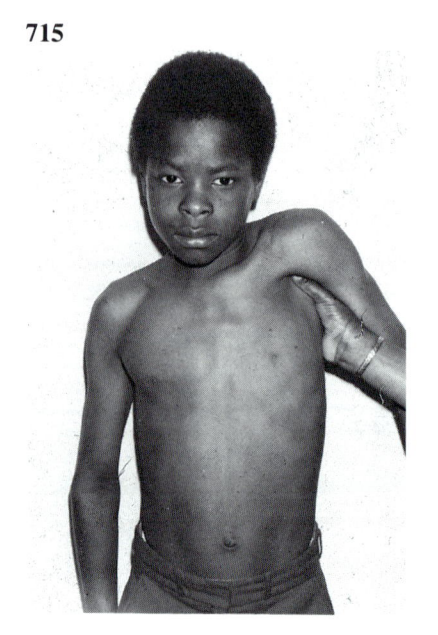

716 Sprengel's shoulder (congenital undescended scapula). Caused by failure of descent of the scapula from the neck. The shoulder on the affected side is elevated. Abduction of the arm may be considerably restricted. May be associated with rib and vertebral anomalies.

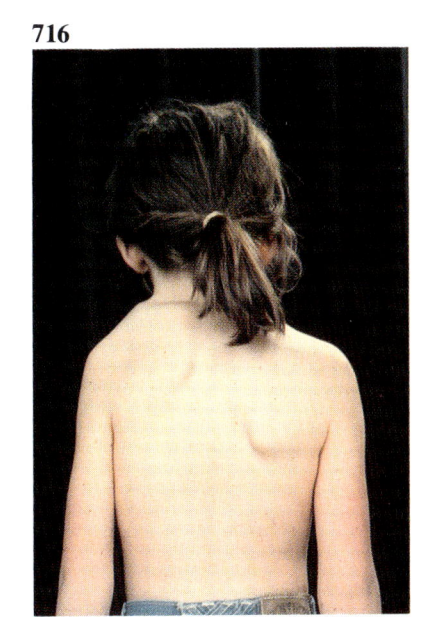

Lower extremities

717 Brachydactyly. There is underdevelopment of one or more digits. In this case the toes are affected. No treatment is required unless there is abnormal shoe pressure.

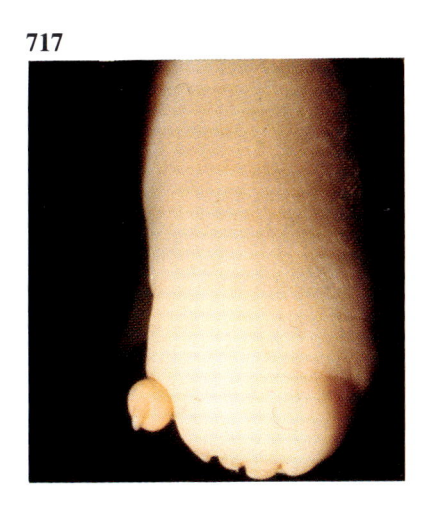

718 Focal gigantism. The second and third toes and their rays are hypertrophied and there is an incomplete syndactyly. May be associated with neurofibromatosis. The pathology consists of a hamartomatous malformation. Treatment consists of amputation of the affected toes and removal of one enlarged metatarsus.

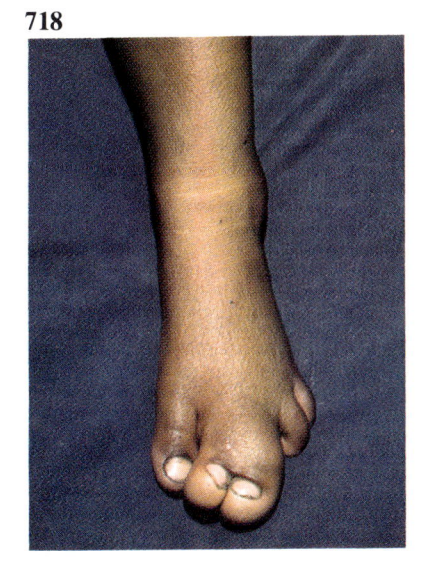

719 Supernumerary fifth toe. The fifth toe, including the metatarsal bone, is duplicated. Treatment consists of excision of the entire ray.

720 Lobster-claw feet (ectrodactyly). Two or three digits and their associated metatarsals are absent. The great toe is generally preserved. Shoe fitting may be difficult because the two parts of the forefoot are widely separated. Reconstruction gives satisfactory results.

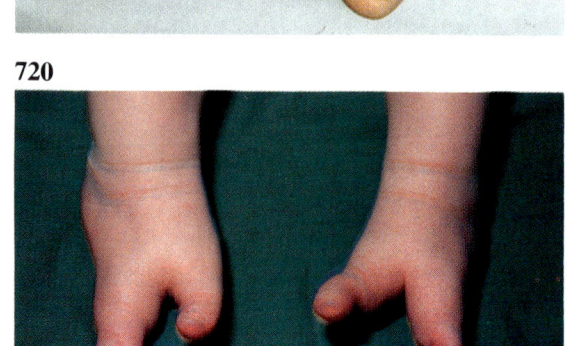

721 Metatarsus primus varus. The head of the first metatarsal is prominent on both sides and there is often redness of the overlying skin caused by shoe pressure. The great toe is deviated laterally. Note also the overlapping right fifth toe (congenital dorsiflexion). At this stage hallux valgus is usually familial.

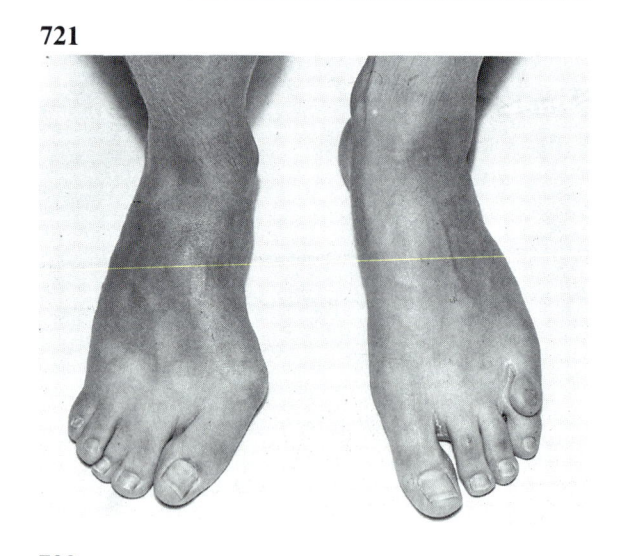

722 Congenital talipes equinovarus (clubfoot). The deformity is severe with plantar flexion of the ankle and a small inverted heel. The forefoot is severely inverted and adducted. Treatment consists of repeated manipulations, strapping and splintage, commencing on second day of life. If full correction is not obtained in 12 weeks, operative correction should be performed.

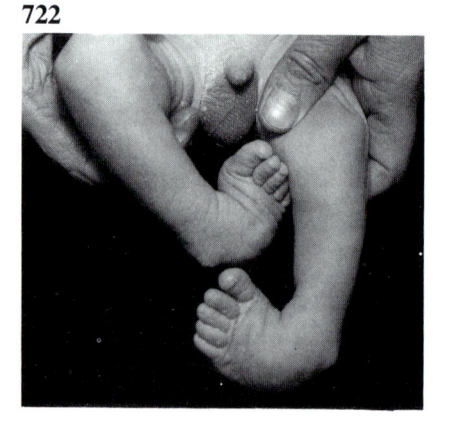

723 Flatfoot (pes planus). Common in infancy caused by instability of the balancing muscle (flexible flatfoot). Usually resolves spontaneously. 'Shoe deformity' may first bring the condition to the attention of the parents. A careful search should be made for anatomical lesions, e.g. external rotation of the hips, genu valgum, tight tendo-achilles, congenital vertical talus. Paralytic conditions, e.g. poliomyelitis, spinal dysraphism, cerebral palsy, may also lead to flatfoot. Excessive joint laxity such as in Marfan's syndrome, Ehlers-Danlos syndrome, osteogenesis imperfecta may also be aetiologically responsible.

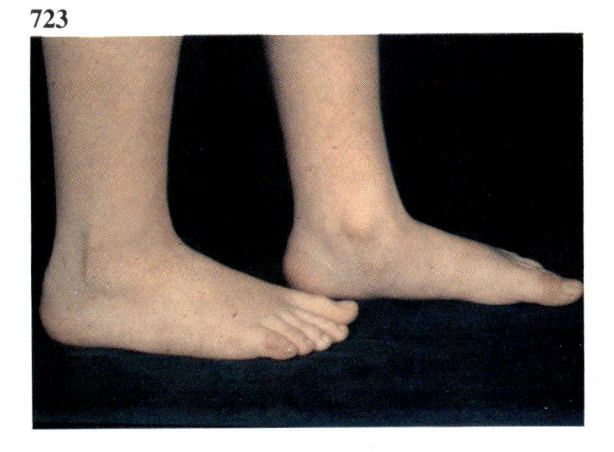

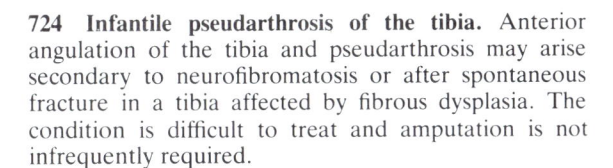

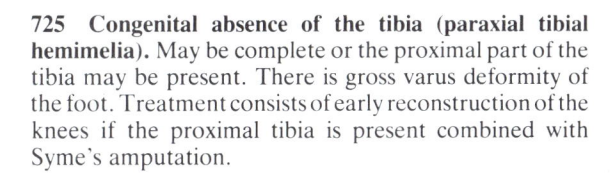

724 Infantile pseudarthrosis of the tibia. Anterior angulation of the tibia and pseudarthrosis may arise secondary to neurofibromatosis or after spontaneous fracture in a tibia affected by fibrous dysplasia. The condition is difficult to treat and amputation is not infrequently required.

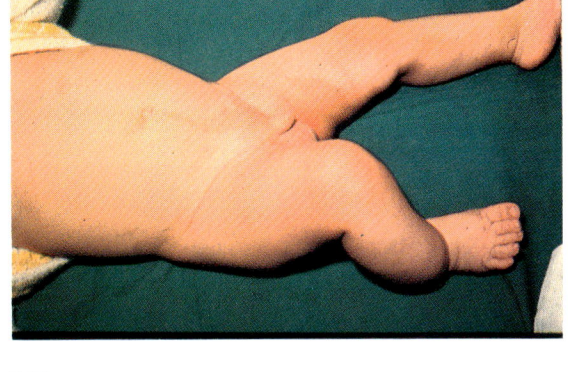

725 Congenital absence of the tibia (paraxial tibial hemimelia). May be complete or the proximal part of the tibia may be present. There is gross varus deformity of the foot. Treatment consists of early reconstruction of the knees if the proximal tibia is present combined with Syme's amputation.

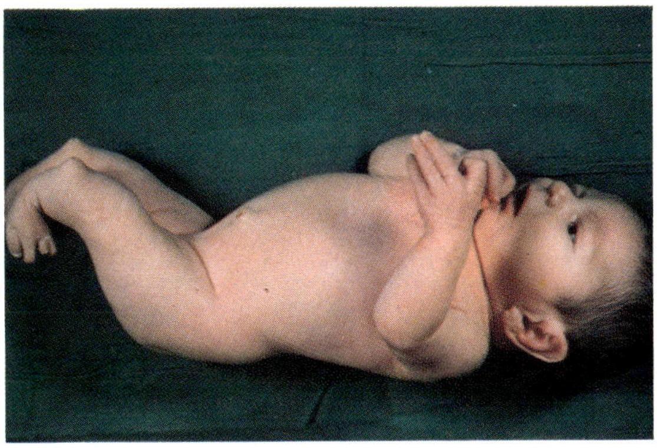

726 Congenital genu recurvatum (dislocation of the knees). The dislocation of the tibia is always posterior. There is marked hyperextension to 120° with restricted flexion of the knees. Associated with severe contracture of the quadriceps muscle.

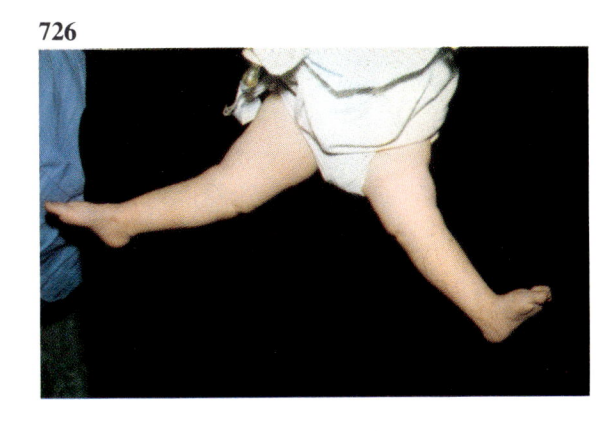

727 and 728 Genu valgum. Usually first brought to attention in child aged three years. a) The child walks and runs awkwardly and there is often a history of frequent falls. The prognosis is excellent. b) Unilateral genu valgum is almost always caused by a previous unrecognised greenstick fracture of the upper end of the tibia.

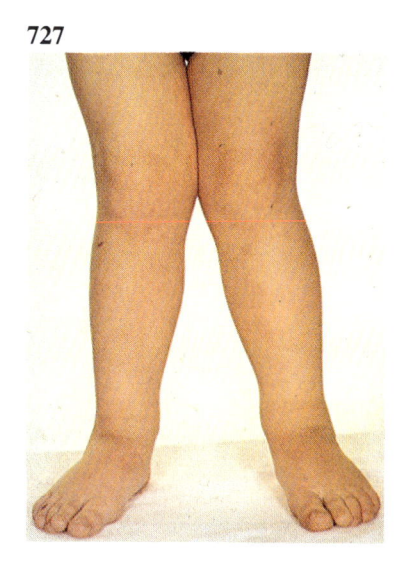

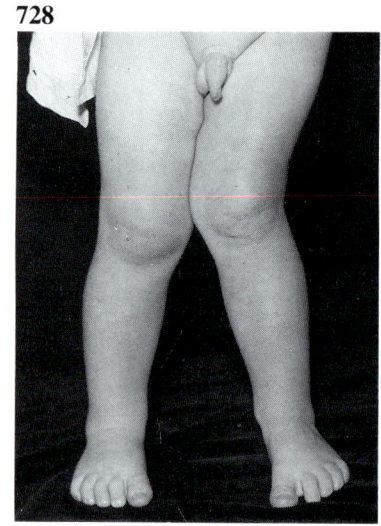

729 Congenital short femur. Presents with shortening of the thigh, with or without lateral bowing of the femoral shaft. Treatment is that for limb inequality if the lesion is unilateral. Femoral lengthening should be performed between 10 to 12 years of age. Suspect spinal dysraphism in this type of case (note wasting below the knee).

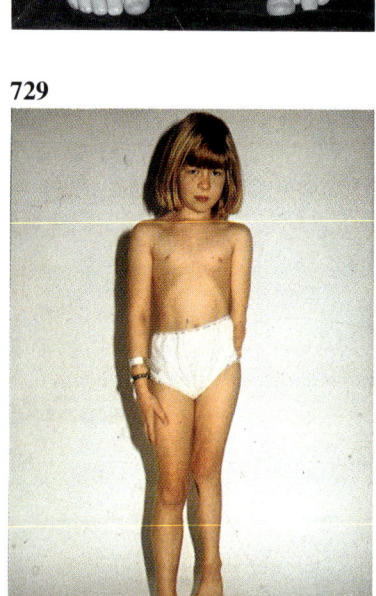

730 Medial femoral torsion (adolescent intoeing). The patellae face medially at an angle of 80°. Bilateral lateral rotation osteotomy is required at nine years of age if no external rotation or compensatory tibial torsion is present.

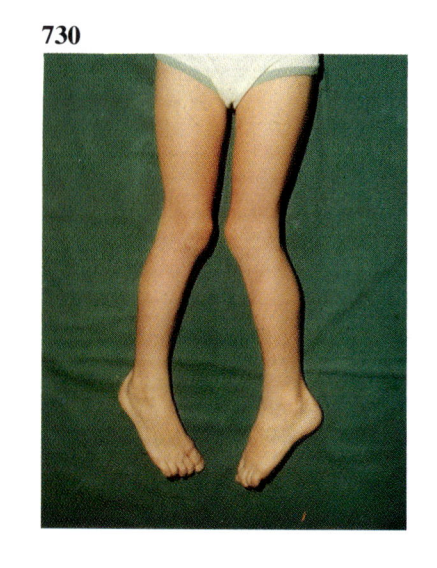

731 Bowleg deformity (genu varum). Commonly caused by a combination of internal torsion and varus of the tibia, together with external torsion of the femur. Usually present at birth and corrects spontaneously. Persistent genu varum may be associated with the various types of rickets.

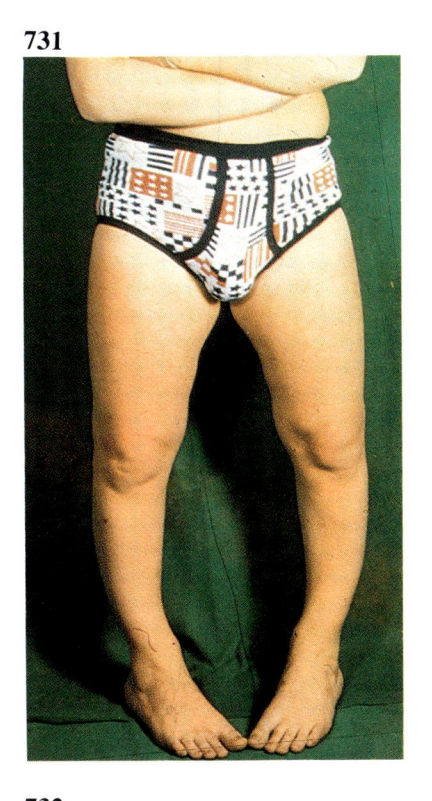

732 Congenital dislocation of the hip. There is limitation of abduction and flexion of the left hip. Note increased number of skin creases (not diagnostic). Ortolani's test is positive when the femoral head can be made to slip in and out of the acetabulum. Diagnosis is confirmed on xray.

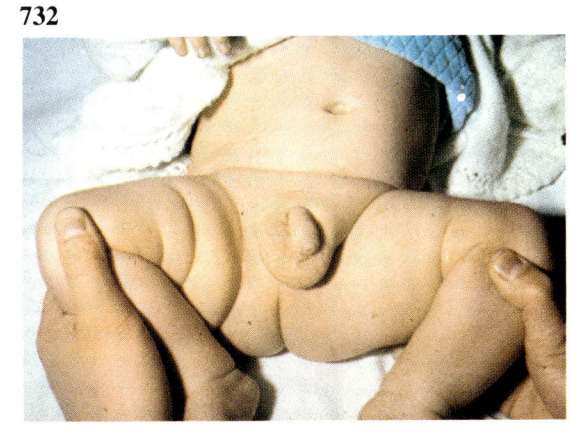

733 Congenital dislocation of the hip. Antero-posterior xray of the pelvis showing underdevelopment of the capital femoral epiphysis on the right, a shallow acetabulum with a steep sloping roof, and a suggestion of a false acetabulum developing above the hip.

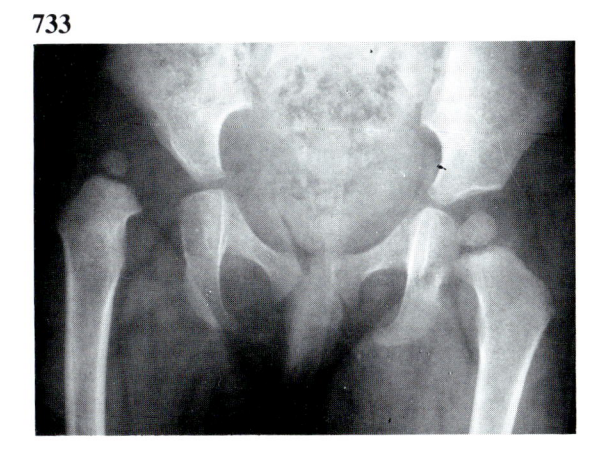

General

734 Phocomelia. Quadriplegic extreme phocomelia. Caused by thalidomide during pregnancy. Associated anomalies of the intestine, eyes and mouth were also present. Most severely affected infants of this variety did not survive.

735 Phocomelia. Most of the humerus is absent. A single bone is present in the forearm and a number of fingers are missing. Function is often remarkably good with or without surgery.

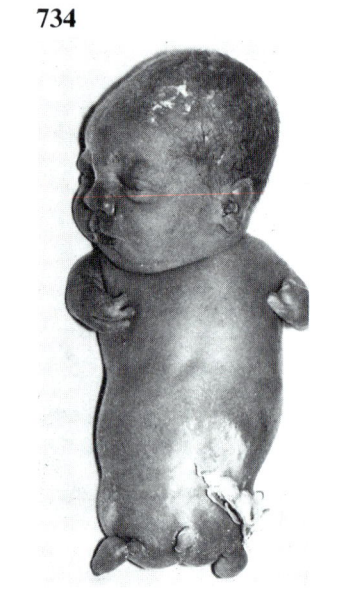

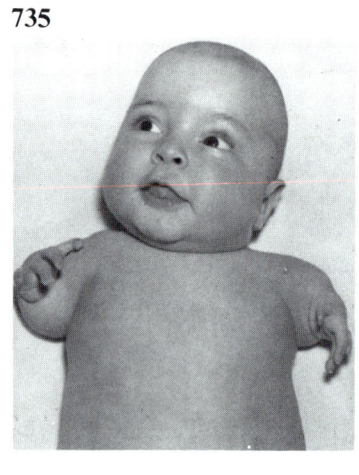

Spinal deformities

1. Scoliosis. Aetiological classification.
A Postural (disappearance in flexion)
  1 Secondary postural as a result of lower limb length discrepancy
  2 Pain and muscular spasm
B Structural (persists on flexion)
  1 Idiopathic (85 per cent of all scoliosis)
  2 Osteopathic, e.g. hemivertebrae, Osteogenesis imperfecta, irradiation, etc
3 Neuropathic, e.g. poliomyelitis, spina bifida, cerebral palsy, etc
4 Myopathic, e.g. muscular dystrophy, arthrogryposis
5 Collagenic, e.g. Marfan's syndrome, Ehlers-Danlos syndrome
6 Neurofibromatosis

736 Thoracolumbar scoliosis. The contralateral shoulder is elevated and there is an obvious curvature of the lower dorsal and upper lumbar spine.

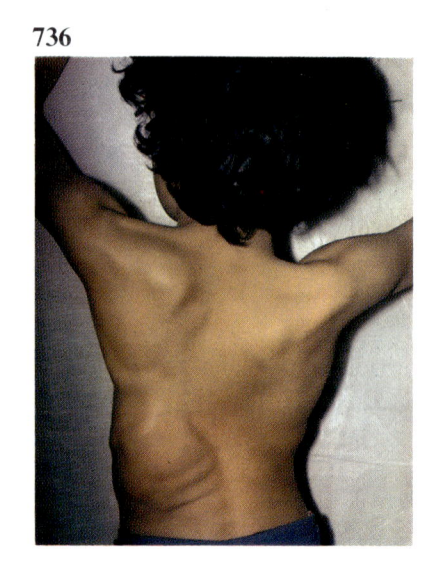

737 **In structural scoliosis** the rotation of the spine is accentuated when the child is told to bend forwards.

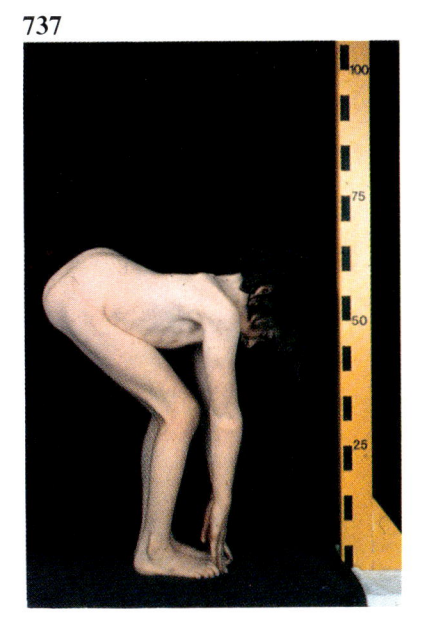

738 Scoliosis. Xray showing curvature of the thoracolumbar spine. The intervertebral disc spaces are wider on the convex side of the curvature. The angle of the curvature is measured by drawing lines perpendicular to the superior surface of the most proximal vertebra and to the inferior surface of the most distal vertebra involved in the scoliosis. The angle formed by these two intersecting lines is the angle of the curve. Note the vertebral deformity of the lumbosacral spine – spina bifida.

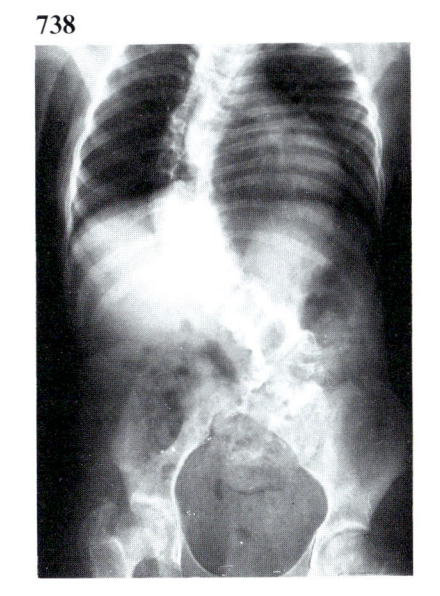

739 Paralytic scoliosis. Caused by muscular imbalance in a neglected athetotic spastic child. Scoliosis, dislocation of the hips and lexion deformity of the knees is evident. Early soft-tissue surgery with muscle balancing procedures and physiotherapy could have prevented many of the stigmata.

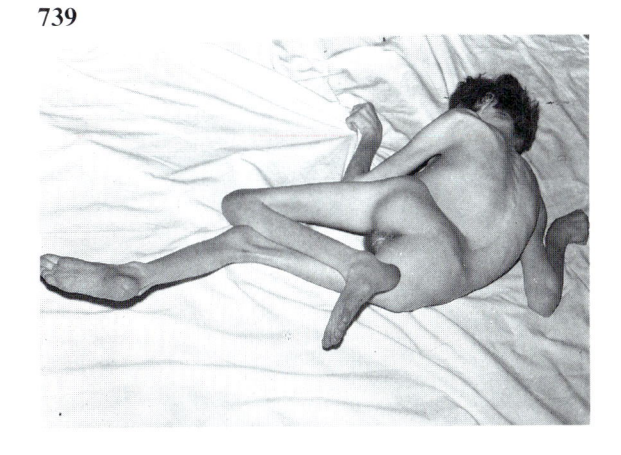

740 Kyphosis. The various types of kyphosis may be classified as follows:
A Osseous type, i.e. secondary to a lesion or anomaly of the vertebra, e.g. anterior hemivertebra, tuberculosis, spina bifida.
B Muscular type (postural) in children with poor physical development, e.g. Morquio cretin.
C Adolescent type (Scheuermann's disease).
The girl shown has a marked lumbar kyphosis secondary to myelomeningocoele.

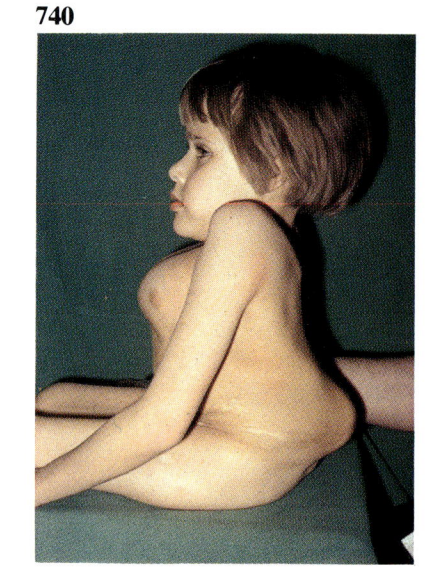

741 Lumbosacral agenesis. There is a characteristic gibbus in the lumbar region. The pelvis is small and underdeveloped and the distance between the ribs and iliac crests is foreshortened. May be associated with neurological deficits of the lower limbs as well as bladder and bowel dysfunction.

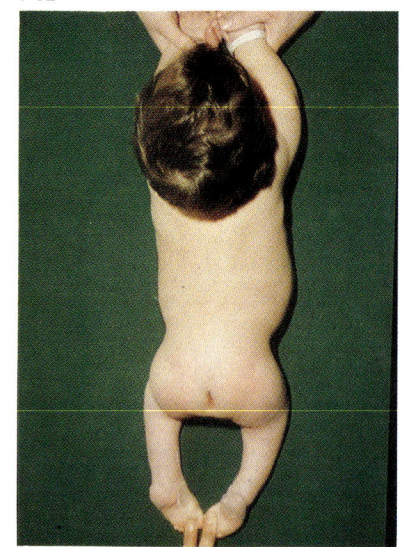

742 Spinal tuberculosis. The intervertebral disc space between L5 and S1 is narrowed. No wedging or forward angulation of the vertebral bodies have occurred. The resulting deformity is slight. May present with an abscess in the buttock or with lesions higher in the lumbar vertebra with a psoas abscess presenting in the groin.

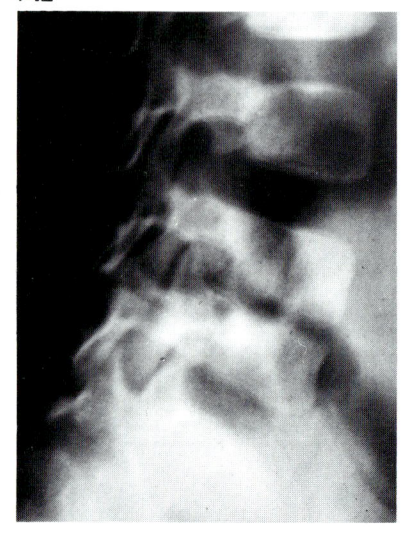

General abnormalities of skeletal development

743 Osteogenesis imperfecta. Hereditary disorder characterised by a fragile skeleton, thin skin and sclera, poor teeth, macular bleeding and hypermobility of joints. Caused by failure of maturation of collagen. Child sustains multiple fractures with minimal trauma. A severe example in a 10-year-old girl with marked dwarfism caused by scoliosis and multiple limb deformities.

744 Osteogenesis imperfecta. Blue sclera caused by intraocular pigment visible through the thin transparent sclera deficient in collagen. The blueness of the sclera is less marked in the severe cases. Vision is not impaired.

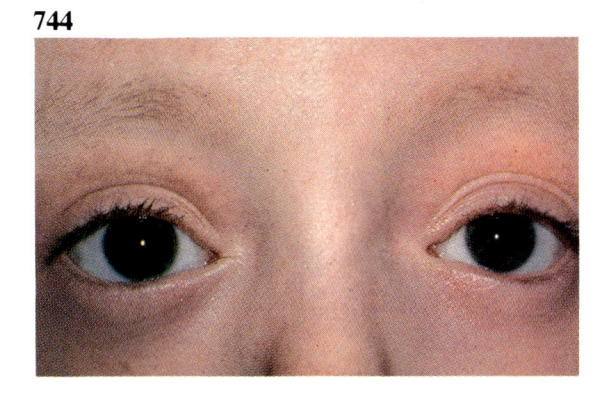

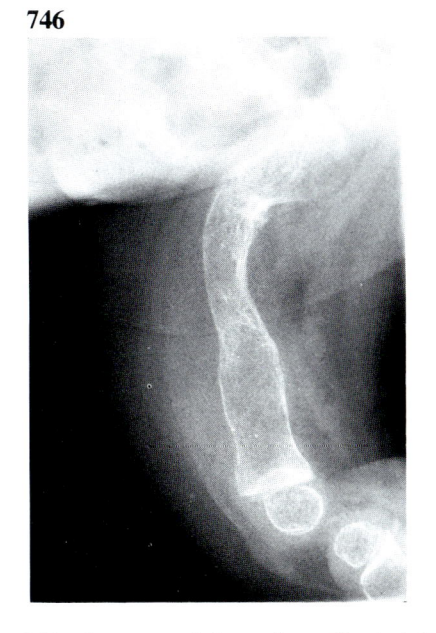

745 Osteogenesis imperfecta. Skull xray in a severe case showing multiple Wormian bones. The skull is thin, enlarged and soft.

746 Osteogenesis imperfecta. Typical deformity of the femur caused by multiple fractures with resultant angulation.

747 Hurler's syndrome (gargoylism, mucopolysaccharidosis 1–H). Autosomal recessive condition caused by an inherited enzyme defect. There is abnormal storage of mucopolysaccharides which are excreted in the urine. The classical facial appearance (large head, wide-set eyes, prominent supraorbital ridges, dark coarse eyebrows, large tongue) is associated with kyphosis, hepatosplenomegaly and deformities of the upper and lower limbs. Mental deficiency and corneal opacities. Death occurs in early childhood.

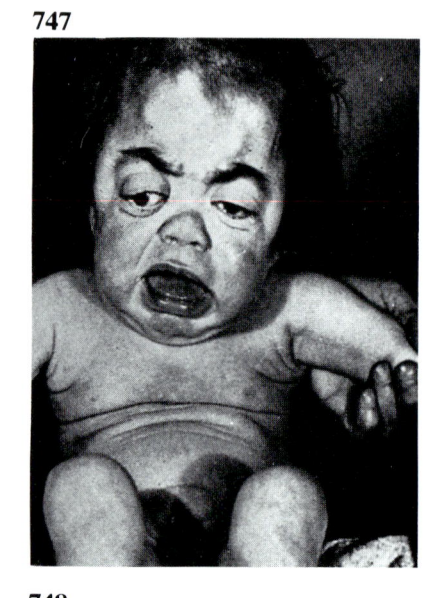

748 Achondroplasia. Commonest type of dwarfism associated with short limbs, normal trunk and a trident hand deformity. Most cases arise spontaneously as mutation but it may be caused by autosomal dominant inheritance. The cause of the inadequate cartilage development is unknown.

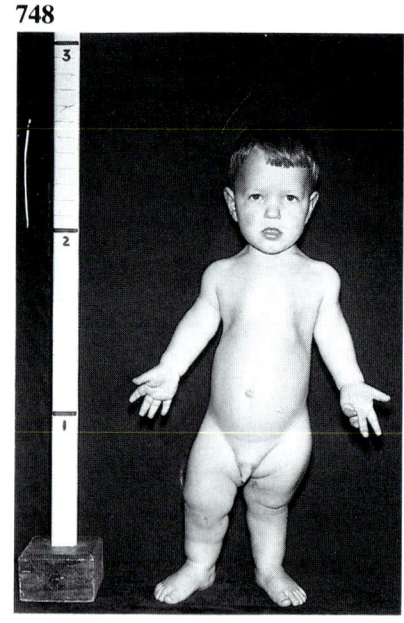

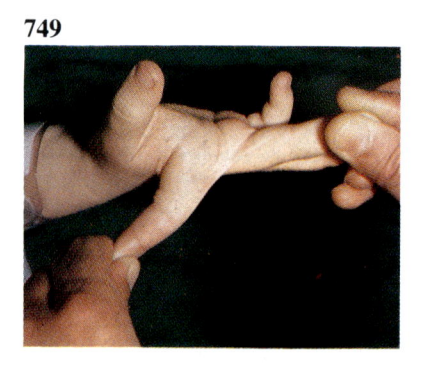

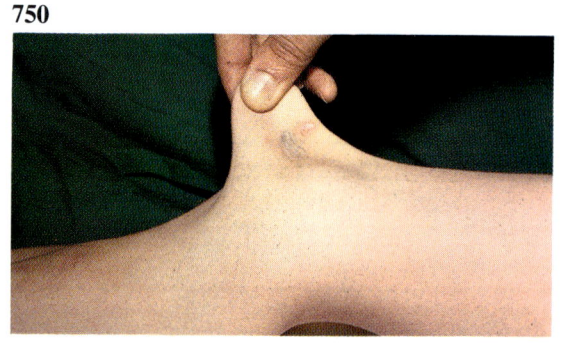

749 and 750 Ehlers-Danlos syndrome. Excessive laxity of the joints a) and skin b) with a liability to subcutaneous haemorrhages. The skin is hyperextensible but not lax. Minor trauma results in wide gaping wounds. Dislocation of various joints (especially hips) occur and kyphoscoliosis may develop.

Arthrogryposis. Condition of obscure origin, possibly caused by intrauterine myopathy or neuropathy which has arrested.

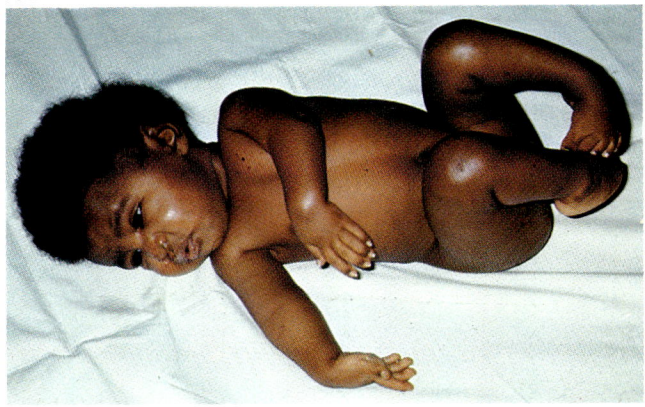

751 Myopathic type. Less common than neuropathic type. Severe flexion contractures of the knees and hips which are fixed in abduction and flexion. There is often an associated kyphoscoliosis and deformity of the chest.

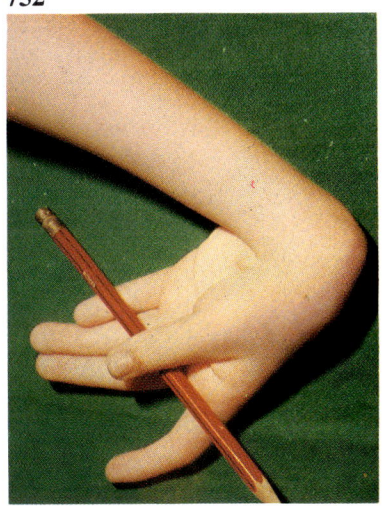

752 Neuropathic type. There is paralysis of the wrist extensors. Function may be improved by excision of the proximal row of carpal bones and transplantation of flexor carpi ulnaris to the dorsum.

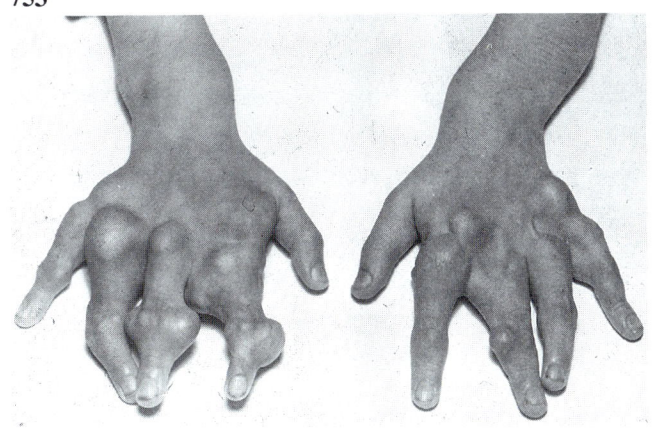

753 Enchondromatosis (Ollier's disease). Multiple enchondromata are present from birth and increase in size progressively throughout life. The lesions are essentially hamartomatous malformations of cartilage cells within the metaphysis. Treatment consists of excision of individual enchondromata with bone grafting.

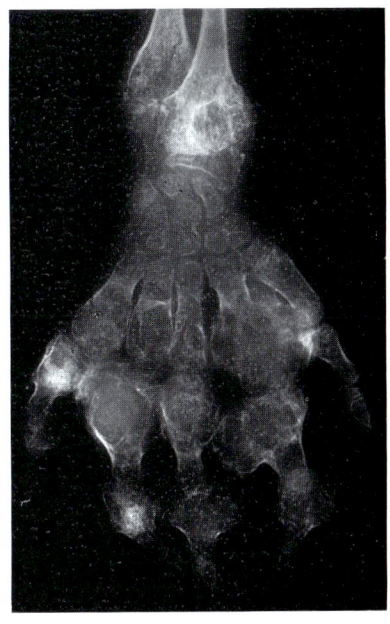

754 Enchondromatosis. Xray showing extensive involvement of the long bones (metacarpals and phalanges) and the metaphysis of the radius and ulna. The affected bones are expanded and characteristically contain fine punctate areas of calcification.

755 Haemophilia. Disorder of clotting mechanism caused by deficiency of Factor VIII. Spontaneous petechiae or haemorrhages are rare, but bleeding into muscles and joints follows minor trauma. Recurrent bleeding may occur at any time unless full healing has taken place. Severe joint destruction and ankylosis can be prevented by appropriate treatment of the coagulation disorder.

756 Popliteal cysts. Presents as a painless swelling on the posteriomedial aspect of the knee. Do not usually cause joint dysfunction. The cyst lies between the gastrocnemius laterally and the semimembranosus and semitendinosus tendons medially. Surgical excision is attended by a high recurrence rate. Spontaneous remissions are common.

757 Perthes' disease (Pseudocoxalgia). One of the causes of an irritable hip. The child presents with pain and a limp. Differential diagnosis includes transient synovitis, tuberculosis, chronic synovitis (rheumatoid) and slipped epiphysis. Pseudocoxalgia is an example of a crushing osteochondritis – aetiology is unknown. The xrays show progressive flattening and increasing density of the left femoral head.

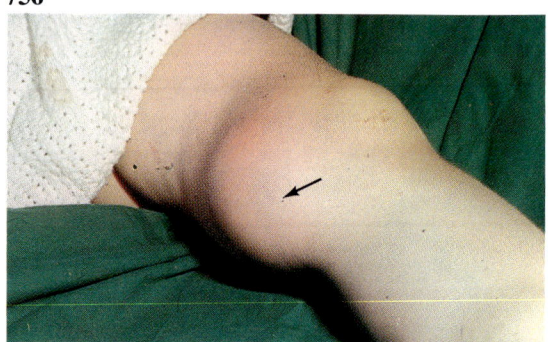

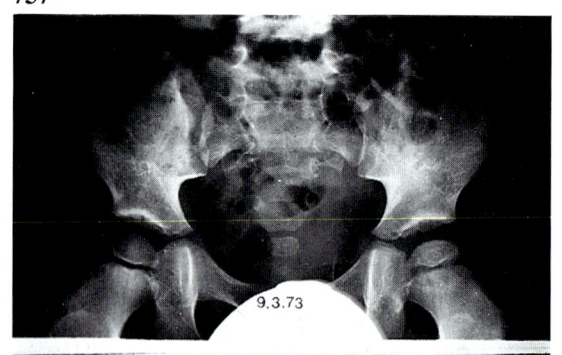

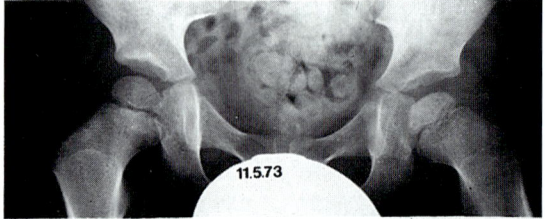

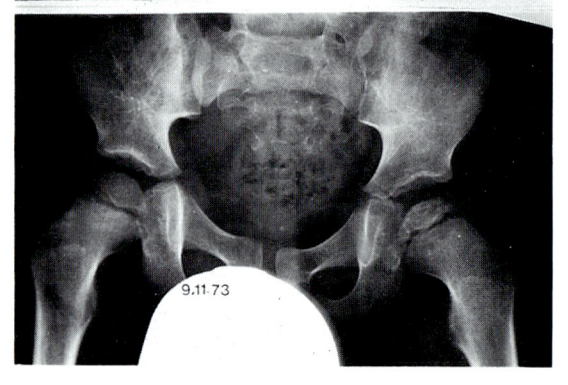

758 Septic arthritis of the hip. Acute purulent arthritis is usually confined to infants under two years of age and is generally secondary to a neighbouring bone lesion or to septicaemia. Infecting organism most commonly Staph. aureus. Less commonly haemolytic streptococcus or E. coli. There is rapid onset of high pyrexia and loss of spontaneous movement of the involved joint. The hip joint is fixed in flexion. Blood culture is often positive. Xray shows lateral dislocation of the left femoral head accompanied by a large inflammatory soft-tissue mass.

759 Rheumatoid arthritis (Still's disease). Combination of rheumatoid polyarthritis and severe visceral involvement, particularly of the spleen and lymph nodes. Characterised by periarticular osteoporosis, soft-tissue swelling and periosteal reaction around some of the metacarpals. Destruction of joints may lead to ankylosis. Fifteen per cent of children with rheumatoid arthritis are left with severe and permanent disability.

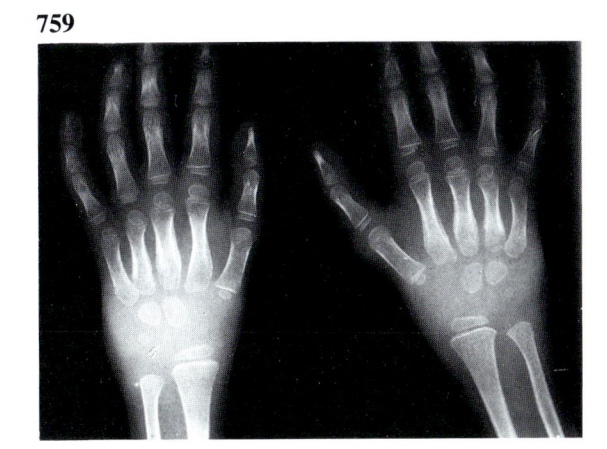

760 Ganglion. Cystic swelling in the vicinity of a joint or tendon sheath. Sites most commonly affected are the wrist, foot and knee. Presents with a painless tensely cystic lump which may be transilluminable. Symptoms caused by nagging ache or weakness may develop. The cyst is usually unilocular and contains a clear gelatinous material. The lesion may disappear spontaneously. Rupture of the cyst with dispersal of the contents in the subcutaneous tissue may effect a cure. Surgical excision with care to ligate any communication with the joint or tendon capsule is usually curative.

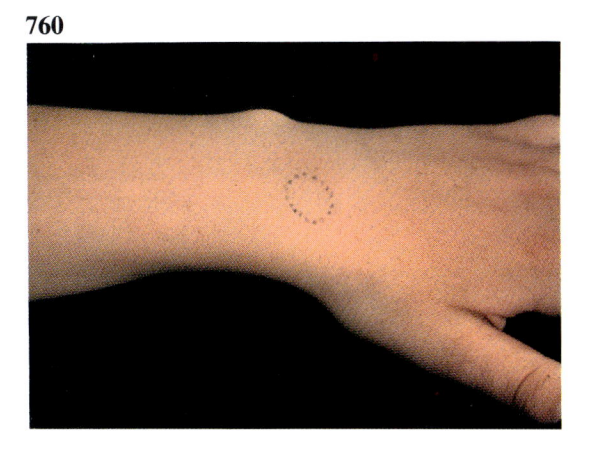

Bone tumours

I. Benign tumours
A Osteogenic – osteoid osteoma, osteoma, benign osteoblastoma.
B Chondrogenic – osteochondroma, enchondroma, benign chondroblastoma.
C Collagenic and other tumours – lipoma, angioma, neurofibroma, desmoblastic fibroma.

II. Malignant tumours
A Osteogenic – osteosarcoma, osteoblastoma.
B Chondrogenic – chondrosarcoma, chondroblastoma.
C Collagenic and other tumours – fibrosarcoma, angiosarcoma, liposarcoma.
D Myelogenic – plasma-cell myeloma, Ewing's tumour, reticulosarcoma, lymphosarcoma, Hodgkin's disease.

III. Osteoclastoma (giant-cell tumour)

761 Osteoid osteoma. Consists of a small round core of osteoid tissue (seldom larger than 1 cm in diameter) surrounded by reactive bone. Characteristically presents with mild nagging pain particularly noticeable at night and relieved by analgesics such as aspirin. Xray of the hip shows a smoothly thickened cortex distal to the lesser trochanter. Tomography reveals a lucent central nidus of the lesion. Treatment consists of complete excision including a small margin of surrounding bone.

762 Osteochondroma (osteocartilaginous exostosis). The lesion consists of an outgrowth of bone and cartilage which forms a prominent lump. The lesion always arises from the metaphyseal region commonly involving the lower end of the femur, upper end of the tibia and upper end of the humerus. The radiolucent cartilaginous cap accounts for the lesion appearing much larger clinically than radiologically. Multiple lesions are seen in diaphyseal aclasis.

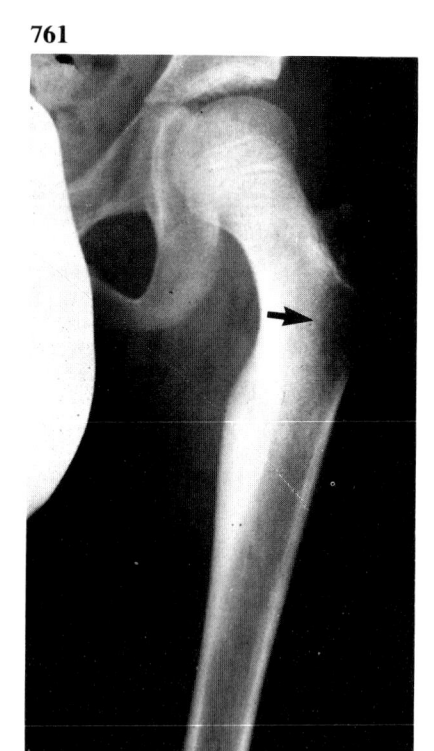

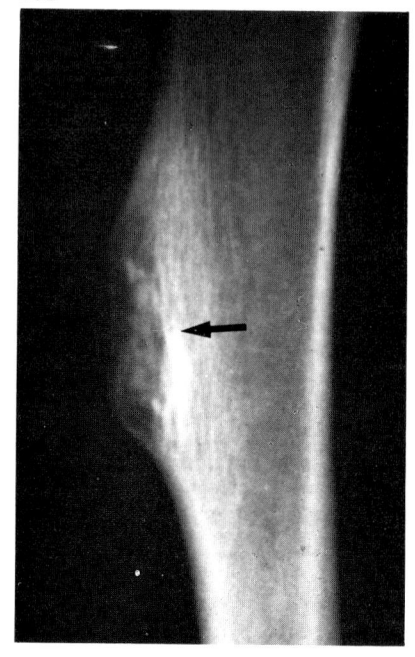

763 Solitary bone cyst (simple bone cyst). Most frequent sites affected are the upper end of the humerus, femur or tibia or lower end of the radius. Cortical bone is resorbed from the inner surface, but periosteal reactive bone on the outer surface contains the lesion. Presents with a pathological fracture resulting from minor trauma. Treatment consists of curettage of the cystic cavity and replacement with bone grafts.

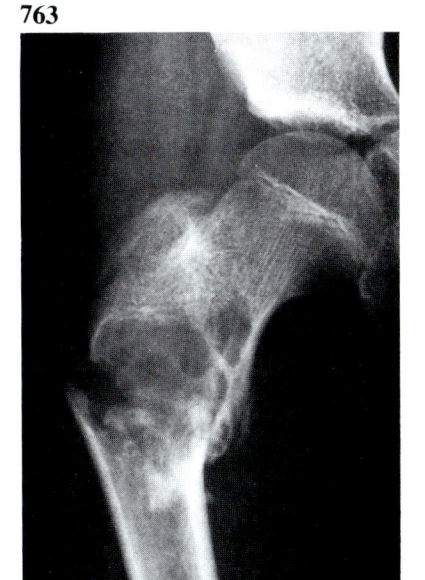

764 Aneurysmal bone cyst. Mainly involves the spine or the metaphysis of long bones. It is a rapidly expanding lesion causing erosion of cortical bone from the medullary surface leading to thinning of the cortex. Usually painful because of rapid expansion of the bone. May present with a pathological fracture. Treatment is by curettage and replacement with bone grafts.

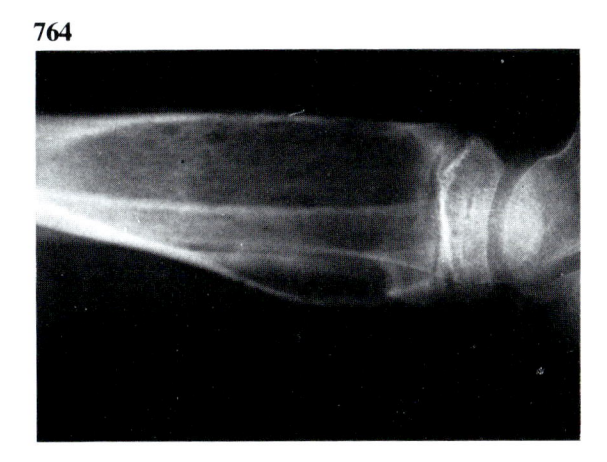

765 Osteogenic sarcoma. Malignant tumour arising in the metaphyseal region of a long bone especially around the knee. Highest incidence is between the ages of 10 to 20 years. Pain which is constant, worse at night and of increasing severity, is the presenting symptom. The involved region is prominent, tender and the overlying skin is warm and shiny. The superficial veins are often dilated.

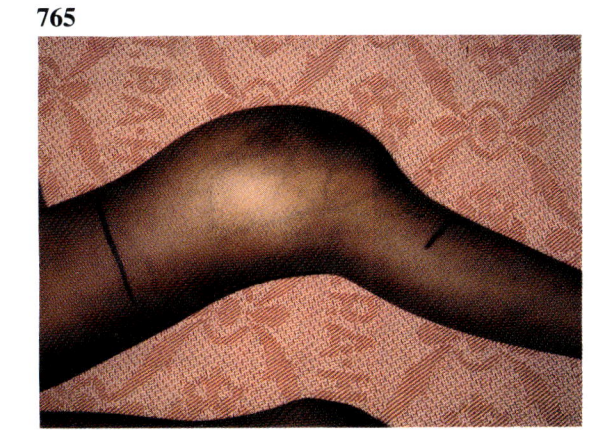

766 Osteogenic sarcoma. Radiologically there is a combination of bone destruction and new bone formation. Reactive periosteal new bone formation occurs where the periosteum has been raised from the underlying cortex (Codman's triangle). The periosteum may show 'sunray' spicules where the tumour has ruptured through the periosteum.

767 Ewing's sarcoma. Second most common bone malignancy in childhood after osteogenic sarcoma. Presents with pain followed by localised swelling of the affected bone. Most commonly involves upper end or midshaft of femur, pelvis, tibia, fibula, humerus, scapula or ribs. Radiologically there is a combination of destruction and sclerosis surrounded by multiple laminae of periosteal new bone ('onion-skin' layers). When the tumour breaks through the periosteum, a 'sunray' appearance occurs. Surgical resection should be carried out when feasible, but amputation is reserved for patients surviving at least six months without distant metastatic spread.

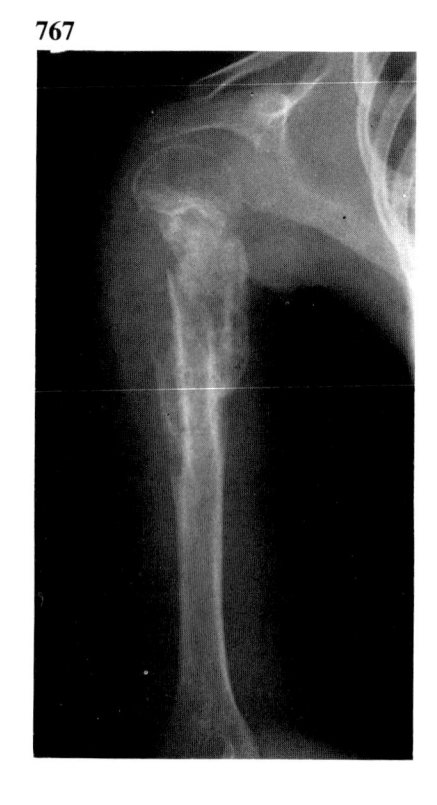

48 Miscellaneous conditions

Accessory limbs

768 Accessory digit overlying the mid-dorsal region of the spine. Usually associated with an underlying vertebral defect.

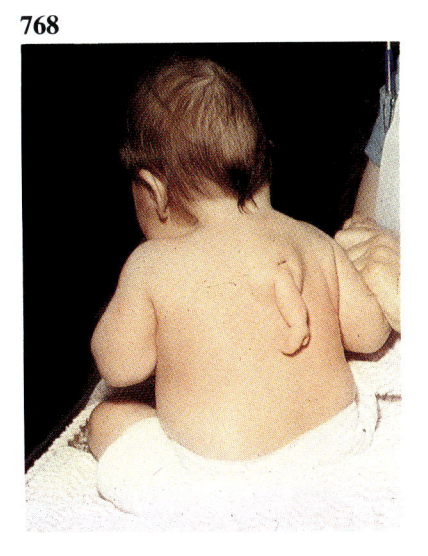

769 Accessory lower limb in association with a major exomphalos (unruptured). The limb is attached to the xiphisternum.

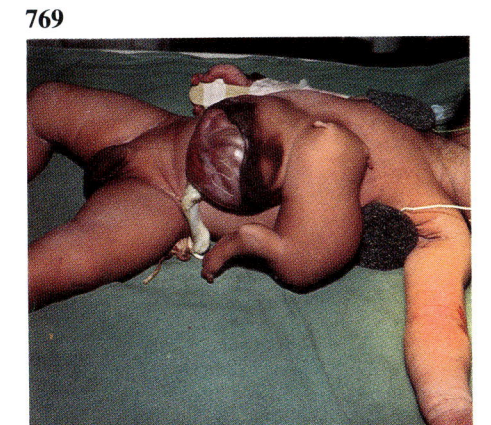

770 Accessory lower limbs (caudal duplication, dypigus). In addition there was a ruptured exomphalos, anorectal agenesis, two sets of external genitalia and an epispadias. Only the laterally placed limbs have any movement or sensation.

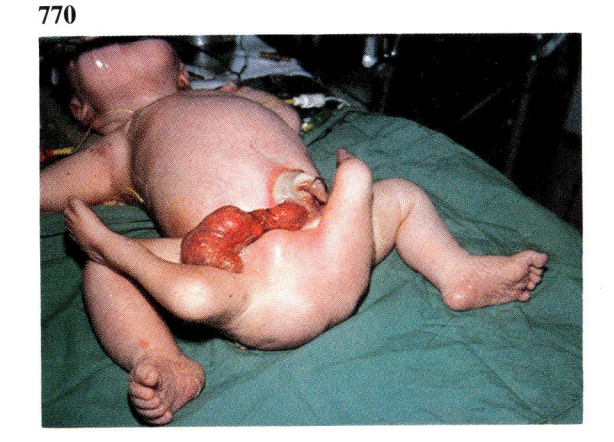

771 and 772 Conjoined twins. Symmetrical twins are classified according to the parts of the body which are attached or shared, i.e. a) thoracopagus where the attachment is over the sternal region. The infants may share a common heart, liver or parts of the gastro-intestinal tract.

b) craniopagus where the attachment is by the heads. The brains are usually separate. Attachment may be in the region of the vertex, occiput or parietal areas.

c) pyopagus (back-to-back), ischiopagus (lower pelvis), etc.

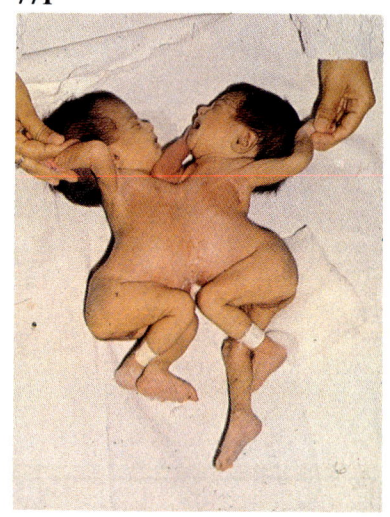

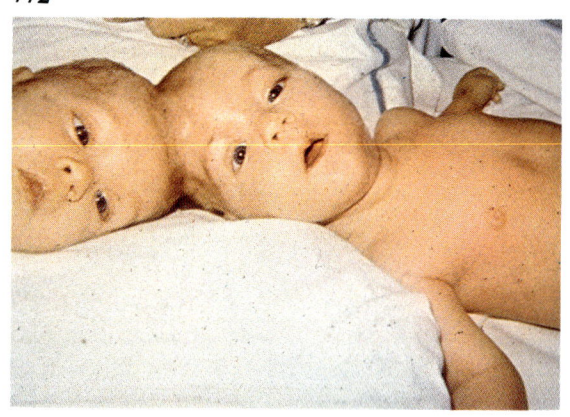

Index

Index

All references are to illustration numbers

Abdominal distension, 17
— muscles, agenesis, 591
— visceral, trauma, 16
Abdominal wall, 244–257
— erythema, 392
— herniation, 270
— oedema, 279, 280
Abscess
— breast, 168
— cervical, 142
— incisional (Crohn's), 371
— liver, 479
— retropharyngeal, 133, 134
Acalculous cholecystitis, acute, 474
Accessory digit, 768
— lower limb with major exomphalos, 769
— lower limbs (caudal duplication, dypigus), 770
— spleen, 493
Accidents in childhood, 34–47
Achalasia, oesophagus, 196
Achondroplasia, 748
Adamantinoma, 97
Adenoma, islet cell, 484
Adhesions
— eyelids, 58
— labial, 644
Adrenal gland, 501–509
— calcification, 19, 502
— haemorrhage, 19, 501
— hyperplasia, 507
Adrenogenital syndrome, 506, 651
Agenesis, abdominal muscles (prune belly syndrome), 591
— lumbosacral, 741
— renal, 551
Amastia (congenital absence of breast), 172
Ameloblastoma (Adamantinoma), 97
Ammoniacal dermatitis (nappy rash), 613
Amoebic colitis, 423, 424
Amputation, congenital of forearm, 711
Anaemia, jaundice in sickle-cell, 478
Anal 'pit', posterior, 452
— stenosis, covered in female, 440
— tag, 'sentinel', 451
Angina, Ludwig's, 84
Angiosarcoma of parotid, 124
Aniridia, 512
Ankyloglossia inferior (tongue tie), 100
Annular pancreas, 305, 485
Anopthalmos, 62
Anosia, 73
Anocutaneous fistula with covered anus, 434, 435
Anorectal agenesis, with hamartomatous malformation, 443
— with rectourethral fistula, 433
— and rectovaginal fistula, 437
Anorectal, anomalies, 428–447
— supralevator, 428, 430, 431
— translevator, 429, 432
Anotia (absence of ears), 108
Antral mucosa, oedema of, 57
Anus and rectum, 428–454
Anus, anterior perianal, 439
— covered with anocutaneous fistula, 434, 435
— ectopic with anovulvar fistula, 438
Apert's disease (Crouzon's, craniofacial dysostosis), 113

Appendix, 384–389
— appendicolith, 386, 387
— carcinoid, 389
— gangrenous, 385
— perforated, 388
— suppurative, 384
'Apple-peel syndrome' ('Christmas-tree' deformity), 318
Arteriovenous aneurysm, 695
— malformation, 694
Arthritis, rheumatoid (Still's disease), 759
— septic of hip, 758
Arthrogryposis, myopathic type, 751
— neuropathic type, 752
Ascariasis (round worms), 376, 378
— with volvulus, 377
Ascites, 284
— chylous, 282, 283
— urinary, 568
Atresia, biliary, 460, 462
— biliary and choledochal cyst, 463
— choanal, 74
— colonic, 415, 416
— duodenal, 303, 304
— hepatic duct, 457
— ileal, 4
— intestinal, 313, 314, 315, 316, 319
— jejunal, 312
— multiple, 317
— oesophageal, 187, 188, 189, 190, 191, 192
— rectal, 441
— vaginal, 643
Auricle, accessory, 111
— protruding ('bat ears'), 112

Balanoposthitis, 610
Barium enema (for Hirschsprung's disease), 403, 404
'Bat ears', 112
B-cell lymphoma (non-Hodgkins), 383
Beckwith–Wiedermann syndrome (EMG), 107, 277
Bifid scrotum, 631
Bile, inspissated bile syndrome, 459
— stained vomit, 301
Biliary tract and liver, 455–480
Biliary atresia, 460, 462
— and choledochal cyst, 463
Biopsy, suction rectal, 407
— Hirschsprung's, 410
— normal, 408, 409
Birth trauma, 5–20
Bladder, 583–598
— diverticulum, 587
— duplications, 586
— exstrophy, 588
— neuropathic, 594
— rhabdomyosarcoma, 595, 596
Bone cyst, solitary (simple), 763
— aneurysmal, 764
Bone metastases, neuroblastoma, 533
Bone tumours, 761–767
Bowleg deformity (genu varum), 731
Brachycephaly, 680
Brachydactyly, 717
Brain tumours, 681–685

Branchial cyst, 153, 154
— fistula, 151
— remnant, 152
— sinus, 150
Breast, 167–174
— abscess, 168
— congenital absence (amastia), 172
— enlarged neonate (mastitis neonatorum), 167
— galactocoele, 174
— haemangioma, 169
— lymphangioma, 173
— pubertal hypertrophy, 171
Breech delivery, 9
— extraction, 18
Bronchogenic cyst, 212
Bruising, buttocks, 9
— face, 8
— multiple, 21
— neck, 22
— periorbital, 34, 36
— scalp, 12
'Bucket handle' tear of metaphysis of humerus, 30
Bulbar urethra, rupture of, 604
Burns, 48–55
— arm and hand, 50
— cigarette, 23
— face, 51
— friction, 45

Calcification, adrenal, 502
Calculus, staghorn, 570
— submandibular, 129
— urinary, 569
— ureteric, 582
Capillary haemangioma, 689
Caput succedaneum (extreme moulding), 5
Carcinoid appendix, 389
Carcinoma, hepatocellular, 471
Carinatum, pectus (pigeon chest), 181
Cataract, 68
'Cat's eye reflex' (leukokoria), 69
Cauda equina, lipoma of, 664
Cavenous haemangioma, 691, 692
Cellulitis, facial, 119
Central nervous system, 653–685
Cephalhaematoma, 6, 7
Cerebellar astrocytoma, 681
Cerebral cortex, laceration of, 38
— damage to, 39
Cervical abscess, anterior, 142
— cleft, midline, 147
— lipoma, 162
— lymphadenopathy, acute, 157
— — chronic, 158
— — tubercular, 159
— meningocoele, 665
— teratoma, 164
Chalasia, 198
Cheek, pellet injury, 47
Cherubism, 99
Chest wall, 175–181
Choanal atresia/stenosis, 74
Cholangiogram, normal, 456
Choledochal cyst, 458, 461
— and biliary atresia, 463
Cholecystitis, acute acalculous, 474
Cholelithiasis, 476, 477
Chordoma, 544, 545
'Christmas-tree' deformity ('Apple-peel syndrome'), 318

Chylothorax, 228
Chylous ascites, 282, 283
Cigarette burn, 23
Cleft, lip, 77
— sternal, distal, 176
— sternal, upper, 175
Cleft lip and palate, 85–89
Cloaca, 436
Cloaca, ectopia (vesicointestinal fissure), 276
Clubfoot, 722
Colitis, amoebic, 423, 424
— Crohn's, 374
— ulcerative, 425, 426, 427
Coloboma, eyelid, 59
Colon, 390–427
— atresia, 415, 416
— duplication cyst, tubular, 336, 337
— polyposis coli, 422
— polyp, 419, 420
— tubular duplication, 336, 337
Common bile duct, spontaneous perforation, 475
Congenital, absence, radius, 712
— tibia, 725
— amputation of forearm, 711
— cystic adenomatoid malformation of left lung, 225
— constriction rings (Streeter's), 714
— dermal sinus, 116
— lung cyst, 223, 224
— epulis (granular cell myoblastoma), 92
— genu recurvatum (dislocation of the knees), 726
— scalp defect, 115
— talipes equinovarus (clubfoot), 722
Cordis, ectopia, 177
Corrosive oesophagitis, 207
Craniofacial dysostosis, 113
Craniopharyngioma, 684
Craniosynostosis, 679, 680
— in hypertelorism, 61
Crohn's disease, 375
— colon, 374
— ileocolic, 373
— perianal lesion of, 369
— incisional abscess, 371
— multiple fistulae, 372
— stomatitis, 370
Crouzon's disease, 113
Cullen's sign, 13, 16
Cushing's syndrome, 505
Cyst, aneurysmal bone, 764
Cyst, branchial, 153
— bronchogenic, 212
— choledochal, 458, 461
— congenital hepatic, 465
— — lung, 223
— dermoid of scalp, 117
— — external angular, 65
— duplication
— — duodenal, 307
— — ileal, 334
— — intestinal, 331, 332
— — jejunum, 333
— — oesophageal, 209–211, 329
— — tongue, 327
— — transverse colon, 338
— eruption cyst, upper gum margin, 91
— external angular dermoid, 65
— giant branchial, 154
— hydatid, 480
— hydatid, lung, 227
— infected thyroglossal, 138
— mucus of lower lip, 82

— mucus of tongue, 104
— multilocular liver, 466
— ovarian, 635
— solitary bone, 763
— pancreatic, 481
— popliteal, 756
— mesenteric, 285, 286
— omental, 287
— splenic, 486, 487, 488
— sublingual, 101
— spinal dermoid, 663
— thyroglossal, 137
— urachal, 253
Cystic dysplastic kidney, 552
Cystic hygroma, 148, 149, 213

Dacrocystitis, acute, 66
Dermal sinus, congenital, 662
Dermatitis, ammoniacal (nappy rash), 613
Dermoid cyst, external angular, 65
— spinal, 663
Diaphragm, 232–243
— eventration, 240
Diaphragmatic hernia, congenital posterolateral, 232–237
— right, 238, 239
Discharge, vaginal, 645
Disease, Crouzon's (Apert's), 113
— Hirschsprung's, 400–414
— Hodgkin's, 494
— infantile polycystic, 554
— Ollier's (enchondromatosis), 753, 754
— Perthes' (pseudocoxalgia), 757
— Still's (rheumatoid arthritis), 759
— Von Recklinghausen's 546
Dislocation, congenital of hip, 732, 733
Diverticulitis, Meckel's, 354
Diverticulum, anterior urethral, 602, 603
— bladder, 587
— Meckel's, 249, 351, 352, 354
— — gangrenous, 356
— — intestinal obstruction secondary to, 251
— — perforated, 250
Diverticulum, pharyngeal pouch, 136
— urachal, 585
Dog bite, of face, 44
Duct, omphalomesenteric (vitelline), 248
— — abnormalities of, 244
— — patent, 247
Duodenal atresia, 302, 303
Duodenal diaphragm, 304
— duplication, 306
— — cyst, 307
— haematoma, 308
Duodenum, 301–310
Duplex kidney, 563, 565
Duplication cyst, duodenal, 307
— ileal, 334
— intestinal, 331, 332
— jejunum, 333
— oesophageal, 209–211, 328, 329
— tongue, 327
— transverse colon, 338
Duplication, bladder, 586
— caudal, 770
— complete ureteric, 564
— tubular, colon, 336, 337
— tubular, ileum, 335
— ureteric with hydronephrosis, 565, 566
— urethra, 601

Ear, 108–112
— absence of (anotia), 108
— 'bat ears', 112
— miniature (microtia), 108
Ecchymosis, periorbital, 72
— scalp, 12
Ectopia cloaca (vesicointestinal fissure), 276
Ectopia cordis, 177
— crossed renal, 555
Ectopic kidney, pelvic, 557
— ureter, 571–573
— ureterocoele, 574
Ectrodactyly, 708, 720
Ectromelia, upper limb, 713
Ehlers-Danlos syndrome, 749, 750
Elbow, pulled, 28
Electric burn, palm, 53
— lower lip, 55
Electric shock, 54
Elephantiasis, 698
EMG – (exomphalos-macroglossia-gigantism), 277
Emphysema, lobar, 221, 222
Encephalocoele, anterior, 64
— frontal, 668
— nasal, 76
— occipital, 670
— parietal, 669
— sincipital, 666, 667
Endodermal sinus (yolk-sac) tumour, 639
Endotracheal intubation, 51
Enchondromatosis (Ollier's disease), 753, 754
Enema, barium (in Hirschsprung's disease), 403, 404
Enterocolitis, 398, 399
— necrotising, 390–399
Ependymoma, 682
Epidermal necrolysis toxic, 703
Epididymo-orchitis, 626
Epiglottitis acute, 135
Epispadias, female, 606
— male, 619
Epulis, congenital (granular cell myoblastoma), 92
— giant, 93
Erosions, acute gastric, 295
Eruption cyst, 91
Erythema, anterior abdominal wall, 392
— periumbilical, 278
Escalator, injury from unprotected grid, 43
Eventration of diaphragm, 240
Ewing's sarcoma, 767
Excavatum, pectus, 178, 179, 180
Exomphalos (omphalocoele), 265–277
— complex, 272
— major, 268, 269, 271
— minor, 266, 267
— ruptured, 273, 275
Exstrophy, bladder, 588
— cloaca (vesicointestinal fissure), 590
— with rectal prolapse, 589
Eye, 56–72
— cataract, 68
— coloboma, 59
— congenital absence, 62
— haemangioma, 63
— hypertelorism, 61
— hyphaema, 56
Eyeball, vestigial in microphalmos, 62
Eyelids, adhesions, 58
— congenital ptosis, 60
— dermoid cyst, 65
— strabismus, 67
— neuroblastoma, 72

— retinoblastoma, 69
— rhabdomyosarcoma, 70
— tumours, 68–70

Face (and skull), 113–124
Face, haemangioma, 118, 121
— lymphangioma, 122
Facial cellulitis, 119
— clefts, 61
— palsy, 13
— trauma, 35
Feet, flatfoot (pes planus), 723
— lobster-claw, 720
Female genital organs, 635–646
— pseudohermaphrodite, 649
Femoral hernia, 263
Femoral torsion, medial, 730
Femur, congenital short, 729
Fibrous dysplasia, 99
Fissure, vesicointestinal (exstrophy of cloaca), 590
Fistula, anocutaneous, 434, 435
— anovulvar, 438
— branchial, 151
— in-ano, 453
— intestinal, 4
— omphaloileal, 349, 350
— rectourethral, 333
— rectovaginal, 437
— urachal, 483
Fistulae, multiple (Crohn's), 372
'Flowerpot sign', 17
Focal gigantism, 718
Foetoamniography, injury, 3
Fontanelle, 27
Forceps, injury, 13
Forearm, congenital amputation, 711
Foreign body, gastric, 300
— ingested, 418
— inhaled, 231
— oesophageal, 204
Fracture, compound depressed, skull, 26, 38
— depressed of skull, 10, 11
— elbow, 29
— long bones, 20
— multiple linear, skull, 25
— orbital, 57
— ribs, 31
— skull, 36, 37
Frenulum, haemorrhage into haemophilia, 94
— upper lip, 81
Frontal encephalocoele, 668
Frostbite, 699
Fundal varices, gastric, 499

Galactocoele, left breast, 174
Gall bladder, absent, 472
— septate, 473
Ganglion, 760
Gangrene, 700–702
Gangrenous appendicitis, 385
— intussusception, 362
— Meckel's diverticulum, 356
Gas in portal venous system, 394
Gastric duplication, 330
— erosions, acute, 295
— foreign body, 300
Gastric fundal varices, 499
— perforation, neonatal, 288–290
— 'spontaneous', 291

— ulcer, 296, 297
Gastroschisis (ruptured exomphalos), 273, 274
Genital organs, female, 635–646
— male, 620–634
Genitalia, ambiguous, 650
Genu recurvatum, congenital, 726
— valgum, 727, 728
— varum (bowleg deformity), 731
Giant epulis, 93
Gigantism, focal, 718
Goitre, 146
Granuloma, umbilical, 245
Graves' disease, 143

Haemangioma, breast, 169
— capillary, 689
— cavernous, 691, 692
— chin, 120
— eye, 63
— face (Kasabach-Merritt syndrome), 121
— involuting, 693
— lip, 80
— nose, 75
— occipital region, 161
— parotid, 128
— tongue, 102
Haemangiolymphangioma, of left maxillary region, 95
— right submandibular region of tongue, 103
Haemangiomata of face, 118
Haematoma, duodenal, 308
— extradural, 40
— perineal, 634
— scrotal, 16
— subcapsular, of liver, 18
— subdural, 27, 39
Haemoperitoneum, 16
Haemophilia, 94, 755
Haemorrhage, adrenal, 19, 501
— intraventricular, 14
— petechial, 8
— subconjunctival, 36, 41, 56
— subperiosteal, 6, 7
Hairy naevus, 687, 688
Hamartoma, of liver, 467
— vulva, 646
Hamartomatous anorectal malformation, 443
Hand deformities, 705–710
Hanging, accidental, 42
Hemihypertrophy, 511
Hemimelia, paraxial tibial, 725
— transverse, 711
Henoch-Schonlein purpura, 365
Hepatic cyst, congenital, 465
— duct, atresia of, 457
Hepatitis, neonatal, 464
Hepatoblastoma, 468, 469, 470
Hepatocellular carcinoma, 471
Hermaphrodite, true, 647, 648
Hernia, bilateral inguinal, 258
— diaphragmatic, 232–237
— femoral, 263
— hiatus, 197–203
— inguinal, 257–260
— — in girl, 264
— into umbilical cord (exomphalos minor), 266
— ischial, 454
— Morgagni, 241–243
— perineal, 633
— right diaphragm, 238, 239
— supraumbilical, 256

— umbilical, 254
Hiatus hernia. 197–203
— paraoesophageal (rolling hernia), 201
— sliding with reflux oesophagitis, 199
— — stricture, 200
Hip, congenital dislocation, 732, 733
— septic arthritis, 758
Hirschsprung's disease, 400–414
Hodgkin's disease, 494
Horseshoe kidney, 556
Hurler's syndrome, 747
Hydatid cyst, liver, 480
— lung, 227
Hydatid of Morgagni, torsion of, 625
Hydrocephalus, 671, 672, 678
— mild, 674, 675
— progressive, 14
Hydrocoele, communicating, 257, 261, 262
Hydrocoeles and inguinal hernias, development of, 257
Hydrocolpos, 641, 642
Hydronephrosis, 558–561
— with ureteric duplication, 566
Hyperplasia, adrenal congenital, 507
Hypersplenism, 490
Hypertelorism, 61
Hypertension, portal, 486–500
Hyperthyroidism, 143, 144
Hyphaema, blood in interior chamber of eye, 56
Hypospadias, 615–618
Hypothyroidism, 145
Hygroma, cystic, 148, 149, 213

Idiopathic scrotal oedema, 622
Idiopathic thrombocytopenic purpura, 491, 492
Ileal atresia, 4
— duplication cyst, 334
Ileitis, acute, 366
Ileocolic Crohn's disease, 373
Ileo ileal intussusception, 361
Ileum, tubular duplication of, 335
Ileus, meconium, 339–343
Ileocaecal lymphoma, 381, 382
Incompetence of lower oesophageal sphincter, 202
Incubator, 1, 2
Inguinal hernia, 257–264
— bilateral, 258
— complete indirect, 257b
— development of, 257
— incomplete indirect, 257c
— in girl, 264
— irreducible right indirect, 260
— left incomplete indirect, 259
Inhaled foreign body, 231
— fumes, 52
Injuries, full thickness tissue injury from electric burn, 53
— head, 37
— non-accidental, 21–33
— pellet, 47
— perinatal, 3–20
— wringer injury of forearm, 45
— — hand, 46
Inspissated bile syndrome, 459
Inspissation, milk, 346, 347
Intestinal, atresia, 311–319
— duplications, 327–338
— malrotation, 320–326
— small, 311–383
Intestinal duplication cyst, 331, 332
Intestinal obstruction in newborn, 251, 311, 355
Intersex, 647–652

Intubation, endotracheal, 51
Intussusception, 357–365
Intraventricular haemorrhage, 14
Involuting haemangioma, 693
Ischial hernia, 454
Islet cell adenoma, 484

Jaundice, 455
Jaundice in sickle-cell anaemia, 478
Jaws, 90–99
Jejunal atresia, 312
Jejunum, duplication cyst of, 333

Kidney, 548–570
— cystic dysplastic, 552
— duplex, 563, 565
— horseshoe, 556
— multicystic, 553
— pelvic ectopic, 557
— ruptured, 548–550
Klippel-Feil syndrome, 165
Knees, dislocation of (congenital genu recurvatum), 726
Kyphosis, 740

Labial adhesions, 644
'Lacunar' skull, 676
Larynx (and pharynx), 132–136
— oedema of, 51
Leukokoria ('cat's eye reflex'), 69
Lip, frenulum, 81
— haemangioma, 80
Lipoma, cervical, 162
— cauda equina, 664
— thigh, 704
Liver and biliary tract, 455–480
Liver abscess, 479
— cyst, multilocular, 466
— hamartoma of, 467
— rupture, 18
— tumour, 468–471
Lobar emphysema, 221, 222
Lobster-claw feet, 720
— hand, 709
Ludwig's angina, 84
Lumbosacral agenesis, 741
Lung, 221–231
— abscess, 226
— congenital cystic adenomatoid malformation of, 225
— cyst (congenital), 223, 224
— hydatid cyst of, 227
— metastasis, 230
— tumours of, 229
Lymphadenopathy, acute cervical, 157
— chronic cervical, 158, 159
Lymphangioma, breast, 173
— chest wall, 185
— (cystic hygroma), 148, 149, 154, 213
— extensive, 696
— face, 122
— left maxillary region, 95
— localized, 697
— right submandibular region, 96
— tongue, 103
Lymphoma, Burkitt's, 98, 547
— B-cell (non-Hodgkin's), 383
— ileocaecal, 381, 382
Lymphosarcoma, 216

Macroglossia, 106, 107
Macrostoma, (transverse facial cleft), 79
Maldescent of testis, 620, 621
Male pseudohermaphrodite, 652
Malrotation, 320–326
— with volvulus, 325, 326
Malnutrition, nutritional abuse, 24
Mandibulofacial dysostosis (Treacher–Collins syndrome), 114
Manometry, anorectal (normal), 405
— — (Hirschsprung's), 406
Mastitis neonatorum, 167
Meatal ulcer, 614
Meckel's diverticulitis, 354
Meckel's diverticulum, 249, 351, 352
— gangrenous, 356
— intestinal obstruction secondary to, 251
— perforated, 250
Meconium ileus, 339–343
— peritonitis, 345, 417
— plug, 414
— — syndrome, 412, 413
Mediastinal masses, 209–219
— teratoma, anterior, 214
Medulloblastoma, 683
Megalopenis, 609
Megaureter, primary obstructive, 581
Meningocoele, 654–656
Mesenteric cyst, 285, 286
Metastatasis, lung, 230
— pulmonary, 519, 520
Metastatic neuroblastoma, 532–534
Metatarsus primus varus, 721
Micropenis, 608
Micropthalmos, 62
Microstoma, 78
Microtia, 108
Midgut volvulus, 321, 325, 326
Milk inspissation, 346, 347
Mongolian spot, 33
Morgagni hernia, 241–243
— torsion of hydatid of, 625
Mouth, 78–89
Mucoviscidosis, 344
Mucus cyst, lower lip, 82
— tongue, 104
Multicystic kidney, 553
Muscular dystrophy, 60
Myelodysplasia, 660
Myelomeningocoele, 657, 658, 659
Myoblastoma, granular cell (congenital epulis), 92

Naevus, 686–688
Nappy rash, 24
Nasolacrimal duct, obstruction of, 66
Neck, 147–166
Necrolysis toxic epidermal, 703
Necrosis, soft tissue, 3
Necrotising enterocolitis, 390–399
Neonatal nephroblastoma, 513
Nephroblastoma, 510, 513, 514–516, 522–524
— recurrent, 521
Neuroblastoma, 217, 219, 525, 527–530, 536
— as cause of proptosis, 71
— bone metastases of, 532–534
— infantile, 526
— metastatic to orbit, 72
— thoracic, 218
Neurofibroma, 215
Neuropathic bladder, 594
Nipple, accessory (polythelia), 170

Non-accidental injury (child abuse), 21–33
Nose, 73–77

Obstructive megaureter, primary, 581
Occipital encephalocoele, 670
Occipital region, haemangioma of, 161
Oedema, abdominal wall, 279, 280
— antral mucosa, 57
— face, 8
— idiopathic scrotal, 622
— larynx, 51
— periorbital, 41
— pulmonary, 52
Oesophageal atresia, 187–192
Oesophageal duplication cyst, 209–211, 328, 329
Oesophageal sphincter, incompetence of lower, 202
Oesophageal varices, 496, 497
— web, 206
Oesophagitis, corrosive, 207
— reflux, 203
— reflux with sliding hiatus hernia, 199
Oesophagus, 186–208
— achalasia of, 196
— foreign body in, 205
Ollier's disease (Enchondromatosis), 753, 754
Omental cyst, 287
Omphalocoele (exomphalos), 265–277
Omphaloileal fistula, 349, 350
Omphalomesenteric (vitelline) duct, 244, 349–356
— duct patent, 247, 248
Orbital fractures ('blowout'), 57
Orbits, lateral displacement of, 61
Orchioblastoma, 627, 628
Orchitis, epididymo, 626
Osteogenesis imperfecta, 743–746
Osteogenic sarcoma, 765
Osteochondroma (osteocartilaginous exostosis), 762
Osteoid osteoma, 761
Ovarian cyst, 635
Ovarian teratoma, 636–638

Palate, cleft, 87–89
Palsy, facial, 13
Pancreas, 481–485
— annular, 305, 485
Pancreatic cyst, congenital, 481
— pseudocyst, 483
— trauma, 482
Papilloedema, 673
Papilloma of tongue, 105
Paralytic scoliosis, 739
Paraoesophageal hiatus hernia (rolling hernia), 201
Paraxial tibial hemimelia, 725
Parietal encephalocoele, 669
Parotid, angiosarcoma of, 124
— mixed haemangioma of, 128
— sialogram, normal, 126
— teratoma of, 123, 131
Parotitis, recurrent, 125
Patent urachus, 584, 252
Pectoralis major, congenital absence of, 182, 715
Pectus carinatum (pigeon chest), 181
Pectus excavatum, 178–180
Pelvic ectopic kidney, 557
Penile disorders, 607–619
Peptic ulceration, 309, 310
— perforation, gastric, neonatal, 288–290
— spontaneous of common bile duct, 475
— 'spontaneous' gastric, 291

Perianal lesion of Crohn's disease, 369
Perineal anus, anterior, 439
— canal, 442
— lesion of Crohn's disease, 369
Perinatal injuries, 5–20
Perineal defect, 632
— haematoma, 634
— hernia, 633
Periorbital bruising, 34, 36
— metastatic disease, neuroblastoma, 535
— oedema, 41
Peritoneal cavity, 278–287
Peritonitis, meconium, 345, 417
— tuberculous, 367
Periumbilical erythema, 278
Perthes' disease (pseudocoxalgia), 757
Pes planus (flatfoot), 723
Petechiae, of head and neck region, 41
Peutz–Jeghers syndrome, 379–380
Pharyngeal pouch diverticulum, 136
Pharynx (and larynx), 132–136
Pheochromocytoma, 503, 504
Phimosis, 612
Phocomelia, 734, 735
Pierre–Robin syndrome, 90
Pigeon chest (pectus carinatum), 181
'Pit', posterior anal, 452
Pneumatosis intestinalis, 393–395
Pneumomediastinum, 220
Pneumonia, 52
Pneumoperitoneum, 395
Pneumothorax, tension, 15, 32
Poland's syndrome, 182
Polycystic disease, infantile, 554
Polydactyly, 706, 707
Polyp, colonic, 419, 420
— rectal, 421
— umbilical, 246
Polyposis coli, 422
Polythelia (accessory nipple), 170
Popliteal cysts, 756
Portal hypertension, 495
Portal hypertension and spleen, 486–500
Portal vein thrombosis, 500
Portal venous system, gas in, 394
Posterior urethral valves, 599, 600
Preauricular sinus, 109
— tags, 110
Primary obstructive megaureter, 581
Prolapse, rectal with exstrophy, 589
Proptosis, unilateral in rhabdomyosarcoma, 70
Prostate, rhabdomyosarcoma of, 598
Prune belly syndrome, 591–593
Pseudarthrosis of tibia, infantile, 724
Pseudohermaphrodite, female, 649
— male (testicular feminisation syndrome), 652
Ptosis, congenital of left eyelid, 60
Pubertal hypertrophy, breast, 171
'Pulled elbow', 28
Pulmonary metastases, 519, 520
— oedema, 52
Purpura, Henoch–Schonlein, 365
— idiopathic thrombocytopenic, 491, 492
Pyelonephritis, 567
Pyloric stenosis, 292–294
Pyonephrosis, 562

Rabies, 44
Rachischisis, 659
Radius, congenital absence of, 712

Ranula, 83
Rectal atresia, 441
Rectal biopsy, Hirschsprung's, 410
— normal, 408, 409
— suction (normal), 407
Rectum and anus, 428–454
Rectourethral fistula with anorectal agenesis, 433
Rectovaginal fistula with anorectal agenesis, 437
Reflux oesophagitis, 203
Reflux, vesicoureteric, 577–580
Renal agenesis, 551
— angiography, selective, 518
— ectopia, crossed, 555
— trauma, 548, 549
Respiratory distress syndrome, 15
Retained smegma ('smegmal cyst'), 611
Retinoblastoma, 69
Retro-orbital tuberculosis, 71
Retroperitoneal teratoma, 537–539
Retropharyngeal abscess, 133, 134
Rhabdomyosarcoma, 70, 71, 595–598
Rheumatoid arthritis (Still's disease), 759
Ribs, congenital absence of, 183, 184
Round worm, (ascariasis), 376–378
Rubella, congenital rubella syndrome, 68

Sacral sinus, 661
Salivary glands, 125–131
Sacrococcygeal teratoma, 540–543
Sarcoma, Ewing's, 767
— osteogenic, 765, 766
Scalds, 48, 49
Scalp, congenital defect, 115
— dermoid cyst of, 117
Scaphocephaly, 679
Scintigram, thyroid, 139
Scoliosis, 736–739
Scrotal haematoma, 16
— oedema, idiopathic, 622
Scrotum and testis, 620–634
'Sentinel' anal tag, 451
Septate gall bladder, 473
Shoulder dystocia, 18, 20
Sialectasis, 127
Sickle-cell anaemia, jaundice in, 478
Sincipital encephalocoele, 666, 667
Sinus, branchial, 150
— congenital dermal, 116, 662
— preauricular, 109
Skull and face, 113–124
Skull fractures, 25, 35–38
— 'Lacunar', 676
— trauma, 26
Smegma, retained ('smegmal cyst'), 611
Sphincter, incompetence of lower oesophageal, 202
Spina bifida occulta, 653
Spinal deformities, 736–742
— dermoid cyst, 663
— tuberculosis, 742
Spleen and portal hypertension, 486–500
— ruptured, 489
— multiple accessory, 493
Splenic cyst, 486–488
Splenoportogram, 498
Sprengel's shoulder, 716
Squint (strabismus), 67, 69
Staghorn calculus, 570
Sternal cleft, 175, 176
Stenosis, covered anal in female, 440
— pyloric, 292–294

Sternomastoid 'tumour', 155
Still's disease (rheumatoid arthritis), 759
Stomach, 288–300
Stomatitis, Crohn's, 370
Strabismus (squint), 67
Strangulation, attempts at, 22
'Strawberry Mark', 690
Streeter's dysplasia, 714
Subconjunctival haemorrhage, 36, 41
Subdural haematoma, 27, 39
Sublingual cyst, 101
Submandibular calculus, 129, 130
Subperiosteal haemorrhage, 6
Suffocation injury, 41
Supernumerary fifth toe, 719
Supraumbilical hernia, 256
Syndactyly, 705

Tag 'sentinel' anal, 451
— preauricular, 110
Technetium scan (TC^{99}), 353
Temporal astrocytoma, 685
Tension pneumothorax, 15, 32
Teratoma, anterior mediastinal, 214
— cervical, 164
— of neck, 163
— ovarian, 636–638
— parotid, 123, 131
— retroperitoneal, 537–539
— sacrococcygeal, 540–543
— testis, 629, 630
— thyroid gland, 140, 141
Testicular feminisation syndrome, 652
Testis, maldescent of, 620, 621
— teratoma of, 629, 630
— torsion of, 623, 624
Testis and scrotum, 620–634
Tetanus, protection against in dog bite, 44
Thigh, lipoma of, 704
Thoracic neuroblastoma, 219
Thoracolumbar scoliosis, 736
Thrombocytopenic purpura, idiopathic, 491, 492
Thumb, floating, 710
Thyroglossal cyst, 137
— infected, 138
Thyroid gland, 137–146
— teratoma of, 140, 141
Thyroid scintigram, 139
Thyrotoxicosis, 143
Tibia, congenital absence of, 725
— pseudoarthrosis of, 724
Toe, supernumerary, 719
Tongue, 100–107
— duplication cyst of, 327
— haemangioma of, 102
— mucus cyst of, 104
— papilloma of, 105
— tie (ankyloglossia inferior), 100
Tonsils, chronically enlarged, 132
Torsion, medial femoral, 730
Torticollis, 156
Tracheo-bronchial cleft, 193
Tracheo-oesophageal fistula and oesophageal atresia, 187, 190
— fistula, 194
— — recurrent, 195
Tracheostomy, emergency, 42
Translevator anorectal anomaly, 444
Transport, of newborn infants, 1, 2
Transverse hemimelia, 711

Trauma, abdominal visceral, 16
— eye, 34
— facial, 35
— pancreatic, 482
— renal, 548, 549
— skull, 26
Treacher–Collins syndrome, 114
Trichobezoar, 298, 299
Tuberculosis, retro-orbital, 71
— spinal, 742
Tuberculous mesenteric adenitis, 368
— peritonitis, 367
— ulceration, 160
Tumour
— bladder, 595, 596
— bone, 761–767
— brain, 681–685
— carcinoid, 389
— chardoma, 544–545
— intestinal, 381–383
— liver, 468–471
— metastatic, lung, 229, 230
— nephroblastoma, 513–524
— neuroblastoma, 525–536
— orbit, 72
— ovarian, 635–640
— pancreatic, 484
— retinoblastoma, 69
— retroperitoneal, 510–547
— rhabdomyosarcoma, eye, 70
— — genitourinary, 595–598, 605
— teratoma
— — abdominal, 537–539
— — facial, 163, 164
— — ovarian, 636–638
— — parotid, 123, 131
— — sacrococcygeal, 540–543
— — testis, 629, 630
— — thyroid, 140, 141
— testis, 626–630
— thoracic, 218
Turner's syndrome, 166
Twins, conjoined, 771, 772

Ulcer, gastric, 296, 297
— meatal, 614
Ulceration, peptic, 309, 310
— tuberculous, 160
Ulcerative colitis, 425–427
Umbilical cord, hernia into or exomphalos minor, 266
— defect, skin-covered, 265
— granuloma, 245
— hernia, 254
— — perforation of, 255
— polyp, 246
Undescended testis, 621
Urachal cyst, 253
— diverticulum, 585
— fistula, 583
Urachus, patent, 252, 584
Ureter, 571–582
Ureteric calculus, 582
— duplication, complete, 564
— — with hydronephrosis, 566
Ureterocoele, 575, 576
— ectopic, 574
Urethra, 599–606
Urinary ascites, 281, 568
— calculi, 569

Vacuum extraction (ventouse), 12
Vagina, rhabdomyosarcoma of, 597
Vaginal atresia, 643
— discharge, 645
Valgum, genu, 727, 728
Valves, posterior urethral, 599, 600
Varices, gastric fundal, 499
— oesophageal, 496, 497
Vascular ring, 208
Vein thrombosis, portal, 500
Ventriculogram, contrast, 677
Vesicointestinal fissure (ectopia cloaca), 276
— (exstrophy of cloaca), 590
Vesicoureteric reflux, 577–580
Viscus, ruptured, 17

Vitelline duct abnormalities, 244
Volvulus, midgut, 321
— with ascariasis, 376
— with malrotation, 325, 326
Vomit, bile-stained, 301
Von Recklinghausen's disease, 546
Vulva, hamartoma of, 646

Waterhouse–Friderichsen syndrome, 508, 509
Wilms' tumour (nephroblastoma), 510, 517

Yolk-sac tumour, 639, 640